OXFORD COGNITIVE S

Face and

C000138935

OXFORD COGNITIVE SCIENCE SERIES

General Editors
MARTIN DAVIES, JAMES HIGGINBOTHAM, JOHN O'KEEFE,
CHRISTOPHER PEACOCKE, KIM PLUNKETT

Forthcoming in the series

FACE AND MIND

ANDREW W. YOUNG

Department of Psychology
University of York

OXFORD UNIVERSITY PRESS

This book has been printed digitally and produced in a standard specification
in order to ensure its continuing availability

OXFORD
UNIVERSITY PRESS

Great Clarendon Street, Oxford OX2 6DP

Oxford University Press is a department of the University of Oxford.
It furthers the University's objective of excellence in research, scholarship,
and education by publishing world-wide in

Oxford New York

Auckland Bangkok Buenos Aires Cape Town Chennai
Dar es Salaam Delhi Hong Kong Istanbul Karachi Kolkata
Kuala Lumpur Madrid Melbourne Mexico City Mumbai Nairobi
São Paulo Shanghai Taipei Tokyo Toronto

Oxford is a registered trade mark of Oxford University Press
in the UK and in certain other countries

Published in the United States
by Oxford University Press Inc., New York

© Andrew W. Young 1998

The moral rights of the author have been asserted
Database right Oxford University Press (maker)

Reprinted 2004

ISBN 0-19-852420-x

Printed in Great Britain by

Antony Rowe Ltd., Eastbourne

PREFACE

Given the fascination of the face for the human species, it has taken scientists a remarkably long time to take seriously the question of how we derive important social information from the faces we see. There were brilliant individual contributions, such as Darwin's book on facial expressions of emotion, but somehow the field didn't seem to become properly established as a research area until the 1970s, when a revitalization of work on facial expression recognition by Paul Ekman and by Carroll Izard, and studies of forensic issues by the Aberdeen group of Hadyn Ellis, John Shepherd, and Graham Davies created widespread interest.

It was Hadyn Ellis who first suggested to me that I should work on face recognition, on a rainy day in 1974 when I confessed to being at something of a loose end in deciding how to spend the rest of my life after completing a PhD in developmental psychology. When I expressed polite interest, he promptly followed through by bundling me, a tachistoscope, and some photographs of faces into the Aberdeen Psychology Department's mobile laboratory van (days before the worst of the cuts in university funding!), driving to a local school, and marooning me there until enough data had been collected for a workable study of hemispheric specialization in children. Then he taught me grammar, punctuation, statistics, and all the other skills needed to see our first joint paper through to publication (Young and Ellis, 1976, *Neuropsychologia*, **14**, 495–8). In retrospect it was a modest effort, which has had no long-term impact, but a useful apprenticeship.

Since then, a number of us have sought gradually to broaden the agenda of face research, moving outwards from an initial interest in recognition of identity to encompass how we interpret other social signals, the patterns of impairment after brain injury, the formation of delusions, and conscious and non-conscious processes. In each case, we have used face perception as a convenient tool for gaining insight into these questions and turning them into tractable research topics.

After 23 years at the 'coal face' of face perception, it seems not a bad moment to take stock of where the seam has taken us. I see no sign yet of it running out, and there are many exciting new shafts to tunnel. So I welcome the opportunity to set down my own thoughts and supplement them by reprinting several papers of recent and less recent origin.

Since 1974, I have had the good fortune to work with many talented colleagues, students, assistants, and collaborators; too many to list individually. I am grateful to all of them for ideas we have worked on together, or which I just stole unashamedly. A number of these people appear as co-authors of papers reprinted here, and I thank them for allowing this to happen without demur. But to some I owe an especial debt.

In the early 1980s, Andy Ellis and Dennis Hay first showed me how it would be possible to begin to approach face recognition from a cognitive neuropsychological perspective, and contributed several key concepts and suggestions to the enterprise. Their ideas have formed the foundation for all subsequent developments. However, it was Freda Newcombe who taught me the practicalities of this type of work and, by her inspirational example, communicated some of the many responsibilities which accompany work with brain-injured people. I have tried hard (albeit with only limited success) to emulate her care not to let the needs of the research take precedence over the needs of the participants who allow us to test them. Even so, I have never managed remotely to approach the selflessness with which she handed over some of the responsibility for part of her own long-term project on the effects of focal brain injury to Dennis Hay and myself. We were then complete novice neuropsychologists, and I still remember with great affection (and some embarrassment) the engaging charm with which she deflected our more preposterous or impractical suggestions and gently steered us toward more workable alternatives.

Although we have not collaborated on many empirical projects, Vicki Bruce has been a constant source of enthusiastic encouragement and ideas, not least through the annual meetings of British researchers working on face perception which we organized together in the 1980s. For a number of us, these meetings were a key factor in developing the shared theoretical perspective and establishing collaborations which have underpinned much of the British research in this area. One of the later recruits to our meetings, Mike Burton, has patiently explained what little I understand of the more technical aspects of mathematical and computational modelling, and spent a lot of time working through many and various random questions I have asked about abstruse aspects of the behaviour of his beautiful simulation.

Above all, though, Hadyn Ellis. Ever since he set me off in this area, I have followed Hadyn's advice on many matters pertaining to scientific direction, and we have continued to collaborate on studies in neuropsychology and more recently neuropsychiatry. For reasons that completely elude me, our personal circumstances have diverged to the point that Hadyn now has power and influence, a Jaguar car, and a house in France, whereas I own a dying Volkswagen and a bicycle, but still we have managed somehow to remain friends and to keep the collaboration going. The neuropsychiatry of delusional misidentification, in particular, has been mainly driven by Hadyn's initiative. It was he who saw the importance of the topic, recognized the opportunity to try a quasi-neuropsychological approach, generated the neat hypothesis that Capgras delusion might be conceptualized as a kind of mirror-image of prosopagnosia, and enlisted the help of Karel de Pauw and Krystyna Szulecka to ensure that our efforts were placed on solid ground through their extensive professional and historical knowledge of these conditions. And through his inspired decision to work with Karel and Krystyna as our psychiatric collaborators, Hadyn characteristically ensured we would always enjoy the work.

Thanks are also due to the editors of OUP's Cognitive Science Series who came up with the idea for the book, to Tony Stone who convinced me it was a worthwhile project and gave a lot of help, to the various publishers who have allowed me to reproduce material, and to Vanessa Whitting who has seen the project through for OUP. Vanessa has shown almost saintly patience in dealing with my evasive replies to her requests for information on progress, and in agreeing to extend deadlines which were already extensions of extensions. I can only hope that if the day of publishers' judgement ever arrives, the (admittedly belated) appearance of this book may just tip the scales away from damnation with the despised non-deliverers.

Finally, I would also like to record my deep gratitude to the many people who have given so freely of their time to assist our research; as participants in experiments, members of control groups, or participants with brain injuries or psychiatric problems. The essential convention of objectivity in scientific reports means we often have to describe them like butterflies pinned to a board, but behind the dispassionate written façade we do try never to forget the generosity which drives many people to undertake what are often tedious tasks for us solely in the hope that eventually the information gained might benefit others. They are the heroes of neuropsychology.

Andy Young
August 1997

CONTENTS

1

Finding the mind's construction in the face

In 1878 Francis Galton presented a paper to the Anthropological Institute in which he described his investigations of composite portraits. By superimposing images of people's faces on top of each other he considered that he could arrive at a photograph which would show their typical characteristics whilst reducing or eliminating unusual variation.

Galton's (1879, 1883) method involved aligning photographs of faces in terms of some prominent feature (such as the eye region), and then overlaying exposures on to the same photographic plate. He expected that composite portraiture could have many potential uses, some of which are illustrated in Fig. 1.1. It might, for instance, help to arrive at a better idea of the appearance of historical figures, by combining the works of different artists in such a way that their separate stylistic idiosyncrasies would disappear; to this end, Galton showed a composite of six different versions of the profile of Alexander the Great. He thought that the same technique might also be used to illustrate family likeness, or the typical appearance of people in health (demonstrated with a composite of twelve officers and eleven privates from the Royal Engineers), people with different types of disease (56 consumptive cases, and 15 tubercular patients), or the physiognomic types associated with different forms of criminality. Other applications would include animal breeding, and forecasting the appearance of the offspring of different marriages.

Galton was an eminent Victorian scientist and mathematician, but his reputation has had a bumpy ride in the 20th century. He is unpopular in many quarters because his interest in individual differences, including racial differences, and his enthusiasm for the direct application of evolutionary concepts to the study of mankind has allowed him to be seen as one of the fathers of eugenics. Some of the darker implications of Galton's technique can already be found in the discussion which took place at the Anthropological Institute, which included a contribution from Sir Edmund Du Cane, HM Director of Prisons. Sir Edmund had

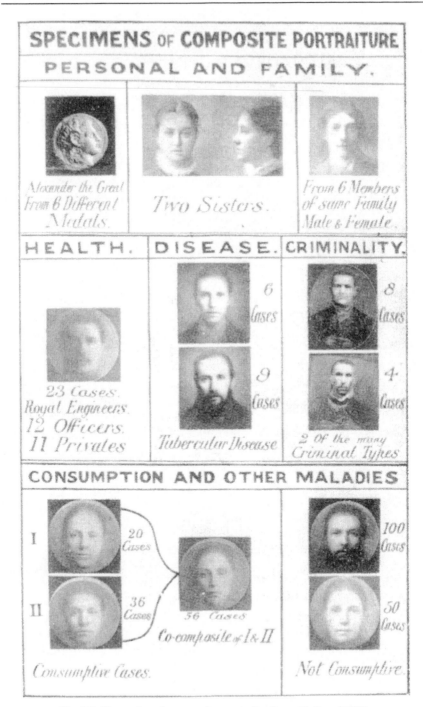

Fig. 1.1 Examples of composite portraits, from Galton (1883).

assisted Galton in collecting photographs of the prison population. He considered that for certain types of criminal

... the tendency to crime is in those persons born or bred in them, and either they are incurable or the tendency can only be checked by taking them in hand at the earliest periods of life. Mr. Galton's process would help to establish this point.

However, despite the distastefulness of some of his views to us now, Galton is still admired by many psychologists because of his ingenuity in opening up important topics to empirical investigation. Before Galton, many of these questions were matters for speculation and discussion. After Galton, it was accepted that informed discussion should take account of evidence. It has been unfortunate for the embryonic police state that measuring people's faces has not provided a neat short cut to the tiresome judicial process, but one senses that Galton would have been willing to revise his preconceptions and accept this when there were sufficient empirical grounds to indicate it would not work.

Politics aside, Galton's agenda for research on composite face portraits gives an interesting example of changes in assumptions. It seems obvious a century later that one cannot reliably tell murderers from non-murderers by their faces, let alone telling murderers from burglars or arsonists, so that it is now hard to credit a scientist of Galton's standing taking the possibility so seriously. This should teach us a certain humility about our own starting assumptions, which will no doubt look just as quaint in much less than another hundred years time. Indeed, advances in understanding of genetics may well give Galton the last laugh, though it still seems unlikely that the relevant genes will also happen to be involved in craniofacial development.

Preview

The present book consists primarily of research and review papers on face perception published by myself and colleagues during the past 12 years. In the present chapter I will explain the basics of our approach, point out why we have investigated the particular questions selected, look at some of the key points which emerge, and pick up their implications. These include broad issues, such as the extent to which our mental lives result from of the operation of discrete components devoted to different purposes, and the differences between conscious and non-conscious processes. Because of the variety of social signals read from the face, it can offer unique insights into some of these questions.

I have grouped the main content of the book so that following this
introductory chapter, the reprinted papers examine faces in their social
and biological context (Chapter 2), and the Bruce and Young (1986)
theoretical framework (Chapter 3). This is followed by chapters
grouped into themes of functional organization (Chapters 4–7), neuropsychiatry (Chapters 8–10), and consciousness (Chapters 11–14). In
each case, I've tried to include papers which make empirical and
theoretical contributions, and which review relevant material. In order
to provide an indication of where things are going, some recent findings
are also incorporated into this introduction.

Why faces?

So why study face perception? The main reason is that the face conveys
to us such a wealth of social signals, and we are so expert at reading
these. In consequence, studies of faces present us with special advantages for answering a range of fundamental questions about human
abilities.

Here is a list of some of the questions scientists have asked about face
perception, taken from Goldstein (1983; p. 224):

Is the facial expression of emotions innately determined so that for each
emotion there exists a corresponding facial behavior common to all people?
Are facial expressions of emotional states correctly identified cross-culturally?
What is the relationship between facial expressions in dogs, monkeys, and
humans? Does the face accurately betray an individual's intelligence, ethnic
membership, or degree of honesty? Are faces innately more attractive than
other visual stimuli to newborn human infants? What role does physical
attractiveness play in person perception? In memory for faces? Are faces more
or less memorable than other visual configurations? Are 'foreign' faces coded in
our memories in the same manner as faces of natives?

This list shows the wide variety of possibilities for research. Many of
them are questions human beings have wondered about since time
immemorial. Not all will be answered here, and some additional
questions will instead assume prominence. But Goldstein's (1983) list
helps in seeing how the face can be used as a vehicle for addressing
many different issues.

A further reason for interest in the face has been its biological
background. The structure of the face has evolved to allow it to contain
organs serving a range of functions; the mouth for eating, nose for
breathing, eyes for seeing, ears for hearing. Some of these then get used
for different purposes too, as in the signalling of emotion by movements

of the facial muscles. And these modified uses can also have long evolutionary histories; the continuity of certain facial expressions between humans, primates, and other mammals was one of the points made by Darwin (1872) in his classic book on the expression of emotions.

Such points have suggested to some authors that there might also be an evolved neural substrate for face perception. Evidence consistent with this speculation has been widely discussed in the research literature, and some of the key findings are reviewed in Chapter 2. These include evidence of innate attentiveness to faces in newborn infants (Goren *et al.* 1975; Johnson *et al.* 1991), studies of other precocious face perception abilities in early infancy (Meltzoff and Moore 1977), our differential sensitivity to face inversion (Valentine 1991; Yin 1969), evidence of right cerebral hemisphere specialization for face recognition (De Renzi *et al.* 1994; Ellis 1983) and involvement of the occipital and temporal lobes (Damasio *et al.* 1982; Meadows 1974), face-specific recognition impairments in some cases of brain injury (De Renzi 1986; McNeil and Warrington 1993), and neurophysiological evidence of face-responsive cells in the temporal lobes of monkeys (Desimone 1991; Gross 1992; Perrett *et al.* 1982, 1992). To this list we can now add studies involving functional imaging of blood flow in the normal human brain, which have both confirmed and extended the neuropsychological and neurophysiological findings (Cabeza and Nyberg 1997; Sergent and Signoret 1992*a*).

As Chapter 2 shows, the sheer volume and diversity of findings pointing to an evolved neural substrate for face perception is impressive, but they need to be carefully evaluated. Each type of study can potentially be interpreted in a number of different ways, but when taken together they now converge fairly convincingly on the conclusion of an evolved substrate. Hence, one can agree that a certain line of evidence (say, infant attentiveness to faces) points to the possibility of an evolved neural substrate for face perception but is subject to caveats A and B, whereas another line of evidence points to the same conclusion but is subject to caveats C and D, and another line of evidence points to the same conclusion but is subject to caveats E and F, and so on. What has to be decided, though, is whether the right conclusion is the one to which all lines of evidence point consistently, or whether caveats A, B, C, D, E, F, and so on all happen to apply simultaneously. Given the number of lines of evidence which can be adduced, the possibility that we are misinterpreting them all is starting to look vanishingly small.

However, even if we accept that there is now compelling evidence pointing toward some form of evolved neural substrate for face perception, we still know remarkably little about it. The infant evidence is exciting, but difficult to relate to adult abilities. The involvement of occipital and temporal lobes needs to be considered in conjunction with their wider contributions to visual recognition (Gross 1992), and the degree of right hemisphere specialization seems less pronounced than the degree of left hemisphere involvement in language (Dr Renzi *et al* 1994). Cases of specific inability to recognize faces after brain injury are exceptionally rare in what is itself an uncommon disorder (prosopagnosia); the more usual observation is that deficits affecting other visual categories can be revealed by formal testing (de Haan *et al.* 1991*a*).

The concept of expertise has become central to evaluating such findings, for several reasons. Carey and her colleagues have drawn attention to the fact that the social and biological importance of faces is such that we are all highly expert face perceivers (Carey 1992; Diamond and Carey 1986). In contrast, there are other categories of visual stimuli for which only some people bother to acquire more than a rudimentary expertise; these would include birds, trees, cars, and railway engines.

The importance of expertise was neatly illustrated in a study by Diamond and Carey (1986), who examined the effect of turning stimuli upside down on our ability to recognize them as having been seen before. They studied expert dog breeders and people who were not especially interested in dogs, and showed that whereas everyone was poor at recognizing upside-down faces, only the dog breeders showed a decrement in performance for inverted as compared to upright pictures of dogs. The disruption due to inversion thus seems to be a side-effect of the fact that our perceptual mechanisms have become tuned to the particular (upright) orientation we usually encounter. For faces, all of us have developed finely tuned expert skills that are vulnerable to inversion, whereas for dogs only the people with a specialist interest have acquired them.

One of the important features of this focus on expertise is that it shows the complexity of the interactions between any evolved neural substrate for face perception and our day to day learning of faces. It is not just a question of having a ready-wired face module and exposing it to a few people it will need to recognize. A more interesting hypothesis is that the infant comes into the world with a mechanism which makes it attentive to faces, and that this attentiveness then ensures that any system for learning visual stimuli gets a strong face input (Johnson and Morton 1991).

The extent to which functional specialization can be moulded through interaction with environmental demands is shown in impressive studies which demonstrate that neurones in the inferotemporal cortex of the monkey will show selective responses to previously novel objects the animal has been taught to recognize (Logothetis and Pauls 1995). An analogous finding in cases of human prosopagnosia may be that acquired visual expertise with other categories is often lost alongside face recognition, as is described here in Chapters 2 and 4. For instance, Bornstein (1963) described a bird watcher who became prosopagnosic and found she had lost the ability to recognize birds. She could see they were birds, but could not identify the species. Similarly, Bornstein *et al.* (1969) reported the case of a prosopagnosic farmer who could no longer identify his individual cows; yet like the bird watcher, he still knew they were cows.

Closely related to the point about expertise are the demands of face recognition. In our daily lives, we need to identify individual faces, rather than assign them to the generic category 'face'. In contrast, the recognition of other objects is often more flexible; you need to recognize *your* coat if you left it hanging next to someone else's, but if you are at a jumble sale it may suffice to know that an item is *a* coat. Moreover, there is evidence that the typical entry level in object recognition is to basic categories of objects, each with their own distinctive appearance (coats, cars, ships, shoes, sealing wax), and that superordinate or subordinate categories can take longer to access (Rosch *et al.* 1976). In these terms recognition of an individual face requires access to a subordinate of the basic category of faces, and in circumstances where the possible range of within-category differences (i.e. the variation between the faces of different individuals) is fairly tightly delimited.

This was not lost on Galton (1883), who remarked that faces form such a homogeneous class of visual stimuli that we must become attuned to quite minor variations in order to differentiate them. He expressed it thus (Galton 1883, p. 3):

The differences in human features must be reckoned great, inasmuch as they enable us to distinguish a single known face among those of thousands of strangers, though they are mostly too minute for measurement. At the same time, they are exceedingly numerous. The general expression of a face is the sum of a multitude of small details, which are viewed in such rapid succession that we seem to perceive them all at a single glance. If any one of them disagrees with the recollected traits of a known face, the eye is quick at observing it, and it dwells upon the difference. One small discordance overweighs a multitude of similarities and suggests a general unlikeness.

In this extract Galton touched on two of the ideas that have become central to the study of face recognition. First, the point that faces demand identification of individual members of a relatively homogeneous stimulus class (Damasio *et al.* 1982; Ellis 1975). Second, the idea that we take in a seen face as a whole, or as Galton put it, 'at a single glance' (Carey and Diamond 1977; Farah 1991). These themes are picked up here in Chapters 2–4.

A further interesting property of face recognition is that the relation between surface form and identity is not fixed. The structure of most manufactured objects and many natural objects is directly linked to the functions they must perform, so that if a visitor in a flying saucer left behind some photographs of things from the planet Zog, we might well be able to tell which were Zoggian tools and which were Zoggian animals on the basis of their appearance alone. With faces, matters are quite different. People's appearances do not correspond exactly to other personal attributes, such as occupations. There are minor constraints (pop singers tend to be younger than politicians, and to have more exuberant hairstyles, etc.), but one cannot usually tell reliably from facial appearance alone whether someone is a banker or a builder.

Psychologists call attributes like occupation 'semantic' information, using a distinction introduced by Tulving (1972) between forms of memory in which we remember specific episodes (such as remembering that you saw Tony Blair giving a speech at the Durham Miner's Gala) and semantic memories which have effectively become part of our conceptual knowledge, and for which we no longer recall how they were initially learnt (e.g. knowing that Tony Blair is a politician). This is rather different to philosophers' use of the term 'semantic'. In terms of the psychological usage, the particular interest of faces is that it is possible to vary independently their visual and semantic properties in a way that cannot be achieved for many other types of visual object.

What also needs to be emphasized, though, is the sheer variety of social signals we get from faces. We use faces not only to recognize people we know, but to assist in determining the age and sex of unfamiliar people, and to monitor the interest, mood, or emotional state of others from their facial expressions, gaze direction, and other cues. In addition, the face forms an important source of social attributions, even though these are often non-conscious and potentially misleading (Lewicki 1986). There is even evidence that seeing the movements of another person's lips contributes to speech perception (McGurk and MacDonald 1976; Summerfield 1992), though the only time we are usually aware of this is through the awkwardness of a badly dubbed film.

The interesting point here is that we are expert decoders of *all* of these signals from the face – not just identity. On this basis, we would expect effects known to be linked to acquired expertise, such as inversion decrements, to apply to these other social signals too. That this is so is clear from a compelling illusion described by Thompson (1980), a variant of which is shown in Fig. 1.2. In this figure, the eyes and mouth have themselves been turned the wrong way up with respect to the rest of the face. When the entire face is inverted, as in the lower panels, this change is barely noticeable, but when the face is the right way up the unusual expression is immediately evident. Like the perceptual processes used in recognizing identity, our analysis of the facial expression has become highly tuned to expect an input signal in the correct orientation.

Because we are all experts at face perception, the face also provides a laboratory stimulus rich in ecological validity. There has been much concern about the artificial nature of many tasks used in psychology experiments. In an experiment on classifying nonsense shapes, for example, one can legitimately wonder to what extent the results reflect

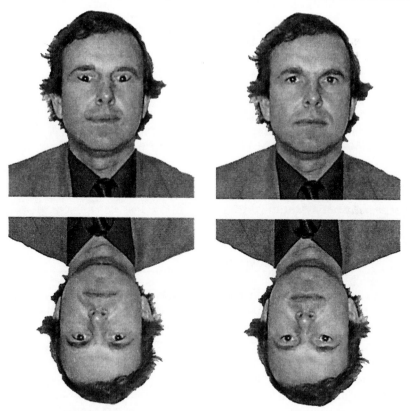

Fig. 1.2 Inversion affects the perception of facial expression (adapted from Thompson 1980).

real-life skills or are simply due to specific strategies created for the particular task employed. Often, research can get bogged down into trying to distinguish such possibilities; ultimately running the risk of slipping into investigating the task itself, rather than the abilities of human beings. Of course, using faces does not give an absolute guarantee that a line of research will not get side-tracked in this way, but with judicious choice of stimuli and tasks it is possible to keep the focus firmly on those abilities people bring to the psychological laboratory, and minimise those they set up in an *ad hoc* manner as responses to peculiar or perverse experimental demands.

In summary, face recognition provides a useful topic for research because of its ecological validity, its intrinsic interest, and its potential utility for addressing more general issues concerning visual cognition. In particular, it has three key properties which can be exploited:

1. Face recognition is a naturally acquired ability which probably represents the acme of perceptual classification skills, since many hundreds of closely similar stimuli (faces) must each be assigned a unique identity.
2. The relation between surface form and identity is relatively arbitrary for faces in comparison to many other types of visual object.
3. Because of their social importance, many types of information can be derived from seen faces (age, sex, expression, etc.), raising interesting issues about how these relate to the recognition of identity.

Variations of these themes feature extensively in modern research on face perception, and all crop up in this book, but the third point forms an especially persistent motif.

Functional organization

We have seen, then, that face research has many intrinsic attractions. However, although there has always been considerable interest in such questions, with a steady stream of scientific publications during the previous 100 years, Goldstein noted that when he reviewed the field in 1983 only a few scientists had developed coherent programmes of face-related research. Instead, for many of the eminent behavioural scientists who had published research on face perception, it tended to be in the form of only one or two articles per person, and in such instances their reputations were not earned as a result of their work with faces.

Goldstein (1983) attributed the disappointing failure of many researchers to stay in the field of face perception to a variety of factors, including the dominating influence of Darwin's (1872) book on facial expressions, certain problems he felt were inherent in Darwin's position, and the sheer difficulty and complexity of the topic. However, I think a more plausible reason lies in the failure of pre-1980s research to develop an overall theoretical perspective. There were some exceptions, the most notable of which concerned recognition of facial expressions, where Ekman (1972; Ekman *et al*. 1972) and Izard (1971) had managed successfully to build on Darwin's insights. But topics like face recognition were dominated by an almost atheoretical approach which sought primarily to manipulate variables and measure their impact. A typical face recognition memory experiment of the time would involve looking at a series of photographs of target faces, and then picking out the exact same photographs when they were mixed with a set of distractor faces a short while later. One could then use this basic paradigm to measure the influence on people's memory of the number of target or distractor faces in the list, the visual similarity of target and distractor items, the stimulus presentation time, the retention interval, the age or sex of the participants, and so on. Nothing wrong with that, except that the number of possible combinations of such variables was very large, and results correspondingly diverse. In reviewing many such studies Ellis (1975) commented on the need for some theoretical structure to impose order on the area and guide studies toward the important issues.

At the time, some of the most exciting developments in cognitive psychology were coming from investigations in which the effects of brain injury were used to test theoretical models; a field now known as cognitive neuropsychology (Ellis and Young 1996; Shallice 1988). The underlying logic was that an adequate account of normal function should be able to account for the patterns of impairment found after brain injury, and that to the extent that it failed to do so it should be revised or abandoned. The field had been kick-started by compelling studies of memory by Shallice and Warrington (1970) and reading by Marshall and Newcombe (1966, 1973).

Shallice and Warrington (1970) studied patient KF, who showed severe impairment of short-term memory, being able to repeat back only one or two digits from a list immediately after it had been said to him. Yet KF's ability to learn and remember material across longer intervals was well preserved. As Shallice and Warrington noted, this pattern of dissociation between impaired short-term memory and preserved long-term memory was flagrantly inconsistent with the then accepted idea that short-term memory acts as a temporary store for items entering long-term memory. On such a theory, it was impossible that damaging the entry route should not also impair long-term storage itself. The view that short-term and long-term recall involve separate, parallel stores therefore gave a more plausible account of the findings.

Marshall and Newcombe's (1966, 1973) work had a similar impact in a different domain. They described cases of reading impairment after brain injury, and carefully analysed the errors made. For example, case GR's errors could be grouped into various types, but a substantial proportion were semantic errors in which a target word was misread as a word with a similar meaning; *ill* read as 'sick', *city* as 'town', and so on. This tendency to make semantic errors in reading words formed the central part of a pattern Marshall and Newcombe (1973) christened 'deep dyslexia'. They saw that deep dyslexia was interesting because the then dominant account of reading involved accessing the word's meaning through a kind of internalized sounding out. But if this account was true, how could a person make reading errors that were primarily based on word meanings? The entirely different view that meaning can be accessed directly from print, without going through sound at all, looked more plausible, and this was also consistent with the fact that GR's semantic errors did not sound like the word he had been shown. On this view, now known as the dual-route theory, the transcoding of print to sound involves a separate process to accessing a word's meaning, and Marshall and Newcombe (1973) showed that this hypothesis was consistent with other forms of acquired dyslexia.

The same theoretical gambit was used by Marshall and Newcombe (1966, 1973) and Shallice and Warrington (1970). They researched an area in which there were reasons to expect some form of sequential, hierarchical organization to prevail, and noted that hierarchic organization predicts an orderly pattern of neuropsychological deficits in which damage to later parts of the sequence can create isolated deficits, but damage to earlier components must affect later components as well. Yet when they studied someone with an impairment caused by brain injury that was severely affecting one of the putative early components, they found that the putatively late component was not abolished. This immediately implied a more parallel, heterarchic form of organization.

It struck my colleagues and me that this logic could be applied to face processing, and that it might form a basis for developing a theoretical model which could underpin research. This enterprise forms much of the meat of Chapters 3–6.

Consider, for example, the following different types of information we can get from faces; we can use the face's physical structure to infer characteristics such as age and sex or to compare the appearance of different people, we can recognize certain emotions from facial expressions, and we can recognize the identities of familiar people. How might access to these different types of information be organized?

There are many possibilities, but Fig. 1.3 shows two different extremes. At one extreme, we can think in terms of a strict hierarchic sequence (Fig. 1.3(a)), in which we first analyse information dependent on the face's physical structure, then compute the expression, and then establish the bearer's identity (if it is known to us). Something like this sequence forms a compelling intuition for many people, because it seems to move from broad to increasingly precise categories, and to require the use of finer and finer visual details. At the other extreme, we might imagine a fully heterarchic organization (Fig. 1.3(b)), in which each ability is simply separate from the others, taking place in parallel.

These possibilities can be tested in neuropsychological studies, by examining the patterns of breakdown of each ability found after brain injury. The ability to perceive the face's physical structure is often tested by asking people to match photographs of unfamiliar faces as being views of the same person or different people; to do this successfully, one has both to see the face clearly and use a number of different cues. Analysis of expression is usually tested by asking for recognition of identifiable emotions, such as those from the Ekman and Friesen (1976) series. Analysis of familiar identity can be tested by requesting recognition of photographs of famous people.

In fact, such tasks had often been used in the neuropsychological literature, and once the issue was framed in this way it was fairly clear that, contrary to intuition, a number of neuropsychological dissociations whose existence favoured the heterarchic model had already been reported (Hay and Young 1982). A review of this literature opens Chapter 6. However, there were also clear limitations to this evidence, and the study reported in Chapter 6 sought to correct some of the deficiencies we identified. It still supported the heterarchic conception, though with some caveats which await further investigation.

What Fig. 1.3 does, though, is to assign face processing abilities to fairly broadly characterized groupings, so it also seemed worth pursuing what would happen if one opted for a finer grained analysis. The topic we chose for this was recognition of a familiar face's identity, for which we distinguished the knowledge that the face belongs to a familiar person; access to identity-specific semantic information about that person (such as their occupation – the term 'identity-specific' is used to separate facts which must be based on personal knowledge from those which can reasonably be deduced from appearance, such as age or sex); and retrieving the person's name. These correspond to recognizably

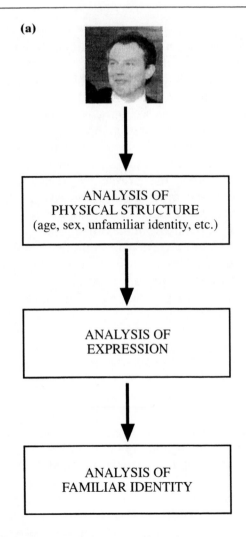

(a)

Fig. 1.3 Examples showing possible hierarchic (a) or heterarchic (b) organization of face processing abilities.

distinct forms of knowledge state (see Chapter 5), but a satisfying sense of full recognition demands that all three types of information are available (Hay and Young 1982).

Again, one can contrast an extreme version of a linear hierarchic model of face recognition (Fig. 1.4(a)) with a fully heterarchic conception (Fig. 1.4(b)), as shown in Fig. 1.4. This time, however, many studies have found data strongly supportive of the linear hierarchy. The typical patterns of failure after brain injury include

(b)

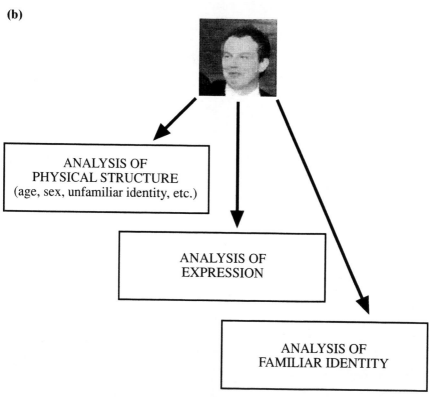

(1) failure to achieve a sense of familiarity combined with problems in retrieving identity-specific semantic information or the name, as in the neuropsychological condition prosopagnosia (de Haan *et al.* 1987*a*);

(2) an adequate sense of familiarity but problems in retrieving identity-specific semantic information or the name (de Haan *et al.* 1991*b*);

(3) inability to recall only the person's name, which corresponds to the neuropsychological condition anomia (Flude *et al.* 1989).

More details are given in Chapter 5 (see Table 5.8). These patterns of error correspond exactly to those to be expected from the linear hierarchy shown in Fig. 1.4(a). However, other possible patterns which might fit a more heterarchic conception of face recognition are not found. These potential patterns are of crucial importance because of their potential for falsifying the linear hierarchic account. For example, a heterarchic model would predict that some people with brain injuries should be able to name familiar faces without being able to provide other forms of identity-specific semantic information. Such a deficit has been widely sought because of its obvious 'black swan' significance, yet

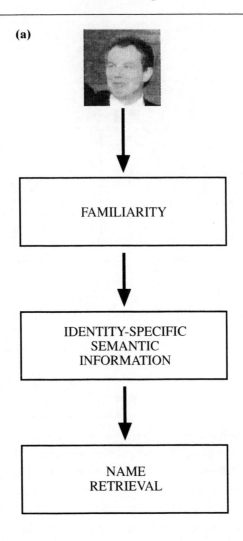

(a)

Fig. 1.4 Possible hierarchic (a) or heterarchic (b) organization of face recognition.

it is almost never reported. The only remotely convincing case in the literature has been DT, a French lady studied by Brennen *et al.* (1996). DT was tested repeatedly with a set of 20 faces of people who were famous in France, and on four occasions she could name Serge Gainsbourg, four times Catherine Deneuve, and once Christine Ockrent without giving appropriate semantic information. However, DT made many other errors (all consistent with the linear model) as well, and she was suffering a dementing illness at the time of testing (scoring 12/30 on the mini-mental state test, probably because of

(b)

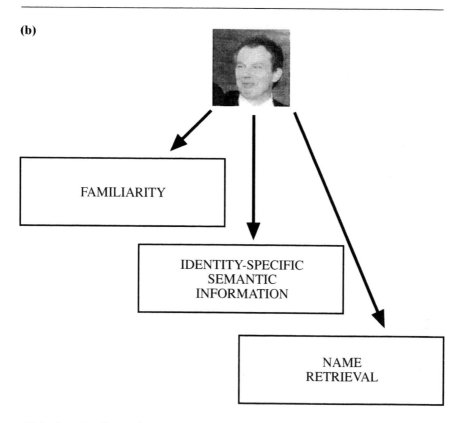

Alzheimer's disease). In contrast, such errors have not been noted in systematic studies of groups of patients with Alzheimer's disease (Greene and Hodges 1996; Hodges and Greene, in press). Therefore, we are faced with the difficulty of interpreting an unusual and infrequent error pattern which is itself untypical of Alzheimer's disease and was not the dominant form of error made by DT. These data therefore need to be considered with caution. In my experience, it can be very tricky to establish that people with advanced dementing illnesses are approaching tasks according to the instructions given to them. As well as deficits which impact directly on face recognition, they often have problems affecting comprehension, attention, and short-term memory.

The research literature to date, then, provides strong but not entirely unequivocal support to a heterarchic model for those abilities shown in Fig. 1.3(b), and a hierarchical model of face recognition itself, as shown in Fig. 1.4(a). If we put these together, we get Fig. 1.5; this gives in simplified form some of the central features of the Bruce and Young (1986) model, which is presented in full in Chapter 3 and discussed extensively in this book.

Facial expression recognition

A theoretical model like Bruce and Young's (1986; reprinted here as Chapter 3) or Fig. 1.5 is not a complete solution to the problem of face processing. It is better thought of as a useful notation – like a map which charts and systematizes our knowledge. The advantages it offers are those of sharpening one's thinking and clarifying the potential agenda for future research. For example, there is still little known from neuropsychological work about our perception of the face's physical structure. Most studies use tests of unfamiliar face matching to probe this ability, and especially the test devised by Benton and his colleagues (Benton *et al.* 1983), but occasionally other attributes such as age perception have been investigated by creative researchers (De Renzi 1989). Even so, basic questions remain almost untouched, such as the relation between deficits on tests of age perception and unfamiliar face matching. There is plenty more to be done!

In general, we can see that the familiar face recognition route has become more elaborated than the other routes in Fig. 1.5. In recent years, my colleagues and I have sought to rectify this imbalance by investigating in more detail impairments affecting the recognition of facial expressions of emotion, and I will briefly summarize some of this work.

In prosopagnosia, the recognition of all familiar faces is affected; one does not encounter people with brain injuries who selectively lose the ability to recognize Tony Blair, or who can recognize politicians but not television presenters, or even men but not women. A natural starting assumption was thus that problems in recognizing facial expressions of emotion would affect all emotions more or less equally severely. This assumption was built into the tests many of us used initially, which provided an overall score for facial expression recognition involving an aggregate across different emotions (Young *et al.* 1993a, 1995, 1996).

Important evidence that impairments of facial expressions recognition might actually affect some emotions more than others was provided by Adolphs and his colleagues in studies of SM, a person with bilateral damage to the amygdala (Adolphs *et al.* 1994, 1995), which is a medial temporal lobe structure widely considered to be involved in emotion. In order to explore this intriguing possibility, we have changed our own procedures and developed tests able to examine recognition of each of the six basic emotions from the Ekman and Friesen (1976) series (happiness, surprise, fear, sadness, disgust, anger).

Stimuli for one such test are shown in Fig. 1.6 (Calder *et al.* 1996; Sprengelmeyer *et al.* 1996). These are computer-manipulated expressions

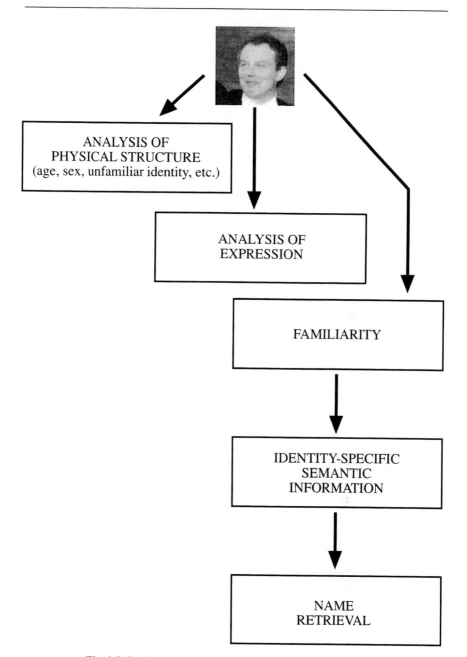

Fig. 1.5 Rudimentary functional model of face processing.

which have been interpolated between prototype images in the Ekman and Friesen (1976) series. Images in the left column contain 90 per cent of one prototype and 10 per cent of the other (e.g. 90 per cent happiness and 10 per cent surprise for the top left image in Fig. 1.6), the next column has 70 and 30 per cent blends, then 50 and 50 per cent, 30 and 70 per cent, and finally 10 and 90 per cent (i.e. 10 per cent happiness and 90 per cent surprise for the top right image in Fig. 1.6).

The procedure used to test recognition of facial expressions was to present the images from Fig. 1.6 one at a time in random order, and ask of each which of the six basic emotions it was most like. This procedure was repeated several times, and results are summarized in Fig. 1.7. The horizontal axes of the sequence, and the vertical axes show the number of times each image was identified as each emotion.

As can be seen in Fig. 1.7, neurologically normal people (top graph in Fig. 1.7) show an orderly progression between discrete regions in which each emotion is perceived. The middle graph in Fig. 1.7 shows averaged data for two people with damage to the amygdala (Calder *et al.*, 1996); they recognize some emotions reasonably well (happiness, surprise, sadness, perhaps disgust), but show noticeable difficulties in recognizing fear or anger. These are comparable to Adolphs *et al.*'s (1994, 1995) findings with SM, who was also particularly poor at recognizing fear, but showed some problems with other emotions, including anger.

The pattern of differentially severe impairment of recognition of anger and fear found after amygdala damage is unlike the type of deficit found in prosopagnosia in two ways. First, prosopagnosia affects recognition of all familiar faces, irrespective of their semantic category; there have been no reports of selectively impaired recognition of, say, politicians' faces. In contrast, the findings for emotion recognition after amygdala damage show that some emotions are more affected than others. Second, recognition from other cues (such as the person's voice) may remain relatively unaffected in prosopagnosia. In contrast, further work on the recognition of emotion after amygdala damage has shown impaired recognition of fear and anger from auditory cues, forming a close parallel to the impairment of facial expression recognition (Scott *et al.* 1997).

We are thus starting to find evidence of different forms of impairment for different types of facial information; recognition of identity can be affected in a way which affects all faces but is specific to the facial domain, as in prosopagnosia, whereas impairments of emotion recognition may compromise the recognition of certain emotions seemingly regardless of the input domain.

Further evidence of this comes from work with people with

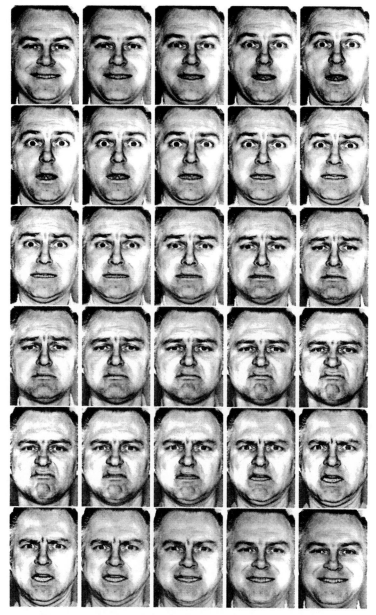

Fig. 1.6 Computer-manipulated images used to test recognition of facial expressions of emotion (Calder *et al.* 1996; Sprengelmeyer *et al.* 1996). The continua shown in each row are happiness–surprise (top row), surprise–fear (second row), fear–sadness (third row), sadness–disgust (fourth row), disgust–anger (fifth row), anger–happiness (bottom row). Moving from left to right, the columns show 90, 70, 50, 30, and 10 per cent interpolations along each continuum.

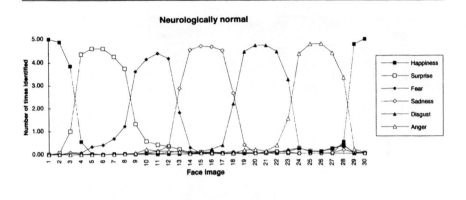

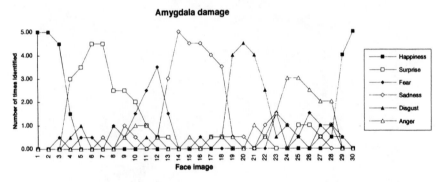

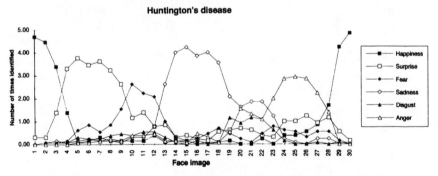

Fig. 1.7 Recognition of the images shown in Fig. 1.6 by neurologically normal people, people with amygdala damage (Calder *et al.* 1996), and people with Huntington's disease (Sprengelmeyer *et al.* 1996). The horizontal axes represent the rows of images from Fig. 1.6 arranged in sequence, and the vertical axes show the number of times each image was identified as each emotion.

Huntington's disease, a hereditary neurodegenerative disorder which initially involves the basal ganglia but eventually leads to widespread brain dysfunction. Average data for a group of 13 people with Huntington's disease (Sprengelmeyer *et al.* 1996) are shown in the lower graph of Fig. 1.7. Again, the recognition of happiness, surprise and sadness does not seem too badly affected. There are distinct problems with fear and anger, but what is most striking is the almost complete inability to recognize disgust. Sprengelmeyer *et al.* (1996) found that for tests of facial and vocal expression recognition, disgust was recognized only at chance level, and was significantly more severely affected than any other emotion.

One of the most tragic features of Huntington's disease is that if one of your parents is affected you have a 50 per cent risk of contracting the disease, but it has an insidious onset which is often not evident until you are beyond child-bearing age. The defective gene was identified in 1993, allowing the possibility of genetic testing for those individuals who are at risk of having inherited the disease, should they wish. Genetic testing is inherently stressful, and not everyone opts for it, but a study of people who presented for genetic testing has shown that the recognition of facial expressions of disgust is affected in individuals who are carriers of the gene for Huntington's disease at a time when they are free from clinically obvious symptoms (Gray *et al.* 1997).

These studies are thus beginning to uncover what neuropsychologists call 'double dissociations' between impairments that compromise the recognition of negative emotions, with recognition of fear and anger especially affected by amygdala damage, and recognition of disgust affected by some other type of brain injury for which the critical lesion has yet to be determined. In a double dissociation, ability A is impaired for one person and spared for another, whereas ability B follows the opposite pattern (relatively preserved in the person who has lost ability A, but impaired in the person who still has ability A). This pattern provides grounds for thinking that these abilities depend on neurologically separable pathways.

A problem with the double dissociation method is that it has become clear that the hypothesis of neurologically separable pathways is not the only possible interpretation, and the evidence needs to be carefully evaluated (Shallice 1988). This is because under certain (restricted) circumstances, different forms of damage to a single system carrying out two different types of operation can produce a pattern akin to a double dissociation. However, such an interpretation seems very forced when there are also neurological grounds for proposing separable pathways; in other words, when each of the dissociable deficits is associated with a different form of brain injury. In this respect, although psychological and neurological models are conceptually distinct, they can enjoy a degree of symbiosis, converging on a common interpretation.

Recent advances in ability to use functional imaging techniques to examine blood flow in the normal human brain provide an additional useful source of information. These have confirmed that the amygdala is responsive to facial expressions of fear (Breiter *et al.* 1996; Morris *et al.* 1996, in press), and that the neural response to facial expressions of disgust involves different brain regions (Phillips *et al.* 1997). The idea of separable neurological pathways underlying our responses to displays of certain emotions by other people is therefore grounded in various lines of evidence.

Such findings may be approached usefully from an evolutionary perspective. Basic emotions, it has often been argued, represent important evolutionary adaptations; Ekman (1992) characterized them as facilitating rapid responses to fundamental life-tasks in ways which have enhanced our fitness to survive. For example, if an animal comes into contact with something dangerous it may become frightened and flee, or it may aggressively stand its ground; danger induces a basic emotion, fear, and a set of preparatory responses that aid in the preservation of life. One can suppose, then, that any animal that can experience fear (or, at least, mobilize a fear response) will be better equipped to survive than one that cannot. Similarly, an animal that is sensitive to perceiving fear in other animals is in a better position to decide when a rapid exit or a display of aggression could pay off. This is not to deny that emotions like fear will also involve learning and cultural influences, but these are probably built upon an evolved substrate. Much the same is true for disgust, whose recognition is impaired in Huntington's disease (Gray *et al.*, in press; Sprengelmeyer *et al.* 1996); the wide range of stimuli which can elicit disgust in humans can be seen as resulting from an accretion of new elicitors to what was originally a rejection response to bad tastes (Haidt *et al.* 1994; Rozin *et al.* 1993).

It is easy to see, then, that basic emotions may have evolved in a piecemeal manner in response to distinct environmental imperatives. However, these evolutionary arguments apply most obviously to the *experience* of emotion, whereas what recent findings demonstrate is impaired *recognition* of emotion in the faces of others. There are already good grounds for thinking that the ability to experience fear is compromised after amygdala damage; one of the most striking effects of amygdala damage in primates is a loss of emotional responsiveness, which can include a willingness to approach previously frightening stimuli (Aggleton 1992; Halgren 1992; LeDoux 1995). The findings of

Adolphs *et al.* (1994, 1995) and Calder *et al.* (1996) go beyond this by showing that there is also impaired recognition of fear in others. This is consistent with the idea that for certain basic emotions there is a close mapping of perceptual mechanisms and corresponding emotional experience (Niedenthal and Halberstadt 1995). Mechanisms for recognizing emotions may be closely linked to those involved in experiencing the equivalent emotions because this has evolved as one of the ways we learn our emotional reactions; many of the things which frighten us do so not because we have direct experience, but because we have learnt from the reactions of others (Brothers 1989). Such a mechanism of emotional contagion has clear biological advantages, since it allows us to learn about different types of danger without being harmed ourselves.

An important aspect of this evolutionary perspective is that it cautions against overenthusiasm for the hypothesis of the amygdala as a kind of fear module. A more plausible idea is that the amygdala is involved in the recognition of fear because it plays a more general role in the appraisal of danger (LeDoux 1995). Further work on the types of appraisal involved in different emotions may provide a fruitful line of enquiry; displays of emotion by other people make an important contribution to our moment to moment evaluation of what is significant in our environment. A useful idea could be that the amygdala's contribution is to recognition of those emotions expressed by others which carry clear signals of the presence of physical danger requiring an immediate response (primarily fear and anger), and that it is less involved in the recognition of emotional responses indicating the presence of noxious stimuli and risk of contamination (disgust).

For present purposes, much of the impact of these findings lies in the clear pointer that the system which recognizes identity from the face may use different organizational principles to the system used to recognize emotion. There are many possible implications to be explored. At the moment, the line of reasoning I have set out here for recognition of emotion is more sketchy than that developed in this book for recognition of identity, and the role of functional models in understanding emotion recognition is less advanced. One of the key tasks for the future will be to put this work on a more solid theoretical foundation.

Testing and refining models

In the previous sections I outlined how neuropsychological evidence can be used to construct the rudiments of a model of face processing.

Table 1.1 Average reaction times (in milliseconds) for deciding the sex or the familiarity of famous men from their faces (Bruce *et al.* 1987)

	Familiar male faces	
	Stereotypically masculine in appearance	Less obviously masculine in appearance
Sex judgement	558	682
Familiary judgement	911	883

However, one point that is abundantly clear from the chequered history of psychology is that there is no royal road to understanding, even though many have sought it. All of the techniques we have available to us are subject to certain drawbacks and limitations; this applies as much to inferences based on neuropsychological associations and dissociations as to any other method. The optimal solution is therefore to seek converging evidence from different methods pointing to the same conclusions – just as we did when evaluating the evidence pointing to an evolved neural substrate for face perception.

Fortunately, other techniques are readily to hand, as Chapters 3–5 make clear. Some of the most powerful involve laboratory experiments. For example, if the hierarchic schema shown in Fig. 1.3 were correct, we would expect that anything which makes the earlier stages of the hierarchy difficult for normal perceivers would have an equivalent (or greater) impact on later stages. Bruce *et al.* (1987) tested this by measuring the time taken to decide whether faces were male or female (an early stage in the putative hierarchy) and the time taken to decide whether faces were familiar or unfamiliar (a late stage in the putative hierarchy). Included in the experiment were two critical sets of famous men's faces – one set of 'hunks' with stereotypically masculine appearance, and the other set of 'wimpish', less obviously masculine appearance. Obviously, it was expected that being a hunk or a wimp would have a pronounced effect on deciding whether or not the face was masculine, and as Table 1.1 shows, this was so (with an advantage of around 120 milliseconds). But how would hunkiness affect the judgement of familiarity? If the hierarchical schema is correct, the difficulty of deciding the face's sex for the wimps should have a knock-on effect on deciding these faces are familiar; but as Table 1.1 shows, there was no hint of this (there was a non-significant difference of around 30 milliseconds, in the wrong direction for the hypothesis). Therefore, the results of Bruce *et al.* (1987) go against the hierarchical model shown in Fig. 1.3, and instead are exactly in line with neuropsychological findings pointing to the heterarchic conception.

The linear sequence of access to familiarity, identity-specific semantic information, and the person's name from a seen face can also be tested in the laboratory. Possibilities include measuring reaction times for decisions which require each type of information (Johnston and Bruce 1990; Young et al. 1986a, b, 1988a), or examining the relative difficulty of learning them. The latter paradigm was introduced by McWeeny et al. (1987), who reasoned that if name retrieval occurs at a later stage of face recognition than does access to identity-specific semantic information, then it should be correspondingly more difficult to learn names to faces than it should be to learn occupations (which are a form of identity-specific semantic information) for faces. To create a particularly stringent test of this hypothesis, McWeeny et al. (1987) used several trials with items which could be either names or occupations (Farmer, Carpenter, Baker, etc.). They showed that it is harder to learn that a face is Mr Baker than it is to learn that a face is a baker, indicating that the source of the difficulty lies in how the information is being learnt (as a name or as an occupation), not in the items themselves.

Many other applications of the experimental method are given in Chapters 3–5, and they consistently support the type of model shown in Fig. 1.5. Support can also be derived from studies of everyday errors (see Chapter 5), which have been used to examine the organization of the face recognition route. The naturalistic diary procedure for investigating everyday errors can also be supplemented and considerably strengthened by investigating errors provoked under laboratory conditions, to examine what types of error occur (Hay et al. 1991), and what types of cue can resolve them (Hanley and Cowell 1988). As Chapter 5 shows, such studies are again consistent with the basic model shown in Fig. 1.5.

We have seen, then, that it is not difficult to put together a basic model of the functional organization of human face processing abilities – it is almost deceptively easy. The tricky part is to arrive at something which is non-trivial. Three criteria have been used to try to ensure this.

1. *The model should account for a wide range of evidence.* We have sought to do this by taking evidence from different types of study (neuropsychology, laboratory experiments, everyday errors) and by considering a wide range of phenomena within each domain. Chapters 3 and 4 elaborate the point.

2. *This evidence should be as solid as possible.* Experiments need to be soundly designed, and neuropsychological case studies in particular must meet stringent criteria (Shallice 1979, 1988). Further developments in techniques for neuropsychological inference are discussed in Chapter 6, and Chapter 7 introduces new methods for distinguishing between different forms of face recognition impairment.

3. *Counterintuitive or falsifiable predictions should be identified and tested.* We have already considered counterintuitive patterns of reaction times for face classification (Table 1.1) and potentially falsifiable claims that certain patterns of neuropsychological deficit will not occur. Several other examples can be found in Chapters 3–5.

However, it remains the case that such models have clear limitations; they represent a beginning in our understanding, not the final answer. But one of their advantages is that because the intention is to chart the relevant domain, once one has a reasonably satisfactory chart it becomes possible to remedy some of the obvious deficiencies by tinkering with parts of it.

A good example concerns 'front-end' face processing. Many people find it unsatisfying that the functional modelling approach essentially ducks the question of how we actually do the job of recognizing faces, facial expressions, and so on and asks instead how these different processes relate to each other. But we all want to know *what type* of visual analysis is involved, *which* facial features are used, *how* they are extracted from images seen in different orientations or lighting conditions, and so on. This point is picked up in Chapter 4, which discusses some of the things we know about how the visual system does this job. The area is one which is now developing rapidly, led by advances in image manipulation and mathematical analysis. Some of the more recent developments in our understanding of the visual analysis of the facial image have been reviewed by Bruce (1994).

One important source of information discussed in Chapter 4 involves the configuration of facial features; we are very sensitive to small changes in the relative positioning of features. Equally importantly, though, this applies not just to the relative positions of eyes, nose, and mouth with respect to each other, but to their own positioning within the face. Figure 1.8 shows a face in which the positions of internal features (eyes, nose, mouth) are simply moved upwards or downwards within the face frame. The effect on appearance is profound.

It has also become clear that the visual system needs to do more than just find the boundaries (edges) of facial features. The development of techniques for creating computer-drawn cartoon images demonstrates

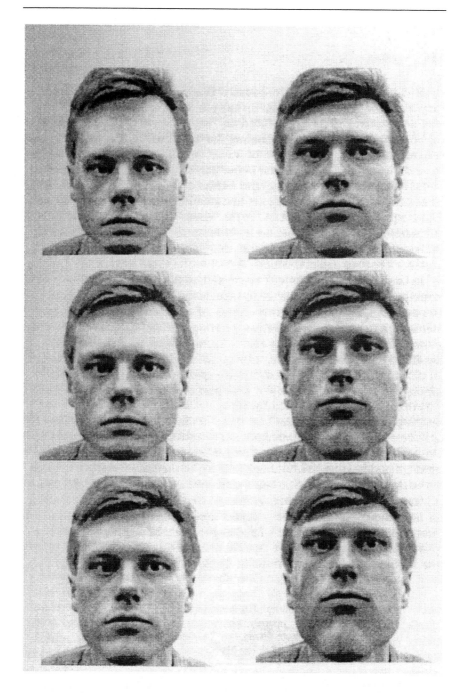

Fig. 1.8 Internal features (eyes, nose, mouth) moved upwards or downwards within the face frame. Reproduced from Bruce (1994, p. 21, Fig. 4).

this nicely (Pearson 1992). The original impetus for this research came from a desire to send complex visual images along telephone lines, to allow deaf people to use the telephone network to communicate by lip-reading and sign language.

Figure 1.9(a) shows a drawing of Michael Caine made by using standard image-processing algorithms to find the edges in a photograph; although it is a faithful rendition of edge information, the result is not particularly easy to recognize. A much better result is achieved if a second 'threshold' process is employed to find regions in the photograph that are darker than a certain level of grey (Fig. 1.9(b)). These regions are then rendered as black. When the edge and threshold images are combined (Fig. 1.9(c)) the result is much better; recognition of such images has been found to be almost as good as recognition of the photographs from which they were derived (Bruce *et al.* 1992).

The benefits of this thresholding technique might derive from at least two possible sources; it marks regions of strong shadow to allow easier recovery of information about the face's three-dimensional shape from patterns of shading, and it also intensifies patterns of surface pigmentation, for example in the eyebrows and hair. Of course, the visual system may use both types of cue, but Bruce (1994) discusses several lines of evidence suggesting that surface pigmentation is especially important in face recognition. One of the most striking of these is shown in Fig. 1.10. The upper row of images in Fig. 1.10 shows the shape of a person's head in a computer image derived from a three-dimensional laser scan; the image is artificially lit in three different ways. Such images show the three-dimensional shape of the head accurately, but lack natural surface pigmentation. They are very difficult to recognize (Bruce *et al.* 1991). One of the people in the lower row of face photographs in

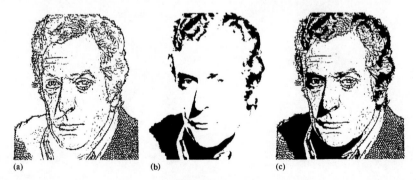

(a)   (b)   (c)

Fig. 1.9 Edge-based (a) and 'thresholded' (b) components of a computer-generated cartoon image of Michael Caine, and (c) a combination of images (a) and (b). Reproduced from Bruce (1994, p. 12, Fig. 1).

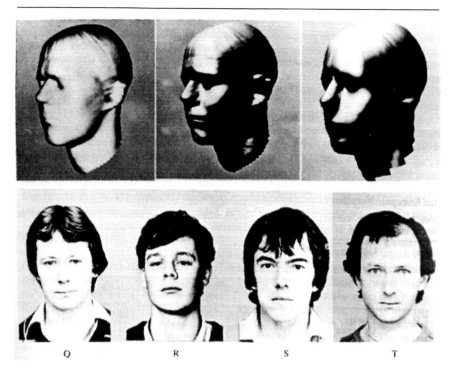

Fig. 1.10 Laser-scanned three-dimensional head model with three different types of lighting)top row) and line-up of four face photographs (bottom row). It is not easy to see that the three-dimensional model matches face R. Reproduced from Bruce *et al.* (1991, p. 759, Fig. 1).

Fig. 1.10 is actually the model who was laser-scanned to create the upper row images, yet it is difficult to see who it is. Similar problems in recognizing such images are found even with highly familiar people (Bruce *et al.* 1991). Performance is usually above-chance, showing that three-dimensional information is of some use, but it is far from ceiling, showing the importance of the missing pigmentation.

Powerful ways of analysing pigmentation and shape based on the mathematical technique of principal components analysis are now being developed, and show considerable promise for developing automated procedures with properties able to account for some aspects of human face processing abilities (Hancock *et al.* 1996; O'Toole *et al.* 1994; Turk and Pentland 1991). The important point here, though, is that researchers pushing these techniques forward recognize that they can be seen as an extension of the functional modelling approach, not a separate or antipathetic enterprise; in effect, they represent attempts to open up the boxes and specify how each component does its job.

The other obvious limitation of a model like Fig. 1.5 is its imprecision. It is easier to follow than a purely verbal account, but it does not really specify how the components interact. This limitation was recognized at an early stage, and the aim was always to move to a version which was implemented as a computer program. A successful implementation of the recognition route part of the model was achieved by Burton *et al.* (1990), using an interactive activation and competition network. The basics of this implementation are discussed in Chapter 4, where its structure is shown in schematic form in Fig. 4.3, but the model has been substantially developed in recent years by Burton and his colleagues (Burton 1994; Burton and Bruce 1993). One of its most important applications can be found in Chapters 11 and 13, which examine how it can be used to account for some of the effects of brain injury.

The reason behind implementing a model as a computer simulation is to make the underlying theory as explicit as possible. This has nothing to do with the idea that the mind is some kind of symbol-manipulating computer program, so elegantly dismissed by Searle (1984), and in my opinion for good reason. The advantage of an implemented model is simply that it provides a step forward because a computer program will not run until everything it has to do has been spelt out. It provides a kind of minimal test that the model is properly specified, with the added advantage that one can now run the simulation to check whether it behaves as one thinks it should (often it doesn't). In the case of Burton *et al.*'s (1990) simulation, certain changes had to be made to the account offered by Bruce and Young (1986; reprinted here as Chapter 3) before it would work properly – details are given in Chapter 13. The fact that these changes were necessary shows the value of a simulation.

Nowadays, then, a computer simulation often follows the presentation of data in many fields of psychology. The current interest in connectionism, coupled with the easy availability of tools for building connectionist models, means that the simulation is often of this (connectionist) form. However, simulation is not a panacea; it needs to be carefully grounded in evidence. In a carefully reasoned critique of the role of connectionist models in cognitive science, McCloskey (1991) has pointed out that to count as implementations of psychological theories, connectionist models must make explicit which features are theory-relevant and which are theory-irrelevant implementational choices, and they must explain exactly how the theoretically relevant parts do what they set out to do. These points follow naturally from the discussion of the different levels at which simulation is possible (or even desirable) initiated by Marr (1982).

This is important because a clear difference in style has emerged between a minority of connectionist models whose intention is to implement accounts that could have been (or which were previously) expressed in box and arrow form (Burton *et al.* 1990; Coltheart *et al.* 1993) and a majority of models representing a more radical connectionist approach which often rejects such concerns, preferring to start from first principles (Farah 1994; Seidenberg and McClelland 1989). We can see this contrast in the case of face recognition, because a different simulation to the Burton *et al.* (1990) approach has been offered by Farah *et al.* (1993). Burton and his colleagues (1990) sought to implement the properties of a model which had been developed primarily to account for a wide range of data on face recognition (Bruce and Young, 1986 – reprinted here as Chapter 3), whereas what Farah *et al.* (1993) wanted to do was to show that some of the effects found after brain injury would be an emergent property of damage to a highly interactive network relying on distributed representations. Their model was thus 'intended to illustrate some very general, qualitative aspects of the behaviour of damaged neural networks in the kinds of tasks used with prosopagnosic patients' (Farah *et al.* 1993, p. 576).

The basic structure of the Farah *et al.* (1993) model is shown in Fig. 1.11(a). It derives from *a priori* theorizing about face recognition, in line with their intention to explore emergent properties of a generic model with minimal specific commitments. There are pools of face input units to act as the initial visual representation of faces, and name units serving to represent names. The semantic units represent semantic information about people, including their occupations, which can be accessed either by names or faces. In addition to these representational units, there are two 'hidden layers' of units, one set between name units and semantic units, and one set between face input units and semantic units. Each pool of units uses fully distributed representations, and units are interconnected via links with variable weights set according to a learning rule.

I have given only a brief description of Farah *et al.*'s model (1993) because this is a fairly standard type of model in the radical connectionist literature – only the particular learning procedure they chose was a trifle unusual, but that does not matter here. What we are interested in is the particular strategy of constructing a deliberately underspecified generic model to explore its emergent properties.

At first sight, this seems very attractive. But I think it entails real dangers. Consider Fig. 1.11(b). This is the first connectionist model of an entire personality; SAMSON (Young 1994*a*). Conveniently, we happen to know quite a lot about SAMSON's behaviour because it is the same model as that of Farah *et al.* (1993), but with the labels changed. In this

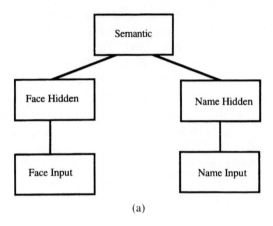

(a)

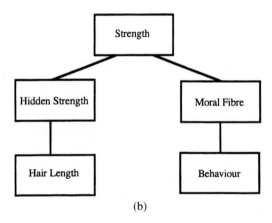

(b)

Fig. 1.11 (a) Structure of a radical connectionist model of face recognition (Farah *et al.* 1993), with pools of units for face input, semantics, and name input, connected by pools of hidden units; (b) SAMSON (Young 1994*a*) – a simulation of alopecia and masculine strength with an organized network.

model, we can simulate the effects of shaving SAMSON's head by reducing the activations of the hair length units. When we do this the model's strength will begin to fall, and it can no longer engage in Delilah-lusting or temple-shattering behaviours. Yet if the hair length units can subsequently gain in activation, its strength returns.

As SAMSON shows, the level of description at which an interpretation is attempted is as crucial in simulation as it is in any other form of psychology. There is a risk of overinterpreting what computer models are doing, as Searle (1984, 1992) has pointed out. We so easily project our own ideas on to boxes with labels like 'face input units' in connectionist models that we can be cajoled into thinking they actually do these things. Some models do actually do them, of course, and it is a desirable goal, but the overwhelming majority are simply mimicking part of the process, and need to be evaluated as more or less good mimics, not mistaken for the real thing. This certainly applies to the models we are discussing here; neither Farah *et al.* (1993) nor Burton *et al.* (1990) take real faces as input at present – they just try to recreate some potential organizational properties of the face recognition system.

This might be thought unfair to Farah *et al.* (1993). Surely, given that neither model is yet able to input real faces, we could just as readily swap the labels on Burton *et al.* (1990) and say mischievous things about that too? To some extent, yes. But there is an important difference, which is that the intention of the Burton *et al.* (1990) account has only been to provide an implementation of an independently motivated theoretical framework – it stands or falls by its ability to mimic a wide range of data from studies of face recognition, and makes no other claims. In contrast, Farah *et al.*'s (1993) focus on examining emergent properties using a generic model has left their account relatively distant from the bulk of the evidence, and there are several standard effects in the literature on face recognition which it is simply unable to handle (Young and Burton, in preparation).

The point is this. Connectionist models provide a powerful tool for implementing and exploring potential accounts of certain patterns of psychological findings. But they do not substitute for evidence. It is evidence which must determine the correct choice of components to be modelled, and a simulation can only be judged by the extent to which it is compatible with a broad range of existing evidence and capable of generating predictions to be tested (Young and Burton, in preparation).

This does not mean that a model which starts out by mimicking effects cannot be taken through to a full implementation. Again, the Burton *et al.* (1990) account provides an example. From its modest beginnings, this model has been broadened to include not only the ability to simulate a wider range of data from neuropsychological case studies (Burton *et al.* 1991; reprinted here as Chapter 13) and laboratory experiments (Burton and Bruce 1993), but also a plausible learning mechanism (Burton 1994). There is no in principle reason why in future the model could not be developed to include a working front-end, based on principal components analysis (Hancock *et al.* 1996; O'Toole *et al.* 1994; Turk and Pentland 1991) or some equivalent technique.

Neuropsychiatry

The agenda I have set out so far is one of conventional behavioural science. We identify a topic area (human face perception), create a simple schema for systematizing what is known, test and refine this against a wide range of evidence, including counterintuitive or falsifiable predictions, and begin to construct a computer-implemented version of our account. This agenda forms much of the content of Chapters 2–7.

Chapters 8–13 take a rather different tack, in which the aim is to broaden the range of topics which can be encompassed. Chapters 11–13 are concerned with recognition and awareness, and Chapters 8–10 with neuropsychiatry. In both cases, the strategy is to use our knowledge of face processing to find an empirical angle on these difficult issues.

First, neuropsychiatry. The initial rationale was to see how far we could push the logic of cognitive neuropsychology, in which models of normal function are tested against their ability to account for the effects of brain injury (Ellis and Young 1996; Shallice 1988). Our interest was in whether the same ground rules might apply with problems that were more obviously 'psychiatric' – why shouldn't an adequate model of normal function be able to account for *any* pattern of impairment in the relevant domain?

Since we had already studied errors in face and person recognition made by neurologically normal people and by people with brain injuries (Chapter 5), delusional misidentification seemed a good place to start. Psychiatrists have described various forms of delusional misidentification, in which other people are systematically misrecognized. Hadyn Ellis and I tried considering how these might be fitted to the Bruce and Young (1986) model – our account (Ellis and Young 1990) is reprinted here as Chapter 8. I no longer find it fully convincing – perhaps it was too much to expect to get something so ambitious right first time – but it contains some interesting ideas and the kernel of work we have subsequently developed on the Capgras delusion.

The Capgras delusion is one of the principal forms of delusional misidentification. It involves the extraordinary claim that certain close relatives have been replaced by near-identical impostors (Capgras and Reboul-Lachaux 1923). Although usually considered a rare phenomenon (Enoch and Trethowan 1991), it has probably been under-diagnosed, and there are now hundreds of descriptions of cases in the psychiatric literature, including many reports that this delusion can follow brain injury.

At first, it is hard to take this delusion seriously – the claim that relatives are impostors, clones, robots or Martians seems so blatantly preposterous. But it is no joke, and is now recognized to carry a significant risk of violence against the alleged impostors (de Pauw and Szulecka 1988). Violence can be extreme, including decapitating the impostor to find the wires, but this is fortunately exceptional.

Psychiatric definitions of delusions emphasize a combination of their unacceptability and implausibility to other people with a similar cultural background and their resistance to reasoned argument or counterevidence. In practice, though, clinical delusions are often not tested against this gold standard, or do not live up to it (Maher 1992). We have had similar experiences, especially with persecutory delusions, where some of the things people say have to be fairly carefully checked before you recognize their unbelievability. In contrast, the claim that your relatives have been replaced is immediately recognizable as most likely to be delusional, despite recent advances in cosmetic surgery, cloning, robotics, and even the possible evidence of simple life forms on Mars. It thus forms a model delusion which meets the standard definition, and is found in many cultures throughout the world. In addition, the Capgras delusion is often noted to follow brain injury, and therefore forms a useful testing ground for theories concerning the interplay of organic and psychological factors (Fleminger 1994; Fleminger and Burns 1993).

In reading many of the case reports and talking to people who have experienced the Capgras delusion we have been struck by the consistency of certain features. Capgras delusion patients can be otherwise rational and lucid, able to appreciate that they are making an extraordinary claim. If you ask 'what would you think if I told you my wife had been replaced by an impostor?', you will often get answers to the effect that it would be unbelievable, absurd, an indication that you had gone mad. Yet the same patients will claim that, none the less, this is exactly what has happened to their own relative. If you ask for evidence that it is an impostor, the patients often tell you that they can *see* the difference, yet they find it hard to express this difference in words. Further probing will sometimes reveal more pervasive feelings that many things seem strange, unfamiliar, almost unreal. Behaviour to the alleged impostor may range from complaint acceptance through puzzlement to outright hostility or physical violence, but there is usually an accompanying mood of noticeable suspiciousness.

These facts suggested to us that Capgras delusion might be a consequence of some form of visual perceptual impairment. Given the nature of the expressed delusion, an obvious tactic was therefore to test perception and recognition of faces. The performance of eight people who had experienced the Capgras delusion on tasks assessing per-

ception of face identity and recognition memory is therefore
summarized in Table 1.2. These data are taken from various sources
(Ellis, Young, Quayle and de Pauw, 1997; Wright, Young and Hellawell,
1993; Young, Ellis, Szulecka and de Pauw, 1990; Young, Reid, Wright
and Hellawell, 1993b), with performance on each test converted into a z
score expressing the degree of impairment in comparison to age-
matched control data; the higher the z score, the more impaired,
whereas negative z scores lie above the control mean. An indication of
maximum possible and chance-level (guessing) performance of each
test is also given.

As Table 1.2 shows, face processing impairments are a common
correlate of Capgras delusion, and everyone except case VD was
significantly impaired on at least one test. In contrast, only one person
showed an impairment on a test of verbal memory, as shown in the last
column of Table 1.2.

Further evidence of visual involvement comes from the closely
related problem of reduplication – the conviction that people or things
have exact or nearly exact duplicates (Weinstein and Burnham 1991).
Reduplication is very similar to the Capgras delusion, but the impostor
claim is not made. For example, case PT (Young *et al.* 1994*a*, reprinted

Table 1.2 Performance of people with Capgras delusion (Ellis *et al.* 1997;
Wright *et al.* 1993; Young *et al.* 1990, 1993*b*) on tasks assessing perception of
face identity and recognition memory

	Face identity				Recognition memory			
	Familiar face recognition (Max = 20 or 30) (Chance close to 0)		Unfamiliar face matching (Max = 54) (Chance = 25)		Faces (Max = 50) (Chance = 25)		Words (Max = 50) (Chance = 25)	
	Acc.	z	Acc.	z	Acc.	z	Acc.	z
GS	15/20	2.39**	43	1.67*	38	1.61	49	−0.90
MC	8/20	9.44***	39	1.70*	41	0.37	41	0.31
ML	13/20	5.10***	35	3.00**	27	3.50**	49	−1.39
KH	17/20	0.54	50	−0.46	33	3.16**	44	1.33
HS	23/30	2.19*	42	1.35	41	0.96	48	−0.13
VD	27/30	0.59	45	0.67	41	0.96	49	−0.49
IN	30/30	−0.61	48	−0.01	33	3.16***	43	1.69*
VL	11/30	6.99***			39	1.51	46	0.60

Acc. = accuracy.
z = number of SDs below control mean.
Asterisked scores are significantly below the control mean: * $z > 1.65$, $p < 0.05$; ** $z < 2.33$,
$p > 0.01$; *** $z > 3.10$, $p < 0.001$.

here as Chapter 9) maintained there were two distinct consultants looking after him. The first consultant (who he called John Smith) was 'a nice bloke', whereas the second (a Dr J. Smith) was someone who was 'distant and aloof'. PT was insistent that these were two separate individuals, both psychiatrists who could be 'brothers or cousins'. When his ability to recognize famous faces was tested, PT made spontaneous comments about duplicates – for example, he identified a photograph of Jimmy Savile as 'one of them Jimmy Saviles' – yet he never did this when asked to recognize famous people's voices. Such observations suggest a visual basis for PT's reduplication; it seems that the origin of his strange claims is in something aberrant about the visual input, not in defective knowledge or logic (which would apply equally to voices). Similar phenomena have also been noted for the Capgras delusion; Hirstein and Ramachandran's (1997) patient claimed that his parents were impostors when he was looking at them, but not when speaking to them on the telephone!

But what kind of visual impairment could create such bizarre delusions? Different possibilities are discussed in Chapters 8–10; the one we favour is that there is a loss of appropriate emotional orienting reactions to visual stimuli with personal affective significance.

The orienting reaction is a concept from Russian psychology; it refers to automatic preparatory responses to stimuli with high signal value to an organism. The idea is that when we meet people we know well, there are automatic emotional responses which will set the initial tone of the subsequent encounter. This conception had been tellingly applied to cases of prosopagnosia (inability to recognize familiar faces after brain injury) by Bauer (1984); he showed that despite the loss of conscious recognition in prosopagnosia, certain types of response to familiar faces were preserved, and these can be indexed through electrodermal changes (skin conductance response, or SCR) created by autonomic nervous system activity. The SCR is usually measured by recording electrical conductivity from the finger or the palm of the hand. When we have an emotional response to something, the secretions from sweat glands caused by activity of the autonomic nervous system alter skin conductance; even very small degrees of emotional arousal can be measured in this way.

The wider implications of Bauer's (1984) findings are discussed in Chapters 11–14, for now we will simply note that our hypothesis has been that Capgras delusion might form a kind of mirror image of prosopagnosia, in which overt recognition is relatively preserved (but not necessarily completely preserved, as Table 1.2 shows) whereas orienting responses are severely diminished. The consequence will be that faces which can be recognized fail to provoke appropriate reactions; the impostor claim represents the patient's hypothesis as to what is behind the resultant sense of things not being as they should. The delusion is primarily centred on close relatives because it is these for which the discrepancy between continuing overt recognition and absent orienting reactions will be most noticeable.

It was immediately apparent to us that this could be tested by measuring SCRs to familiar faces, but it took some time to get the methods right. Our account, based on a lack of emotional orienting responses, predicts loss of SCR to familiar faces in Capgras delusion, whereas this is not predicted by any of the other various hypotheses that have been offered to try to explain this delusion. We are therefore considerably encouraged that two recent studies have produced findings consistent with this prediction; Hirstein and Ramachandran (1997) tested a single patient and found no SCR to personally familiar faces, and we (Ellis *et al.* 1997) tested five patients and found no SCR to famous faces. Figure 1.12(a) shows mean SCR amplitudes to familiar (famous) and unfamiliar faces for normal controls, five people with Capgras delusion, and for psychiatric controls taking similar medication (Ellis *et al.* 1997). Only the people with Capgras delusion show no differential response to familiar compared to unfamiliar faces. However, the people with Capgras delusion also show a lack of responsiveness to all faces, so Fig. 1.12(b) gives range-corrected scores which take account of this, showing that the pattern of loss of SCR to familiar faces in Capgras delusion is still found when measured in this way. In contrast, the SCRs of people with Capgras delusion to an auditory tone were normal in magnitude and rate of habituation (Ellis *et al.* 1997).

Note especially that Ellis *et al.* (1997) showed abnormal SCRs to famous faces for which the patients they tested had not expressed any particular delusional beliefs. Lack of responsiveness is found to all faces in Capgras delusion, not just to the faces of people who have been subjected to the impostor allegation. This is exactly as Ellis and Young's (1990) hypothesis predicts.

Evidence can therefore be found to suggest the utility of this general approach. However, it now seems to us that the original statement of our ideas (Ellis and Young 1990; reprinted as Chapter 8 here) lacked something. Even if one accepted the premise that the Capgras delusion represents a person's attempt at explaining powerfully abnormal perceptual experiences, nothing was said about why such a bizarre (impostor) explanation should be offered. Why didn't a person in the grip of such an experience just say something to the effect that 'things seem very strange, but I'm not sure what's causing it'?

(a)   **SCR to faces**

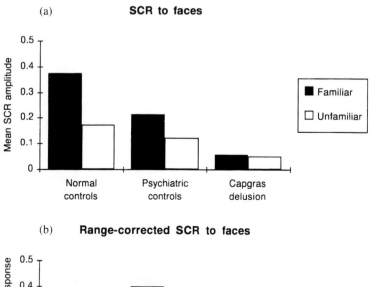

(b)   **Range-corrected SCR to faces**

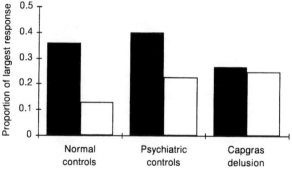

Fig. 1.12 Mean SCR amplitude to familiar and unfamiliar faces for normal controls, psychiatric controls, and five people with Capgras delusion (Ellis *et al.* 1997). (a) Amplitudes in μS; (b) range-corrected responses.

In fact, many people do say such things; they just get less attention from psychiatrists, neurologists, and psychologists. The Capgras delusion represents the tip of a large iceberg of plausible and less plausible personal explanations of anomalous experiences. We think that what characterizes people with Capgras delusion is that they have additional problems which serve to create conditions under which extravagant explanations can be formed and sustained. This idea is explained in Chapter 10 (Young 1994*b*), which draws particular attention to the importance of the suspicious mood that so often accompanies this delusion. Suspicious moods create biases which focus the person's attention on to seeking external causes for their problems (Kaney and Bentall 1989), and allow conclusions to be reached on the basis of insufficient evidence (Dudley *et al.* 1997; Garety *et al.* 1991). Other recent work has also shown that people become (not unnaturally) preoccupied with their delusions and find it difficult to take their attention away from anything which seems relevant to the delusional belief (Leafhead *et al.* 1996). This heightened attention to delusion-related material may serve to make the world seem to throw up evidence consistent with the delusion, serving further to increase the bias to find relevant information, creating a vicious circle which can make a delusion become almost a self-fulfilling prophecy.

From this perspective, the Capgras delusion reflects an interaction of different impairments, and this has important implications for the logic of extending the cognitive neuropsychology approach to try to create a cognitive neuropsychiatry. Cognitive neuropsychology has worked well in analysing single, selective, often stable deficits, but this is not like what we are doing here and a rather different rule-book may be needed. Chapter 10 discusses the relation between the Capgras delusion and certain other forms of neuropsychiatric phenomenon, including the equally extraordinary and bizarre claim that you are dead, described in a classic report by Cotard (1882).

People experiencing the Cotard delusion will admit that they are still able to walk and talk, yet insist they are dead; detailed subjective accounts are given by Young and Leafhead (1996). Sometimes they refuse to eat, or make preparations for the funeral they imminently expect. One of the people we investigated, KH, was brought to hospital after he stabbed himself to show that he had no blood (Wright *et al.* 1993). He was depressed at the time, and was given appropriate medication and subsequently discharged. Some months later, however, he had to be readmitted to hospital in an agitated and paranoid state, believing among other things that his father had been replaced by an impostor. On this later admission KH also maintained that some of the hospital staff he knew from his previous visits had been replaced by ill-intentioned 'dummies'. Because of this subsequent episode of Capgras delusion, data pertaining to KH's face processing abilities are summarized in Table 1.2.

As Chapter 10 discusses, there are a number of parallels between the Capgras and Cotard delusions, including evidence that they can be associated with similar forms of brain injury, defective face processing abilities (Young *et al.* 1994*b*), and similar feelings of strangeness and unfamiliarity. The striking difference is in the patients' moods; depressed for people voicing the Cotard delusion, suspicious for the Capgras delusion. A plausible hypothesis is therefore that these two delusions represent different interpretations of fundamentally similar perceptual abnormalities, but that people in suspicious moods blame others for these abnormalities whereas depressed people correctly (but exaggeratedly) attribute the change to themselves.

Cognitive neuropsychiatry thus presents interesting opportunities, and these are being actively pursued by a number of research groups (David 1993; Frith 1992; Halligan *et al*. 1994), but I suspect it is going to need some careful attention to basic principles to get it right.

Face recognition and awareness

When we recognize a familiar face we know who it is; we can act appropriately (or inappropriately if we wish) based on our past personal knowledge of that person, introduce them to others if necessary, and so on. Overt recognition of this sort seems so integral to our concept of what it means to recognize someone that functional models such as Bruce and Young (1986; reprinted as Chapter 3) did not draw any distinction between face recognition and awareness of recognition.

However, Bauer (1984) reckoned just such a distinction was necessary. He measured the skin conductance response (SCR) of prosopagnosic patient LF when he was shown a face and a series of names was read out. If the name was the same person as the face, LF's skin conductance changed. Yet if LF was asked simply to choose the correct name, he performed at chance level. The basic technique is an adaptation of the guilty knowledge test used in lie detection, but Bauer wasn't suggesting that LF was lying. Instead, it seemed there was a difference between his inability to recognize the face overtly, consciously, and some form of covert, non-conscious recognition which could be picked up in the SCR.

I found this result most surprising. Having worked with a few people with prosopagnosia, I had never seen anything in their behaviour or test results to suggest anything other than a total inability to recognize familiar faces. Although cognitive psychology had loosened some of the corsets of behaviourism, it was also the case that certain topics were still considered a little distasteful in polite psychological circles. Conscious-ness was one of these. My colleagues and I read and re-read Bauer's (1984) report, examining every detail of the method to see what was wrong, but we found nothing. We were organizing a conference on faces and took the opportunity to invite Bauer to make a presentation. He proved to be careful, cautious, conscientious in his approach; just entirely plausible. When a confirmatory report by Tranel and Damasio (1985) appeared, it was clear that this effect had to be taken very seriously.

With hindsight, we should not have been so taken aback. The results of Weiskrantz and his colleagues from their studies of blindsight – preserved responses to stimuli presented in subjectively blind parts of the visual field – were well known at the time (Weiskrantz 1980; Weiskrantz *et al.* 1974). The reason we did not immediately see the parallel to Bauer's (1984) work was that blindsight was widely believed to be mediated by subcortical visual pathways, even though Weiskrantz himself was obviously sceptical that this was all there was to it; it has taken a lot of further research on the neurophysiology of blindsight to establish that this was indeed an oversimplification (Cowey and Stoerig 1992).

Bauer (1984) thought that his results showed that orienting responses to emotionally significant stimuli and conscious, overt recognition of the same stimuli are mediated by neurologically dissociable pathways. We have already seen how Ellis and Young (1990; reprinted as Chapter 8) developed this view into an account of the Capgras delusion. A further possibility that also followed from it was that a similar effect might be present in normal people if a face was presented under conditions which would prevent conscious recognition. This was investigated by Ellis *et al.* (1993); the study is reprinted here as Chapter 12. Differential SCRs to familiar (compared to unfamiliar) faces were indeed found for faces presented to normal people at exposures too brief to permit conscious recognition, and there was no further increase in the SCR to faces presented for sufficient time to allow conscious recognition.

Bauer (1984) also proposed neuroanatomical pathways which might be involved in orienting responses and overt recognition, but this has proved more contentious (Hirstein and Ramachandran 1997; Tranel *et al.* 1995). This dispute, though, has been over getting the neurology right, not over the separate pathways hypothesis itself. It is a good example of how, even though they can often be usefully combined, psychological and neurological hypotheses can have some degree of independence from each other. Both Bauer and his critics are in agreement that at the psychological level one needs to distinguish functional pathways involved in overt recognition and orienting responses; they disagree on where these are realized in the brain.

A crucial question concerning Bauer's (1984) findings was whether such effects were restricted to the SCR, or could they be demonstrated in other ways? The existence of a report by Bruyer and his colleagues which used learning techniques (Bruyer *et al.* 1983) suggested to us that behavioural indices of covert recognition in prosopagnosia might be developed if we could find tests which examined face recognition in-directly, by measuring its influence on some other task. This spawned a number of studies, reviewed by Young (1994*c*), which forms Chapter 11.

Table 1.3 summarizes findings from 20 studies of covert recognition and related effects in cases of prosopagnosia. As the table makes clear, a wide range of such phenomena has been reported; further details of the paradigms can be found in Chapter 11 or in the papers cited in the third column of Table 1.3. Importantly, such effects are evident even when overt recognition of individual faces is absent, with face naming, ability to give the occupation or other identifying information, and assessment of face familiarity all at chance level (see Chapter 11).

The existence of covert recognition in prosopagnosia is therefore no longer disputed; the focus has shifted on to how it is best interpreted. Our initial efforts centred on the notion of some form of neurological disconnection between face recognition and awareness of recognition (de Haan *et al.* 1987*a*), and this had the advantage that Schacter *et al.* (1988) showed how the same approach could be applied to a number of different neuropsychological deficits. But problems became increasingly apparent. There was no detailed account of what 'signals to awareness' might be, and attempts to describe some of the phenomena in box and arrow terms (Young and de Haan 1988) began to reach an almost Byzantine complexity, as Chapter 13 demonstrates (see Figure 13.2, and associated discussion).

A definite step forward was therefore achieved with the discovery that a simple and plausible form of damage to Burton *et al.*'s (1990) interactive activation model could simulate some of these behaviours. If the connection strengths of the links connecting the model's 'face' units to more central parts of the system were halved, it became unable to recognize any inputs via that route yet still showed priming and interference effects from now unrecognized faces (Burton *et al.* 1991). These simulations are described in detail in Chapter 13; they work because a model of this type can continue to pass activation around the system at sub-threshold levels.

The implications of this type of simulation need to be considered carefully. It does not prove that this is why covert recognition is found in prosopagnosia. What it does is to show that this is a plausible candidate mechanism, subject to the limitation that other candidates may also be discovered in due course. But because we now have a candidate mechanism for covert recognition, and because it derives from such a simple modification to Burton *et al.*'s (1990) account of normal recognition, it helps to demystify the phenomenon.

Recently, Mike Burton and I have been assessing just how strong a candidate this actually is (Young and Burton, in preparation). We had shown that it can simulate associative priming and interference effects (Burton *et al.*, 1991; reprinted here as Chapter 13), but would other

Table 1.3 Examples of covert recognition of familiar faces and related findings in cases of prosopagnosia. Such effects are reported even when overt recognition of individual faces is at chance level

Effect	Brief description	Reports*	Current status in Burton model
SCR	Skin conductance response to familiar faces or to face paired with correct name	1, 2, 16–18	Model not applicable to SCR
Evoked potentials	Difference between familiar and unfamiliar faces	11	Model not applicable to evoked potentials
Eye movements	Difference between familiar and unfamiliar faces	12	Model not applicable to eye movements
'Mere exposure' effect	Preference for faces seen previously in judging which of two faces is 'more likeable'	9	Unclear what 'preference' would mean in a model of this type
Face matching	Better performance at matching photographs of familiar than unfamiliar faces	5, 14, 15	Simulable with Burton (1994) learning model
Savings in relearning	Faster learning of correct than incorrect face + name or face + occupation pairings	3, 5, 7, 8, 10, 13–15, 19	Simulable with Burton (1994) learning model
Self-priming	A face can facilitate recognition of the subsequently presented name of the same person	4	Easily simulated; same as Burton et al. (1991) account of associative priming
Associative ('semantic') priming	A face can facilitate recognition of the subsequently presented name of a closely associated person	13, 20	Simulated by Burton et al. (1991); see Chapter 13
Interference	Faces can interfere with semantic classification of simultaneously presented names	4–6, 15	Simulated by Burton et al. (1991); see Chapter 13
Cued recognition	Above-chance performance at guessing which of two names is correct for a familiar face	7, 8, 14, 15	Can be simulated (Burton et al. 1991); see Chapter 13
Provoked overt recognition	When faces from the same semantic category are presented together, there can be some overt recognition	7, 8, 14, 15	Cannot be simulated at present (Young and Burton, in prep)

*Research papers cited:
1. Bauer (1984).
2. Bauer (1986).
3. Bruyer et al. (1983)
4. De Haan et al. (1992).
5. De Haan et al. (1987a).
6. De Haan et al. (1987b).
7. De Haan et al. (1991).
8. Diamond et al. (1994).
9. Greve and Bauer (1990)
10. McNeil and Warrington (1991)
11. Renault et al. (1989).
12. Rizzo et al. (1987).
13. Schweinberger et al. (1995).
14. Sergent and Poncet (1990).
15. Sergent and Signoret (1992).
16. Tranel and Damasio (1985).
17. Tranel and Damasio (1988).
18. Tranel et al. (1995).
19. Young and de Haan (1988).
20. Young et al. (1988b).

effects prove as tractable? Our conclusions are summarised in the final column of Table 1.3. There are certain effects which cannot be simulated with this approach because the type of measure used has not been modelled; these form the first 4 rows of Table 1.3. Then there are several effects which can be simulated either with the original Burton *et al.* (1990) model or the extended variant incorporating a learning rule (Burton, 1994). But the bottom row of Table 1.3 shows an effect which has been reported in a number of studies which we were unable to simulate (Young and Burton, in prep.).

The effect in question is a form of provoked overt recognition, rather than covert recognition *per se*, but it seems likely that these are closely related. Although prosopagnosia involves a dramatic deficit of overt recognition, in which even the closest personal acquaintances may not be recognized from their faces in everyday life, it turns out that the deficit need not be absolute. Sergent and Poncet (1990) found that their patient, PV, could achieve overt recognition of some faces if several members of the same semantic category were presented together. This only happened for some semantic categories, and it reflected genuine recognition rather than laborious deduction. It wasn't due to PV thinking things like 'if they're film stars, I guess the blonde one could be Marilyn Monroe', because when PV could not identify the category herself she continued to fail to recognize the faces even when the occupational category was pointed out to her. This observation of overt recognition provoked by simultaneously presenting multiple exemplars of a semantic category has since been replicated with patients PH (de Haan *et al.* 1991*a*), PC (Sergent and Signoret 1992*b*), and ET (Diamond *et al.* 1994). The phenomenon is very striking; the patients themselves tend to be highly surprised at being able to recognize faces overtly.

Sergent and Poncet (1990) suggested that their demonstration shows that 'neither the facial representations nor the semantic information were critically disturbed in PV, and her prosopagnosia may thus reflect faulty connections between faces and their memories'. They thought that the simultaneous presentation of several members of the same category may have temporarily raised the activation level above the appropriate threshold. This account bears a striking resemblance to that of Burton *et al.* (1991) for prosopagnosia with covert recognition, so we thought that the Burton model should be able to reproduce these results.

It turned out that in many analogues of Sergent and Poncet's (1990) procedure that we tried, the 'lesioned' Burton model did not produce such behaviour (Young and Burton, in preparation). The reasons are to be found in the fact that interactive activation and competition networks use within-pool inhibitory links to help stabilize activation in each pool. The advantage which accrues through sharing semantics with other stimuli presented at the same time is therefore balanced, or even outweighted, by the disadvantage which accrues from within-pool inhibition.

This failure to simulate provoked overt recognition seems to us to be a potentially serious weakness of the interactive activation and competition model. Provoked recognition is now a well documented phenomenon, and a complete account of prosopagnosia must provide an explanation. Although the Burton model seems close in spirit in Sergent and Poncet's (1990) account of provoked recognition, at present we cannot get it to simulate this effect. At a minimum, it is clear that further work is needed to overcome this limitation. In the meantime, the Burton simulation remains the principal candidate account of covert recognition because of the good range of phenomena it *can* simulate, and any other model cannot be considered better unless it does all this and more, but the fact remains that it is not yet achieving 100 per cent success.

Psychology and philosophy

In using face perception as a way to explore consciousness and delusional beliefs we have started to enter treacherous philosophical waters. But I think it is worth trying to sail in them – the hazards are there, but so are the potential rewards. What is needed is to bring together philosophical and psychological concerns to achieve a workable synthesis. I am not at all confident of my own ability to do this, but I've managed to get some advice from philosophers. It will take a while, though, to know whether we are sinking or swimming.

Findings such as Bauer's (1984) demonstration of covert recognition of familiar faces in prosopagnosia force us to think about consciousness, but it is a notoriously tricky concept. The issues surrounding consciousness have been discussed by Young and Block (1996), reprinted here in slightly abridged form as Chapter 14. A number of different forms of neuropsychological impairment involving different aspects of conscious awareness are brought together here. They are discussed in relation to distinctions between phenomenal consciousness, access consciousness, and monitoring and self-consciousness. This allows us to clarify how consciousness relates to intentional actions, and to offer the beginnings of an evolutionary account.

An equally intriguing set of issues arises from work in cognitive neuropsychiatry, and these are touched on in Chapter 10. They include what makes our percepts normally seem so real to us? Delusions in which the feeling of things being real seems to be dysfunctional also raise important questions about our sense of self and self-existence.

Dennett (1996) has picked up some of these issues. Using persuasive understatement, he notes of the Capgras delusion that 'this amazing phenomenon should send shock waves through philosophy' (Dennett 1996, p. 111). Dennett's point is that in certain respects neuropsychiatric case studies can be seen as analogues of philosophical thought experiments, such as those that have been popular in philosophical discussions of personal identity (Parfit 1984; Williams 1973). Thought experiments are used on the assumption that they can act as challenges to philosophical theories, but the same goes for neuropsychiatric case studies, and with the extra urgency that these are genuine, real-world phenomena, not something from an imaginary twin-earth. It is a further extension of the logic used pervasively in cognitive neuropsychology, but this time into the province of philosophy.

One way to do this is to look at ideas about the nature of beliefs. I have recently worked on these with Tony Stone, and much of the rest of this section comprises some of our thoughts in summary form, being heavily cribbed from Stone and Young (1977). I am using it here simply to demonstrate the kind of thing that can be done, hopefully showing the potential of the approach.

An example concerns what many philosophers have taken to be the key characteristic of our belief system – its holism. The idea is that the belief system forms a coherent whole and that changing any one belief will also require adjustment of many others. Consider Dennett's (1987) reaction to the idea of attributing to someone the belief that rabbits are birds. Dennett (1987, p. 14) asks

Could anyone really and truly be attributed that belief? Perhaps, but it would take a bit of a story to bring us to accept it.

One way to see why we need 'a bit of a story' is to reflect upon another of Dennett's examples. Dennett (1981) asks us to explain how a future neurocryptographer might insert the false belief that *I have an older brother living in Cleveland* into someone's brain. Dennett argues that this is a more difficult task than might be thought at first. For if this belief is to be inserted successfully, wouldn't lots of other beliefs also have to be inserted? Beliefs that would enable the subject of the experiment to answer questions such as 'What's your brother's name?', 'How old is he?', 'Are you an only child?'. Dennett concludes (1981), p. 44) that this does not show that 'wiring in' false beliefs is impossible, but that 'one could only wire in one belief by wiring in many (indefinitely many?) other cohering beliefs so that neither biographical nor logical coherence would be lost'.

The existence of relatively circumscribed delusional beliefs seems to challenge this conception. In cases of Capgras delusion, shouldn't the introduction of the belief that your spouse has been replaced by an impostor lead on to numerous other false beliefs? Beliefs about where they have gone, beliefs about what explains such strange events, what their significance might be, whether you are now a bigamist, and so on? In practice, this doesn't seem quite like what happens; instead, a few other beliefs may change, but mainly the delusional belief is somehow kept isolated.

In Dennett's (1981) example, the insertion of a false belief was not straightforward because successful insertion seemed to require that other beliefs also be changed. Many philosophers argue that belief fixation is a *conservative* process, striving 'to accomplish the maximum in accommodating data at the minimum cost in overall disturbance to previous cognitive commitments' (Fodor 1987).

Delusional belief formation, however, does not seem to be conservative; the postulation of doubles is by any logical standard a profligate hypothesis.

Stone and Young (1997) therefore argue that conservatism plays a more complex role in belief formation. What delusional and non-delusional bizarre beliefs suggest is that the belief formation system contains within it a tension between *two* principles that can come into conflict; a tension between forming beliefs that require little re-adjustment to the web of belief (conservatism) and forming beliefs that do justice to the deliverances of one's perceptual systems. We can call the latter the need to form beliefs that are *observationally adequate* (Fodor 1989).

So the kind of theory of belief fixation put forward by Fodor, one that stresses that seeing is believing (observational adequacy) and yet incorporates conservatism into the way one alters the web of belief, may provide a way of understanding delusional belief formation. If the belief formation mechanism is to be adaptive, a balance needs to be maintained between these two imperatives, but in a person experiencing a delusion this balance goes too far toward observational adequacy as against conservatism. In Fodor's (1989) view, conservatism and observational adequacy are independent constraints, so there 'is no guarantee that the hypothesis that fits most of the data will be maximally conservative or, conversely, that the maximally conservative hypothesis will be the one that fits most of the data'.

Fodor has also argued that perception plays a special role in belief fixation because it provides the data for our inferences. Without perception the only theories we could have would be truths of logic or those that follow by implication from what we already know. From this perspective it is unsurprising that our perceptions should be given the power to override existing beliefs.

In the above discussion, neuropsychiatric delusions were used to provide evidence for a certain view of belief formation. Psychology informs philosophy. But there are equally important examples where philosophy can help to sharpen the psychology. A case in point concerns the conceptual issues which arise in any account of delusions. These include whether delusions represent genuine belief states, and inconsistencies in emotions accompanying the delusions.

The first issue boils down to whether patients really believe their delusions, and so what it means to call something a belief. The view that delusions are false beliefs is inherent in the way psychiatrists usually define them, and it was unquestioningly adopted in the nineteenth century. However, the idea of delusions as false beliefs has not been universally popular since (Berrios 1991; Sass 1994), and theorists have pointed out that the status of delusional beliefs as beliefs is cast into doubt by the fact that deluded individuals do not always act in ways that we might consider to be appropriate to the content of their delusions. This point has been particularly eloquently made by Sass (1994), in his discussion of schizophrenia. Sass's (1994) position is that the idea that the person with schizophrenia takes the imaginary as real is incorrect; he regards it as wrong to think that a person with schizophrenia has formed a false belief about the actual world. Instead, Sass points out that people with schizophrenia often fail to act on their delusions. His line of argument (Sass 1994, p. 42) is that they are best thought of as living in a solipsistic universe where

to act might feel either unnecessary or impossible: unnecessary because external conditions are at the mercy of thought, since the world is idea . . . impossible because real action, action in a world able to resist my efforts, cannot occur in a purely mental universe.

Although Sass (1994) was primarily concerned with schizophrenia, his position is relevant to present concerns because people with the Capgras delusion can also fail to act in ways that we would think of as appropriate. They often do not, for example, report the fact that their spouse has been replaced to the police, and they have been known to live companionably with the impostor.

However, Stone and Young (1997) show that Sass's (1994) argument from inappropriate action does not work. There has been some empirical progress in identifying those factors which make it more likely that delusions will be acted on (Buchanan 1993; Buchanan *et al.* 1993); it would be incorrect to imply that absence of actions is characteristic or inevitable. In addition, there is no single action that is *intrinsically* appropriate to a belief. An action is only appropriate or inappropriate to a belief relative to some project that an agent has (Williams 1973). Consider the failure to report the impostor to the police. Why would any person experiencing the Capgras delusion not do that? In fact, Williams' (1973) analysis can help us to see the potential appropriateness of this kind of (in)action. For example, the person who acts in accordance with a delusion – even where the action is just the speech act of asserting his or her bizarre belief – will cause distress to others and may experience recriminations or unwanted attentions of the medical profession. It is surely a perfectly understandable project to try to avoid these consequences.

A more difficult problem which arises in considering delusions as false beliefs is that they often seem to lack appropriate accompanying emotion (Sass 1994). Using the example of Capgras delusion, it is easy to see that if some of your relatives were replaced by impostors, you would probably be very concerned about the fate of the original relatives. If you had grounds for suspecting they were dead, you might well grieve. However, people experiencing the Capgras delusion seldom seem to show such concern, and may even experience inappropriate emotions. For example Alexander *et al.*'s (1979) patient, who experienced the Capgras delusion after a brain injury sustained in an accident, did not seem concerned about what had happened to his real wife, and instead expressed his gratitude that she had located a substitute who was now looking after him.

Stone and Young (1997) acknowledge that absent or inappropriate emotions require explanation, and that they do not as yet have a complete answer. It is an interesting issue for future work, but some relevant observations can be offered.

The most obvious way to deal with the point is to hypothesize that emotional deficits may contribute to the formation of delusions. To some extent, this has been Ellis and Young's (1990) position anyway, since the particular form of perceptual impairment they proposed to account for the Capgras delusion involved a loss of affective reactions; whether one sees this as primarily a perceptual deficit or primarily emotional is in part a question of which label is preferred. Given that affective reactions to visual stimuli are thought to be lacking, it is less surprising that the delusion will show some abnormal emotional features, and it is also of course possible that some Capgras delusion patients may in addition suffer more widespread emotional impairments.

However, there is a further counterintuitive aspect of the Capgras delusion which may be instructive. Intuitively, we tend to think that identification comes before emotional reaction; first you recognize your spouse, then you experience the relevant emotions. The Capgras delusion cases suggest that this intuitive thought is incorrect; they fit with a line of reasoning advocated by Zajonc (1980), who has queried the widely adopted assumption that affect is post-cognitive. Zajonc (1980) notes that affective reactions are often our very first reactions to stimuli, and that they can sometimes be made even when cognitive judgements like recognition are not possible (Kunst-Wilson and Zajonc 1980). From such evidence, Zajonc (1980) concludes that affect and cognition are under the control of separate and partially independent systems. Ellis and Young's (1990) account of the Capgras delusion is, of course, exactly in line with this claim. Asynchronies between expressed delusions and accompanying emotions may therefore be both expected and potentially explicable.

These points touch on another area where I think a very useful contribution might come from philosophy. This concerns the notion of 'familiarity', which is discussed briefly in Chapter 10.

Familiarity is a key concept in the face recognition literature, and with good reason. In everyday life, we encounter both familiar and unfamiliar people, and we need to be able to assign faces to the categories of those we know or those we do not know. In addition, the experience of familiarity can occur in relatively pure form; in laboratory and in diary studies it has been noted that normal people sometimes find that they know that a face is familiar but cannot remember where they have seen it before (Hay et al. 1991; Young et al. 1985); this can also happen as a persistent problem after brain injury (de Haan et al. 1991b).

The ease with which we can determine familiarity may be relatively great for faces compared to other naturally occurring visual stimuli, because the ability is of such ecological importance. In contrast to the plethora of familiar and unfamiliar faces we see every day, we seldom encounter anything other than familiar words or familiar types of object; pronounceable non-words (such as 'blunk') or unfamiliar objects are relatively uncommon in people's daily lives. A great deal of the experimental literature on human face recognition therefore relies on the 'face familiarity decision task' (Bruce and Valentine 1985) as a laboratory analogue of this everyday ability; subjects are shown a series of faces, some of which are known to them, and their task is to make a speeded familiar vs. unfamiliar decision to each face.

All of this has to do with familiarity in the sense of knowing that we know someone; a kind of certainty that one has encountered them before. Familiarity in this sense is a relatively basic piece of cognitive information. Researching this cognitive form of familiarity has been a useful tactic, but studies of the Capgras delusion and related conditions show that familiarity may be more complex.

A commonly reported claim of Capgras delusion patients is that people and things seem somehow unfamiliar, and this is also found in other psychiatric and neurological conditions (Critchley 1989; Sno 1994). And of course there are also forms of abnormal experience which involve a kind of hyper-familiarity, or *déjà vu* (Sno and Linszen 1990). Yet in the Capgras delusion, at least, there does not seem to be a particularly obvious problem of cognitive familiarity; faces can seem strange or unfamiliar even when they are recognized as those of known people. This is consistent with the position developed by Ellis and Young (1990; Chapter 8 here) that a root cause of the Capgras delusion lies in an absence of appropriate emotional reactions to visual stimuli, if one assumes that these contribute to a kind of emotional familiarity. As is noted in Chapter 10, it may therefore be useful to pay more attention to distinguishing different forms of familiarity, and especially to separate those aspects that involve cognitive familiarity from those that may be more closely linked to emotional and orienting reactions to people, things, and events which have personal relevance (Van Lancker 1991).

Credo

In a paper which struck terror into the hearts of many cognitive psychologists, Newell (1973) offered a trenchant critique of the field as it then existed. His main theme was that you can't play 20 questions with nature and win. He characterized research at the time as being excessively driven by laboratory phenomena. When a potentially interesting experimental effect was found (such as the effect of set size on deciding whether a target item is part of a set held in short-term memory), researchers would ask a question based on some form of binary opposition; for example, is memory search a serial or a parallel process? At first, some progress would seem to be made, but gradually inconsistent results would also arise, and eventually it would become clear that there was something to be said for both points of view. At this point, many researchers would just bring another binary opposition into play (e.g. is memory search an automatic or an effortful process?), and work on that until it too became unworkable. And when this happened, another binary question could be dreamed up (is the set size effect due to encoding or to retrieval?). Finally, if you got really tired of this, you could start applying the same strategy to another laboratory-based phenomenon (perhaps loss of information from short-term memory with an interpolated task). And so on.

These examples are taken from the lengthy lists drawn up by Newell (1973). There may have been an element of caricature, but the points struck home. Rightly, Newell (1973) expressed disappointment that the history of this investigative strategy showed that, far from resolving central issues, it was associated with failure to achieve cumulative impact or build up a coherent overall picture. Worse still, he was depressed at the prospect that if one thought about *n* more studies of the same type, even when *n* could be a very large number indeed it was unclear whether real progress would be made.

Newell's (1973) view was that it was desirable to use a different strategy which would involve building more ambitious models, capable of dealing with complex tasks and ultimately able to handle many different tasks with the same system. Naturally, this was the approach he pursued with great distinction in his own work.

I think Newell (1973) had the right diagnosis of the weaknesses of much of cognitive psychology in the early 1970s, but he handed out the wrong prescription. Certainly it was desirable to shift the focus of theorizing higher than the individual laboratory effect, but the history of psychology shows equally that the opposite danger of creating theories that are abstract and too far removed from the data is just as real. Anyone who can remember the days when undergraduates had to study Hullian learning theory, with its edifice of esoteric and exotic concepts like the fractional antedating goal response, will know what I mean. For a long time this was the dominant theoretical approach to learning and motivation; it was theory in the grand manner, but now it looks like theory for theory's sake.

I therefore think there is a strong case for intermediate-level theories, targeted at a particular domain of expertise but kept tightly under the control of pertinent data. Here, we have used face perception as such a domain, but there are plenty of others where a similar tactic has paid off; working memory (Baddeley 1986) forms one of the most successful examples.

A feature of much of the research subject to Newell's (1973) critique was that it had lost contact with the world outside the laboratory. The phenomena investigated were all generated in highly specific experimental paradigms. Certainly, one could see that short-term memory is a real-world phenomenon, and even follow the theroetical moves which would lead to a study of the effect of set size on searching for information held in short-term memory. But once an experimental paradigm was established to do this, it seemed to take on a life of its own.

A considerable inbuilt advantage of face perception research is therefore the ecological validity of the face as a visual stimulus. In addition, my colleagues and I have tried to keep our research linked to a wider context than the laboratory by studying everyday errors and the effects of brain disease. We like doing experiments too, but we have tried to use them to probe issues thrown up by theoretical or practical issues, rather than as an end in themselves.

The rest of this book consists of reprinted versions of previously published papers. I've tried to make a selection which explores different aspects of each theme, but inevitably there is some repetition of key points. Perhaps that is no bad thing, and an advantage of using papers reprinted from other sources is that it is easy to follow how the line of reasoning underlying the research has developed, if the material is read sequentially. A more important consequence, though, is that each chapter is complete in itself, allowing readers to dip in and explore immediately whichever topics they wish. The choice is yours.

A common theme of the work reprinted here is that of 'finding the mind's construction in the face'. It comes from Act I, scene iv of *Macbeth*, when Duncan is discussing the treachery of someone he had trusted. He reflects that

There's no art
To find the mind's construction in the face;

By this he means that you cannot divine character from appearance. It remains true to this day, and despite the efforts of Galton (1883) and others it will probably always be so. But what Galton did manage, for face perception as for so many other topics, was to show that there are other questions which can be resolved empirically, if you go about it the right way. The claim set out here is that we are now developing a science of face perception which can indeed shed light on certain aspects of mental life. The face may offer a murky and imperfect window to the mind, but we can begin to make out some things through it.

References

Adolphs, R., Tranel, D., Damasio, H., and Damasio, A. (1994). Impaired recognition of emotion in facial expressions following bilateral damage to the human amygdala. *Nature*, **372**, 669–72.

Adolphs, R., Tranel, D., Damasio, H., and Damasio, A. R. (1995). Fear and the human amygdala. *Journal of Neuroscience*, **15**, 5879–91.

Aggleton, J. P. (1992). The functional effects of amygdaloid lesions in humans: a comparison with findings from monkeys. In *The amygdala*, (ed. J. P. Aggleton), pp. 485–503. Wiley-Liss, New York.

Alexander, M. P., Stuss, D. T., and Benson, D. F. (1979). Capgras syndrome: a reduplicative phenomenon. *Neurology*, **29**, 334–9.

Baddeley, A. (1986). *Working memory*. Oxford University Press.

Bauer, R. M. (1984). Autonomic recognition of names and faces in prosopagnosia: a neuropsychological application of the guilty knowledge test. *Neuropsychologia*, **22**, 457–69.

Bauer, R. M. (1986). The cognitive psychophysiology of prosopagnosia. In *Aspects of face processing*, (ed. H. D. Ellis, M. A. Jeeves, F. Newcombe, and A. Young), pp. 253–67. Martinus Nijhoff, Dordrecht.

Benton, A. L., Hamsher, K. S., Varney, N., and Spreen, O. (1983). *Contributions to neuropsychological assessment: a clinical manual*. Oxford University Press.

Berrios, G. E. (1991). Delusions as 'wrong beliefs': a conceptual history. *British Journal of Psychiatry*, **159**, 6–13.

Bornstein, B. (1963). Prosopagnosia. In L. Halpern (Ed.), *Problems of dynamic neurology*, (ed. L. Halpern), pp. 283–318. Hadassah Medical School, Jerusalem.

Bornstein, B., Sroka, H., and Munitz, H. (1969). Prosopagnosia with animal face agnosia. *Cortex*, **5**, 164–9.

Breiter, H. C., Etcoff, N. L., Whalen, P. J., Kennedy, W. A., Rauch, S. L., Buckner, R. L., *et al.* (1996). Response and habituation of the human amygdala during visual processing of facial expression. *Neuron*, **17**, 875–87.

Brennen, T., David, D., Fluchaire, I., and Pellat, J. (1996). Naming faces and objects without comprehension – a case study. *Cognitive Neuropsychology*, **13**, 93–110.

Brothers, L. (1989). A biological perspective on empathy. *American Journal of Psychiatry*, **146**, 10–19.

Bruce, V. (1994). Stability from variation: the case of face recognition. The M. D. Vernon Memorial Lecture. *Quarterly Journal of Experimental Psychology*, **47A**, 5–28.

Bruce, V. and Valentine, T. (1985). Identity priming in the recognition of familiar faces. *British Journal of Psychology*, **76**, 363–83.

Bruce, V. and Young, A. (1986). Understanding face recognition. *British Journal of Psychology*, **77**, 305–27.

Bruce, V. Ellis, H. D., Gibling, F., and Young, A. W. (1987). Parallel processing of the sex and familiarity of faces. *Canadian Journal of Psychology*, **41**, 510–20.

Bruce, V., Healey, P., Burton, M., Doyle, T., Coombes, A., and Linney, A. (1991). Recognising facial surfaces. *Perception*, **20**, 755–69.

Bruce, V., Hanna, E., Dench, N., Healey, P., and Burton, M. (1992). The importance of 'mass' in line drawings of faces. *Applied Cognitive Psychology*, **6**, 619–28.

Bruyer, R., Laterre, C., Seron, X., Feyereisen, P., Strypstein, E., Pierrard, E., and Rectem, D. (1983). A case of prosopagnosia with some preserved covert remembrance of familiar faces. *Brain and Cognition*, **2**, 257–84.

Buchanan, A. (1993). Acting on delusion: a review. *Psychological Medicine*, **23**, 123–34.

Buchanan, A., Reed, A., Wessely, S., Garety, P., Taylor, P., Grubin, D., and Dunn, G. (1993). Acting on delusions. II: The phenomenological correlates of acting on delusions. *British Journal of Psychiatry*, **163**, 77–81.

Burton, A. M. (1994). Learning new faces in an interactive activation and competition model. *Visual Cognition*, **1**, 313–48.

Burton, A. M. and Bruce, V. (1993). Naming faces and naming names: exploring an interactive activation model of person recognition. *Memory*, **1**, 457–80.

Burton, A. M., Bruce, V., and Johnston, R. A. (1990). Understanding face recognition with an interactive activation model. *British Journal of Psychology*, **81**, 361–80.

Burton, A. M., Young, A. W., Bruce, V., Johnston, R., and Ellis, A. W. (1991). Understanding covert recognition. *Cognition*, **39**, 129–66.

Cabeza, R. and Nyberg, L. (1997). Imaging cognition: an empirical review of PET studies with normal subjects. *Journal of Cognitive Neuroscience*, **9**, 1–26.

Calder, A. J., Young, A. W., Rowland, D., Perrett, D. I., Hodges, J. R., and Etcoff, N. L. (1996). Facial emotion recognition after bilateral amygdala damage: differentially severe impairment of fear. *Cognitive Neuropsychology*, **13**, 699–745.

Capgras, J. and Reboul-Lachaux, J. (1923). L'illusion des 'sosies' dans un délire systématisé chronique. *Bulletin de la Société Clinique de Médicine Mentale*, **11**, 6–16.

Carey, S. (1992). Becoming a face expert. *Philosophical Transactions of the Royal Society, London*, **B335**, 95–103.

Carey, S. and Diamond, R. (1977). From piecemeal to configurational representation of faces. *Science*, **195**, 312–14.

Coltheart, M., Curtis, B., Atkins, P., and Haller, M. (1993). Models of reading aloud: dual-route and parallel-distributed-processing approaches. *Psychological Review*, **100**, 589–608.

Cotard, J. (1882). Du délire des négations. *Archives de Neurologie*, **4**, 152–70, 282–95.

Cowey, A. and Stoerig, P. (1992). Reflections on blindsight. In A. D. Milner and M. D. Rugg (Eds.), *The neuropsychology of consciousness*, (ed. A. D. Milner and M. D. Rugg), pp. 11–37. Academic Press, London.

Critchley, E. M. R. (1989). The neurology of familiarity. *Behavioural Neurology*, **2**, 195–200.

Damasio, A. R., Damasio, H., and Van Hoesen, G. W. (1982). Prosopagnosia: anatomic basis and behavioral mechanisms. *Neurology*, **32**, 331–41.

Darwin, C. (1872). *The expression of the emotions in man and animals*. John Murray, London.

David, A. S. (1993). Cognitive neuropsychiatry? *Psychological Medicine*, **23**, 1–5.

de Haan, E. H. F., Young, A., and Newcombe, F. (1987*a*). Face recognition without awareness. *Cognitive Neuropsychology*, **4**, 385–415.

de Haan, E. H. F., Young, A., and Newcombe, F. (1987*b*). Faces interfere with name classification in a prosopagnosic patient. *Cortex*, **23**, 309–16.

de Haan, E. H. F., Young, A. W., and Newcombe, F. (1991*a*). Covert and overt recognition in prosopagnosia. *Brain*, **114**, 2575–91.

de Haan, E. H. F., Young, A. W., and Newcombe, F. (1991*b*). A dissociation between the sense of familiarity and access to semantic information concerning familiar people. *European Journal of Cognitive Psychology*, **3**, 51–67.

de Haan, E. H. F., Bauer, R. M., and Greve, K. W. (1992). Behavioural and physiological evidence for covert face recognition in a prosopagnosic patient. *Cortex*, **28**, 77–95.

Dennett, D. (1981). *Brainstorms: philosophical essays on mind and psychology*. Harvester, Brighton.

Dennett, D. (1987). *The intentional stance*. MIT Press, Cambridge, Massachusetts.

Dennett, D. (1996). *Kinds of minds: towards an understanding of consciousness*. Weidenfeld & Nicolson, London.

de Pauw, K. W. and Szulecka, T. K. (1988). Dangerous delusions: violence and the misidentification syndromes. *British Journal of Psychiatry*, **152**, 91–7.

De Renzi, E. (1986). Current issues in prosopagnosia. In *Aspects of face processing*, (ed. H. D. Ellis, M. A. Jeeves, F. Newcombe, and A. Young), pp. 243–52. Martinus Nijhoff, Dordrecht.

De Renzi, E., Bonacini, M. G., and Faglioni, P. (1989). Right posterior brain-damaged patients are poor at assessing the age of a face. *Neuropsychologia*, **27**, 839–48.

De Renzi, E., Perani, D., Carlesimo, G. A., Silveri, M. C., and Fazio, F. (1994). Prosopagnosia can be associated with damage confined to the right hemisphere – an MRI and PET study and a review of the literature. *Neuropsychologia*, **32**, 893–902.

Desimone, R. (1991). Face-selective cells in the temporal cortex of monkeys. *Journal of Cognitive Neuroscience*, **3**, 1–8.

Diamond, R. and Carey, S. (1986). Why faces are and are not special: an effect of expertise. *Journal of Experimental Psychology: General*, **115**, 107–17.

Diamond, B. J., Valentine, T., Mayes, A. R., and Sandel, M. E. (1994). Evidence of covert recognition in a prosopagnosic patient. *Cortex*, **30**, 377–93.

Dudley, R. E. J., John, C. H., Young, A. W., and Over, D. E. (1997). Normal and abnormal reasoning in people with delusions. *British Journal of Clinical Psychology*, **36**, 243–58.

Ekman, P. (1972). Universals and cultural differences in facial expressions of emotion. In *Nebraska symposium on motivation, 1971*, (ed. J. K. Cole), pp. 207–83. University of Nebraska Press, Lincoln, Nebraska.

Ekman, P. (1992). An argument for basic emotions. *Cognition and Emotion*, **6**, 169–200.

Ekman, P. and Friesen, W. V. (1976). *Pictures of facial affect.* Consulting Psychologists Press, Palo Alto, California.

Ekman, P., Friesen, W. V., and Ellsworth, P. (1972). *Emotion in the human face: guidelines for research and an integration of findings.* Pergamon, New York.

Ellis, H. D. (1975). Recognizing faces. *British Journal of Psychology*, **66**, 409–26.

Ellis, H. D. (1983). The role of the right hemisphere in face perception. In A. W. Young (Ed.), *Functions of the right cerebral hemisphere*, (ed. A. W. Young), pp. 33–64. Academic Press, London.

Ellis, H. D. and Young, A. W. (1990). Accounting for delusional misidentifications. *British Journal of Psychiatry*, **157**, 239–48.

Ellis, A. W. and Young, A. W. (1996). *Human cognitive neuropsychology: a textbook with readings.* Psychology Press, Hove, East Sussex.

Ellis, H. D., Young, A. W., and Koenken, G. (1993). Covert face recognition without prosopagnosia. *Behavioural Neurology*, **6**, 27–32.

Ellis, H. D., Young, A. W., Quayle, A. H., and de Pauw, K. W. (1997). Reduced autonomic responses to faces in Capgras delusion. *Proceedings of the Royal Society: Biological Sciences*, **B264**, 1085–92.

Enoch, M. D. and Trethowan, W. H. (1991). *Uncommon psychiatric syndromes*, (3rd edn). Butterworth-Heinemann, Oxford.

Farah, M. J. (1991). Patterns of co-occurrence among the associative agnosias: implications for visual object representation. *Cognitive Neuropsychology*, **8**, 1–19.

Farah, M. J. (1994). Neuropsychological inference with an interactive brain: a critique of the 'locality' assumption. *Behavioral and Brain Sciences*, **17**, 43–104.

Farah, M. J., O'Reilly, R. C., and Vecera, S. P. (1993). Dissociated overt and covert recognition as an emergent property of a lesioned neural network. *Psychological Review*, **100**, 571–88.

Fleminger, S. (1994). Delusional misidentification: an exemplary symptom illustrating an interaction between organic brain disease and psychological processes. *Psychopathology*, **27**, 161–7.

Fleminger, S. and Burns, A. (1993). The delusional misidentification syndromes in patients with and without evidence of organic cerebral disorder: a structured review of case reports. *Biological Psychiatry*, **33**, 22–32.

Flude, B. M., Ellis, A. W., and Kay, J. (1989). Face processing and name retrieval in an anomic aphasic: names are stored separately from semantic information about familiar people. *Brain and Cognition*, **11**, 60–72.

Fodor, J. (1987). *Psychosemantics: the problem of meaning in the philosophy of mind.* MIT Press, Cambridge, Massachusetts.

Fodor, J. (1989). *The theory of content and other essays.* MIT Press, Cambridge, Massachusetts.

Frith, C. D. (1992). *The cognitive neuropsychology of schizophrenia*, Lawrence Erlbaum, Hove, East Sussex.

Galton, F. (1879). Composite portraits, made by combining those of many different persons into a single resultant figure. *Journal of the Anthropological Institute*, **8**, 132–44.

Galton, F. (1883). *Inquiries into human faculty and its development*. Macmillan, London.

Garety, P. A., Hemsley, D. R., and Wessely, S. (1991). Reasoning in deluded schizophrenic and paranoid patients: biases in performance on a probabilistic inference task. *Journal of Nervous and Mental Disease*, **179**, 194–201.

Goldstein, A. G. (1983). Behavioral scientists' fascination with faces. *Journal of Nonverbal Behavior*, **7**, 223–55.

Goren, C. G., Sarty, M., and Wu, P. Y. K. (1975). Visual following and pattern discrimination of face-like stimuli by newborn infants. *Pediatrics*, **56**, 544–9.

Gray, J. M., Young, A. W., Barker, W. A., Curtis, A., and Gibson, D. (1997). Impaired recognition of disgust in Huntington's disease gene carriers. *Brain*, **120**, 2029–38.

Greene, J. D. W. and Hodges, J. R. (1996). Identification of famous faces and famous names in early Alzheimer's disease. Relationship to anterograde episodic and general semantic memory. *Brain*, **119**, 111–28.

Greve, K. W. and Bauer, R. M. (1990). Implicit learning of new faces in prosopagnosia: an application of the mere-exposure paradigm. *Neuropsychologia*, **28**, 1035–41.

Gross, C. G. (1992). Representation of visual stimuli in inferior temporal cortex. *Philosophical Transactions of the Royal Society, London*, **B335**, 3–10.

Haidt, J., McCauley, C., and Rozin, P. (1994). Individual differences in sensitivity to disgust: a scale sampling seven domains of disgust elicitors. *Personality and Individual Differences*, **16**, 701–13.

Halgren, E. (1992). Emotional neurophysiology of the amygdala within the context of human cognition. In *The amygdala*, (ed. J. P. Aggleton), pp. 191–228. Wiley-Liss, New York.

Halligan, P. W., Marshall, J. C., and Ramachandran, V. S. (1994). Ghosts in the machine: a case description of visual and haptic hallucinations after right hemisphere stroke. *Cognitive Neuropsychology*, **11**, 459–77.

Hancock, P. J. B., Burton, A. M., and Bruce, V. (1996). Face processing: human perception and principal components analysis. *Memory and Cognition*, **24**, 26–40.

Hanley, J. R. and Cowell, E. S. (1988). The effects of different types of retrieval cues on the recall of names of famous faces. *Memory and Cognition*, **16**, 545–55.

Hay, D. C. and Young, A. W. (1982). The human face. In *Normality and pathology in cognitive functions*, (ed. A. W. Ellis), pp. 173–202. Academic Press, London.

Hay, D. C., Young, A. W., and Ellis, A. W. (1991). Routes through the face recognition system. *Quarterly Journal of Experimental Psychology*, **43A**, 761–91.

Hirstein, W. and Ramachandran, V. S. (1997). Capgras syndrome: a novel probe for understanding the neural representation of the identity and familiarity of persons. *Proceedings of the Royal Society, London*, **264**, 437–44.

Hodges, J. R. and Greene, J. D. W. (1997). Knowing about people and naming them: can Alzheimer's disease patients do one without the other? *Quarterly Journal of Experimental Psychology*, (In press.)

Izard, C. E. (1971). *The face of emotion*. Appleton-Century-Crofts, New York.

Johnson, M. H. and Morton, J. (1991). *Biology and cognitive development: the case of face recognition*. Blackwell, Oxford.

Johnson, M. H., Dziurawiec, S., Ellis, H., and Morton, J. (1991). Newborns' preferential tracking of face-like stimuli and its subsequent decline. *Cognition*, **40**, 1–19.

Johnston, R. A. and Bruce, V. (1990). Lost properties? Retrieval differences between name codes and semantic codes for familiar people. *Psychological Research*, **52**, 62–7.

Kaney, S. and Bentall, R. P. (1989). Persecutory delusions and attributional style. *British Journal of Medical Psychology*, **62**, 191–8.

Kunst-Wilson, W. R. and Zajonc, R. B. (1980). Affective discrimination of stimuli that cannot be recognized. *Science*, **207**, 557–8.

Leafhead, K. M., Young, A. W., and Szulecka, T. K. (1996). Delusions demand attention. *Cognitive Neuropsychiatry*, **1**, 5–16.

LeDoux, J. E. (1995). Emotion: clues from the brain. *Annual Review of Psychology*, **46**, 209–35.

Lewicki, P. (1986). Processing information about covariations that cannot be articulated. *Journal of Experimental Psychology: Learning, Memory, and Cognition*, **12**, 135–46.

Logothetis, N. K. and Pauls, J. (1995). Psychophysical and physiological evidence for viewer-centred object representations in the primate. *Cerebral Cortex*, **5**, 270–88.

McCloskey, M. (1991). Networks and theories: the place of connectionism in cognitive science. *Psychological Science*, **2**, 387–95.

McGurk, H. and MacDonald, J. (1976). Hearing lips and seeing voices. *Nature*, **264**, 746–8.

McNeil, J. E. and Warrington, E. K. (1991). Prosopagnosia: a reclassification. *Quarterly Journal of Experimental Psychology*, **43A**, 267–87.

McNeil, J. E. and Warrington, E. K. (1993). Prosopagnosia: a face specific disorder. *Quarterly Journal of Experimental Psychology*, **46A**, 1–10.

McWeeny, K. H., Young, A. W., Hay, D. C., and Ellis, A. W. (1987). Putting names to faces. *British Journal of Psychology*, **78**, 143–9.

Maher, B. A. (1992). Delusions: contemporary etiological hypotheses. *Psychiatric Annals*, **22**, 260–8.

Marr, D. (1982). *Vision*. Freeman, San Francisco.

Marshall, J. C. and Newcombe, F. (1966). Syntactic and semantic errors in paralexia. *Neuropsychologia*, **4**, 169–76.

Marshall, J. C. and Newcombe, F. (1973). Patterns of paralexia: a psycholinguistic approach. *Journal of Psycholinguistic Research*, **2**, 175–99.

Meadows, J. C. (1974). The anatomical basis of prosopagnosia. *Journal of Neurology, Neurosurgery, and Psychiatry*, **37**, 489–501.

Meltzoff, A. N. and Moore, M. K. (1977). Imitation of facial and manual gestures by human neonates. *Science*, **198**, 75–8.

Morris, J. S., Frith, C. D., Perrett, D. I., Rowland, D., Young, A. W., Calder, A. J., and Dolan, R. J. (1996). A differential neural response in the human amygdala to fearful and happy facial expressions. *Nature*, **383**, 812–15.

Morris, J. S., Friston, K. J., Buechel, C., Frith, C. D., Young, A. W., Calder, A. J., and Dolan, R. J. (1997). A neuromodulatory role for the human amygdala in processing emotional facial expressions. *Brain*, (In press.)

Newell, A. (1973). You can't play 20 questions with nature and win: projective comments on the papers of this symposium. In *Visual information processing*, (ed. W. G. Chase), pp. 283–308. Academic Press, New York.

Niedenthal, P. M. and Halberstadt, J. B. (1995). The acquisition and structure of emotional response categories. In *The psychology of learning and motivation: advances in research and theory*, vol. 33, (ed. D. L. Medin), pp. 23–64. Academic Press, New York.

O'Toole, A. J., Deffenbacher, K. A., Valentin, D., and Abdi, H. (1994). Structural aspects of face recognition and the other-race effect. *Memory and Cognition*, **22**, 208–24.

Parfit, D. (1984). *Reasons and persons*. Oxford University Press.

Pearson, D. (1992). The extraction and use of facial features in low bit-rate visual communication. *Philosophical Transactions of the Royal Society, London*, **B335**, 79–85.

Perrett, D. I., Rolls, E. T., and Caan, W. (1982). Visual neurones responsive to faces in the monkey temporal cortex. *Experimental Brain Research*, **47**, 329–42.

Perrett, D. O., Hietanen, J. K., Oram, M. W., and Benson, P. J. (1992). Organization and functions of cells responsive to faces in the temporal cortex. *Philosophical Transactions of the Royal Society, London*, **B335**, 23–30.

Phillips, M. L., Young, A. W., Senior, C., Brammer, M., Andrew, C., Calder, A. J., *et al.* (1997). A specific neural substrate for perceiving facial expressions of disgust. *Nature*, **389**, 495–8.

Renault, B., Signoret, J. L., Debruille, B., Breton, F., and Bolgert, F. (1989). Brain potentials reveal covert facial recognition in prosopagnosia. *Neuropsychologia*, **27**, 905–12.

Rizzo, M., Hurtig, R., and Damasio, A. R. (1987). The role of scanpaths in facial recognition and learning. *Annals of Neurology*, **22**, 41–5.

Rosch, E., Mervis, C. B., Gray, W. D., Johnson, D. M., and Boyes-Braem, P. (1976). Basic objects in natural categories. *Cognitive Psychology*, **8**, 382–439.

Rozin, P., Haidt, J., and McCauley, C. R. (1993). Disgust. In *Handbook of emotions*, (ed. M. Lewis and J. M. Haviland), pp. 575–94. Guilford, New York.

Sass, L. A. (1994). *The paradoxes of delusion. Wittgenstein, Schreber, and the schizophrenic mind*. Cornell University Press, Ithaca, New York.

Schacter, D. L., McAndrews, M. P., and Moscovitch, M. (1988). Access to consciousness: dissociations between implicit and explicit knowledge in neuropsychological syndromes. In *Thought without language*, (ed. L. Weistrantz), pp. 242–78. Oxford University Press.

Schweinberger, S. R., Klos, T., and Sommer, W. (1995). Covert face recognition in prosopagnosia: a dissociable function? *Cortex*, **31**, 517–29.

Scott, S. K., Young, A. W., Calder, A. J., Hellawell, D. J., Aggleton, J. P., and Johnson, M. (1997). Impaired auditory recognition of fear and anger following bilateral amygdala lesions. *Nature*, **385**, 254–7.

Searle, J. (1984). *Minds, brains and science: the 1984 Reith lectures*. British Broadcasting Corporation, London.

Searle, J. R. (1992). *The rediscovery of the mind*. MIT Press, Cambridge, Massachusetts.

Seidenberg, M. S. and McClelland, J. L. (1989). A distributed, developmental model of word recognition and naming. *Psychological Review*, **96**, 523–68.

Sergent, J. and Poncet, M. (1990). From covert to overt recognition of faces in a prosopagnosic patient. *Brain*, **113**, 989–1004.

Sergent, J. and Signoret, J.-L. (1992*a*). Functional and anatomical decomposition of face processing: evidence from prosopagnosia and PET study of normal subjects. *Philosophical Transactions of the Royal Society, London*, **B335**, 55–62.

Sergent, J. and Signoret, J.-L. (1992*b*). Implicit access to knowledge derived from unrecognized faces in prosopagnosia. *Cerebral Cortex*, **2**, 389–400.

Shallice, T. (1979). Case study approach in neuropsychological research. *Journal of Clinical Neuropsychology*, **1**, 183–211.

Shallice, T. (1988). *From neuropsychology to mental structure*. Cambridge University Press.

Shallice, T. and Warrington, E. K. (1970). Independent functioning of verbal memory stores: a neuropsychological study. *Quarterly Journal of Experimental Psychology*, **22**, 261–73.

Sno, H. N. (1994). A continuum of misidentification symptoms. *Psychopathology*, **27**, 144–47.

Sno, H. N. and Linszen, D. H. (1990). The *déjà vu* experience: remembrance of things past? *American Journal of Psychiatry*, **147**, 1587–95.

Sprengelmeyer, R., Young, A. W., Calder, A. J., Karnat, A., Lange, H. W., Hömberg, V., et al. (1996). Loss of disgust: perception of faces and emotions in Huntington's disease. *Brain*, **119**, 1647–65.

Stone, T. and Young, A. W. (1997). Delusions and brain injury: the philosophy and psychology of belief. *Mind & Language*, **12**, 327–64.

Summerfield, Q. (1992). Lipreading and audio-visual speech perception. *Philosophical Transactions of the Royal Society, London*, **B335**, 71–8.

Thompson, P. (1980). Margaret Thatcher – a new illusion. *Perception*, **9**, 483–4.

Tranel, D. and Damasio, A. R. (1985). Knowledge without awareness: an autonomic index of facial recognition by prosopagnosics. *Science*, **228**, 1453–4.

Tranel, D. and Damasio, A. R. (1988). Non-conscious face recognition in patients with face agnosia. *Behavioural Brain Research*, **30**, 235–49.

Tranel, D., Damasio, H., and Damasio, A. R. (1995). Double dissociation between overt and covert recognition. *Journal of Cognitive Neuroscience*, **7**, 425–32.

Tulving, E. (1972). Episodic and semantic memory. In *Organization of memory*, (ed. E. Tulving and W. Donaldson), pp. 381–403. Academic Press, New York.

Turk, M. and Pentland, A. (1991). Eigenfaces for recognition. *Journal of Cognitive Neuroscience*, **3**, 71–86.

Valentine, T. (1991). A unified account of the effects of distinctiveness, inversion, and race in face recognition. *Quarterly Journal of Experimental Psychology*, **43A**, 161–204.

Van Lancker, D. (1991). Personal relevance and the human right hemisphere. *Brain and Cognition*, **17**, 64–92.

Weinstein, E. A. and Burnham, D. L. (1991). Reduplication and the syndrome of Capgras. *Psychiatry*, **54**, 78–88.

Weiskrantz, L. (1980). Varieties of residual experience. *Quarterly Journal of Experimental Psychology*, **32**, 365–86.

Weiskrantz, L., Warrington, E. K., Sanders, M. D., and Marshall, J. (1974). Visual capacity in the hemianopic field following a restricted occipital ablation. *Brain*, **97**, 709–28.

Williams, B. (1973). *Problems of the self: philosophical papers 1956–1972*. Cambridge University Press.

Wright, S., Young, A. W., and Hellawell, D. J. (1993). Sequential Cotard and Capgras delusions. *British Journal of Clinical Psychology*, **32**, 345–9.

Yin, R. K. (1969). Looking at upside-down faces. *Journal of Experimental Psychology*, **81**, 141–5.

Young, A. W. (1994*a*). What counts as local? Commentary on M. J. Farah, 'Neuropsychological inference with an interactive brain: a critque of the "locality" assumption'. *Behavioral and Brain Sciences*, **17**, 88–9.

Young, A. W. (1994*b*). Recognition and reality. In *The neurological boundaries of reality*, (ed. E. M. R. Critchley), pp. 83–100. Farrand, London.

Young, A. W. (1994*c*). Covert recognition. In *The neuropsychology of high-level vision: collected tutorial essays*, (ed. M. J. Farah and G. Ratcliff), pp. 331–58. Lawrence Erlbaum, Hillsdale, New Jersey.

Young, A. W. and Block, N. (1996). Consciousness. In *Unsolved mysteries of the mind: tutorial essays in cognition*, (ed. V. Bruce), pp. 149–79. Erlbaum (UK)/Taylor & Francis, Hove, East Sussex.

Young, A. W. and Burton, A. M. Simulating face recognition: implications for modelling cognition. (In preparation.)

Young, A. W. and de Haan, E. H. F. (1988). Boundaries of covert recognition in prosopagnosia. *Cognitive Neuropsychology*, **5**, 317–36.

Young, A. W. and Leafhead, K. M. (1996). Betwixt life and death: case studies of the Cotard delusion. In *Method in madness: case studies in cognitive neuropsychiatry*, (ed. P. W. Halligan and J. C. Marshall), pp. 147–71. Psychology Press, Hove, East Sussex.

Young, A. W., Hay, D. C., and Ellis, A. W. (1985). The faces that launched a thousand slips: everyday difficulties and errors in recognizing people. *British Journal of Psychology*, **76**, 495–523.

Young, A. W., McWeeny, K. H., Ellis, A. W., and Hay, D. C. (1986*a*). Naming and categorizing faces and written names. *Quarterly Journal of Experimental Psychology*, **38A**, 297–318.

Young, A. W., McWeeny, K. H., Hay, D. C., and Ellis, A. W. (1986*b*). Access to identity-specific semantic codes from familiar faces. *Quarterly Journal of Experimental Psychology*, **38A**, 271–95.

Young, A. W., Ellis, A. W., and Flude, B. M. (1988*a*). Accessing stored information about familiar people. *Psychological Research*, **50**, 111–15.

Young, A. W., Hellawell, D., and de Haan, E. H. F. (1988*b*). Cross-domain semantic priming in normal subjects and a prosopagnosic patient. *Quarterly Journal of Experimental Psychology*, **40A**, 561–80.

Young, A. W., Ellis, H. D., Szulecka, T. K., and de Pauw, K. W. (1990). Face processing impairments and delusional misidentification. *Behavioural Neurology*, **3**, 153–68.

Young, A. W., Newcombe, F., de Haan, E. H. F., Small, M., and Hay, D. C. (1993*a*). Face perception after brain injury: selective impairments affecting identity and expression. *Brain*, **116**, 941–59.

Young, A. W., Reid, I., Wright, S., and Hellawell, D. J. (1993*b*). Face-processing impairments and the Capgras delusion. *British Journal of Psychiatry*, **162**, 695–8.

Young, A. W., Hellawell, D. J., Wright, S., and Ellis, H. D. (1994*a*). Reduplication of visual stimuli. *Behavioural Neurology*, **7**, 135–42.

Young, A. W., Leafhead, K. M., and Szulecka, T. K. (1994*b*). The Capgras and Cotard delusions. *Psychopathology*, **27**, 226–31.

Young, A. W., Aggleton, J. P., Hellawell, D. J., Johnson, M., Broks, P., and Hanley, J. R. (1995). Face processing impairments after amygdalotomy. *Brain*, **118**, 15–24.

Young, A. W., Hellawell, D. J., van de Wal, C., and Johnson, M. (1996). Facial expression processing after amygdalotomy. *Neuropsychologia*, **34**, 31–9.

Zajonc, R. B. (1980). Feeling and thinking: preferences need no inferences. *American Psychologist*, **35**, 151–75.

2

Faces in their social and biological context

Reprinted in slightly modified form from Ellis, H. D. and Young, A. W.
(1989), Are faces special? in *Handbook of research on face processing*,
(ed. A. W. Young and H. D. Ellis), pp. 1–26, North Holland, Amsterdam.
With kind permission of Professor H. Ellis and Elsevier Science – NL,
Sara Burgerhartstraat 25, 1055 KV Amsterdam, The Netherlands.

Interest in the processes underlying the perception and recognition of
faces has become very active. Theories have sprung up where almost
none existed beforehand (Ellis 1975). These include information-
processing models (Hay and Young 1982; Bruce and Young 1986; Ellis
1986); a computer-recognition model (Kohonen *et al.* 1981); a neurophysiological model (Baron 1981); and neuropsychological models
(Damasio *et al.* 1982; Ellis 1983; Rhodes 1985).

Numerous questions have arisen in the course of these various efforts
at determining a clear theoretical base for the understanding of face
processing. In this chapter we shall largely confine ourselves to one of
the questions of interest, but we shall also endeavour to explicate a
general approach to building a model of face processing that
incorporates the essential qualities of most of the apparently different
theoretical positions currently being offered.

Are faces special?

The central theme of this chapter is neatly defined by the question posed
by Teuber in 1978. He asked 'Are faces, with their relatively greater
dependence on the right hemisphere, "special" in a similar way to that
in which speech, with its dependence (in most of us) on the left
hemisphere is said to be "special"?' (p. 890).

Teuber was not the first to wonder about the specialness of faces; nor
indeed was he the first to avoid giving an unequivocal answer to the
question (Ellis 1975). Part of the difficulty lies in the fact that the term
'special' is not clearly defined. In a broad sense, of course, faces are
special: they have been described as the single most important visual

pattern in our environment (Ellis 1981a),and our ability to discriminate hundreds of faces despite the many similarities between individuals probably represents the ultimate in our perceptual classification skills. Galton (1883) drew attention to the way in which for face perception 'one small discordance overweighs a multitude of similarities and suggests a general unlikeness'.

For a more precise definition of the term 'special', however, we must turn to the reviews by Hay and Young (1982) and Blanc-Garin (1984). These authors draw distinctions between the different meanings of 'special' as applied to faces. In particular, Hay and Young (1982) distinguished the notions of 'uniqueness' and 'specificity'. Uniqueness may be viewed as the extreme form of specificity for it implies that not only are faces handled by a system that is separate from that used for recognizing other objects, but that this system works in a different way from other visual recognition systems. The 'weaker' specificity position is that a separate system exists for faces but that this system may or may not work in a similar way to systems used in processing other classes of visual input. Our principal aim in this review is to consider the various lines of evidence that have been employed to examine the question of specificity for processing faces.

Modularity and gnostic fields

Arguments for the existence of specific recognition systems are currently couched in terms of modularity (Marr 1982). Fodor (1983) has presented the most complete justification for believing that cognition requires an underpinning of modules that have 'vertical' properties (i.e. not shared by other modules). Like Teuber, he identifies the language processing mechanism as the prototypical modular system and mentions face recognition as another likely candidate for what elsewhere he terms a domain-specific input system.

Domain specificity implies that only a restricted class of stimuli can activate that particular module. One possible mechanism considered by Fodor for switching in a particular module involves the use of a proto-typical pattern that represents the essential qualities of that class and which may then serve as a means for measuring the deviations from this canonical representation likely to be produced by any individual input pattern. Light et al. (1979) have independently argued for such a system operating in face perception; moreover they have shown that faces which are markedly deviant from the average or prototype are actually better remembered than those that are close to it. There could, of course, be a range of prototypical faces around which individual faces may cluster, but tentative attempts to investigate this possibility using photographically derived composite faces have not been very successful (Ellis 1981*b*). We will return to this point later.

A slightly older approach to the issue of how we recognize patterns from different classes was taken by Konorski (1967). He presented a very comprehensive theory of cognition in which he employed the concept of a 'gnostic area', of which there are a number, each tuned to a different category of input. According to Konorski they are organized in files of related gnostic units. Thus, face analysis may be carried out by a group of separate units that represent faces in general, faces belonging to a particular category (e.g. males, females, children, or grown-up persons), and faces of our acquaintances; together these different gnostic units make up a hierarchically organized gnostic field.

Although many other aspects of Konorski's thinking have attracted the attention and appreciation of Western psychologists (see Dickinson and Boakes 1979), with one notable exception (Martindale 1981) his ideas on pattern recognition have been largely ignored and so we will take this opportunity to relate them in some detail.

Konorski (1967) was concerned to explain what he termed 'unitary perceptions' – that is, the almost instantaneous recognition of already known stimulus objects. He contrasts this with 'complex perceptions' that occur when scrutinizing a given object by shifting attention from one element to another before being able to identify it. Face recognition of course, usually involves unitary perception but it may sometimes occur without any associations (name, biographical details, etc. – see Young *et al.* 1985). Furthermore a face that has undergone some change in one of its constituent elements (e.g. beard removed) may be recognized instantly and the perceiver has only some dim awareness that something is different. Such changes, as well as photographic distortions and the like, may be tolerated because the relevant gnostic unit somehow 'bends' the input to fit the standard form (Ellis 1981*b*).

An important aspect of Konorski's theory is that visual objects are categorized and that only a limited set of categories exist to process the possible range of sensory experience. Ignoring the gnostic areas Konorski proposed for the processing of non-visual patterns, it is interesting to note that he put forward the idea that there are nine categories of visual stimulus objects that are dealt with by separate gnostic fields. These are

(1) small manipulable objects (e.g. cups, keys, watches);
(2) larger, partially manipulable objects (e.g. cars, desks);

(3) non-manipulable objects (e.g. trees, buildings);
(4) faces;
(5) facial expressions;
(6) animated objects (i.e. animals, including human figures);
(7) printed words, signs, and symbols;
(8) handwriting;
(9) positions of limbs.

Thus faces are important enough in their capacity both as conveyors of individual identity and as signallers of emotional expressions to warrant two independent gnostic fields according to Konorski (1967) who argued that 'The category of unitary perceptions elicited by particular faces is in many respects highly specific and different from all other categories of visual perceptions' (p. 118). His argument for the existence of a different gnostic field for analysing facial expressions rests simply on the fact that prosopagnosics, who display a profound inability to recognize faces, are usually able to read emotional expressions – an argument refined and extended by later commentators (Hay and Young 1982; Ellis 1983; Rhodes 1985).

The development of gnostic units involves a learning process in which a number of free neurones are claimed by a particular stimulus pattern so that a degree of redundant coding occurs. This, presumably, preserves cognitive functioning as neurones die.

It is interesting to note that in some ways, Konorski anticipated a contemporary debate on the representation of stored information. He believed that gnostic units are served by 'transit fields' which act as sub-processors, firing when excited by particular pattern elements. Different gnostic units might share certain identical transit units, which is reminiscent of current ideas on distributed memory systems in which pattern recognition is supported by something like a matrix of elements whose pattern of excitation gives rise to the experience of different objects (Hinton & Anderson 1981). The gnostic units, however, become more like 'logogens' (Morton 1969) or 'pictogens' (Seymour 1979) – that is, single neurones that fire in the presence of a specific pattern. Broadbent (1985) has argued, however, that it is erroneous to contrast these two approaches because they may simply involve different levels of explanation. Konorski (1967) seems to have dealt with this problem in a similar way by describing at one level a system for computing visual data by the use of elements that are shared across the population of possible patterns and positing at a higher level individual gnostic units that respond only to a single known pattern. We will return to this aspect of Konorski's theory when discussing models of face recognition.

Konorski (1967), then, identified nine gnostic fields. But on what grounds were these based? It must be admitted that this is the weakest point of his theory because, although most evidence was derived from clinical cases of specific cognitive deficits following brain injury (and here it must be said, Konorski rather uncritically relied upon a limited set of source references), some, he admitted, were the product of educated guesses. It is likely that any category of object may give rise to a specific gnostic area if it proves useful to an individual. Let us illustrate this with an example already used by one of us (Ellis 1981*b*). Bateson (1977) tested the claims of an ornithologist that she was able to identify individually some hundreds of Bewick swans at a wildlife reserve by photographing the swans as she named each one. Bateson was able later to test her recognition accuracy and he found her to be almost perfectly accurate. Now it seems not too fanciful to suggest that for this person (and other similar experts) a 'Bewick swan gnostic field' exists that enables her to perceive and store differences among individual birds that would escape the majority of us.

A similar argument may be used to explain the findings of Assal *et al.* (1984). They observed a prosopagnosic farmer who initially lost his ability to recognize either familiar people or his own cows. Eventually he regained the ability to identify faces but the agnosia for cows remained. Presumably, in the case of this farmer, cow identification was sufficiently important and practised enough for a gnostic field specialized in cow perception to have developed.

Our suggestion is that gnostic fields are formed as a result of cognitive need and by a process of perceptual learning. Their number and their 'purity' may not be completely predetermined but an important question remains as to whether innate factors play any part at all. In the case of faces there is evidence for some degree of pre-wiring which we will now review.

Developmental studies

For this discussion we will confine ourselves to face perception and ask whether the newborn infant arrives in the world with any preformed ability to perceive faces?

The results of a study by Goren *et al.* (1975) are very striking and particularly germane to this chapter. Goren *et al.* worked with infants having a mean age of nine minutes – some of the youngest subjects ever to be observed in a cognitive study. Each infant was shown in turn four stimuli; a schematic face, two scrambled faces, and a blank face. Each stimulus was moved to and fro through a 180 degree arc, and head and eye movements to follow the stimulus were noted.

Goren *et al.* found that their sample significantly preferred to look at the stimulus figure that most resembled a human face, suggesting an innate mechanism both for identifying 'facedness' and for choosing to attend to such patterns. These results are quite remarkable and one naturally wishes to be sure that they are not the consequence of some artefact. One misgiving lies in the fact that newborn babies have relatively poor visual acuity. Indeed the analysis by Souther and Banks (1979) shows that at this stage of development babies are unlikely to perceive a static monochrome photograph of a face at all. It could be argued, however, that the stimuli of Goren *et al.* were high-contrast and moving which should make them much easier to detect (real faces also have colour information which may also aid the immature visual system), but the question of visual maturity at birth is a crucial one.

Such a surprising set of results (at least to some commentators) needs to be replicated before any firm conclusions are drawn. To this end Johnson *et al.* (1991) attempted a partial replication in which the observation and scoring of babies' head and eye movements was achieved from video recordings by independent judges rather than directly by experimenters as in the Goren *et al.* study.

The results shown in Fig. 2.1 strongly support those of Goren *et al.* The infants preferred to follow the face-like pattern significantly more than the scrambled face pattern and both commanded more attention than the blank head-outline stimulus.

What can be the significance of these data? The fact that newborn infants respond to a face-like configuration is unlikely not to be of some biological importance. Tzavaras *et al.* (1970) suggested that parent–infant bonding requires that babies pay attention to their caretakers. This activity would be greatly expedited by some innate concept of facedness, however vague (cf. Conrad 1947). Innate attentiveness to faces would help both in making the parents attached to their baby and in beginning the build-up of information on which the baby will base its own subsequent attachment to and recognition of its caretakers. Moreover the replication of Goren *et al.*'s (1975) finding also supports the idea that some patterns, at least, may be discerned by newborn babies despite the immaturity of their visual systems. It does not, however, address the issue as to whether this attentional mechanism is mediated primarily through cortical or subcortical structures (Bronson 1974).

In addition to their attentiveness to faces, there is also evidence that neonates can discriminate emotional expressions. Field *et al.* (1982) carried out a study in which infants of mean age 36 hours watched an adult who maintained a fixed happy, sad, or surprised expression. They showed that if the expression remained the same over a number of trials

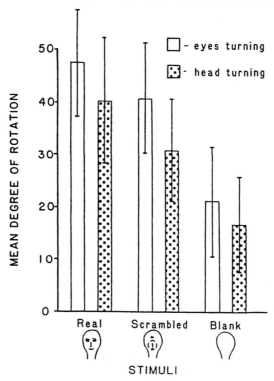

Fig. 2.1 Histograms indicating the extent of both head and eye movements to a schematic face, scrambled face, and blank figure. (Data from Johnson *et al.* 1991, experiment 1.)

the infant lost interest in the face (i.e. looked at it for less time), but that if the expression then changed there was renewed interest (in the form of increased looking). Clearly, infants of this age must be able to discriminate the facial expressions, or such differential visual fixation patterns would not occur.

Field *et al.* (1982) also observed that the infants they studied tended to imitate the expression they were watching. This finding is comparable to the remarkable observations made by Meltzoff and Moore (1977, 1983*a*). They found that very young infants would imitate facial gestures (open mouth, tongue protrusion, lip protrusion). The explanation offered for this behaviour is that it 'involves intermodal matching in which infants recognize an equivalence between the act seen and their own act' (Meltzoff 1981, p. 102). There are, of course, other interpretations for these data and it should be said that, while some replications have been reported (Jacobson 1979; Vinter 1985), others have failed to do so (Hayes and Watson 1981; Koepke *et al.* 1983;

McKenzie and Over 1983). Meltzoff and Moore (1983b), however, suggest a number of methodological niceties that were not always observed in these failed replications.

Meltzoff and Moore's (1977, 1983a) observations add support to the idea that neonates have fairly sophisticated routines not only for perceiving faces but for matching the movements of a face before them by their own facial musculature. It should be added, however, that the capacity for imitation is not restricted to facial gestures. Meltzoff and Moore (1977) also found that young infants imitate finger gestures, suggesting that the innate imitation capacity is not face-specific. But our interest in their claims does concern the evidence for facial imitation because it goes beyond evidence for mere attention to facial patterns and implies an even greater innate capacity for processing facial information and organizing facial responses.

The facts that neonates pay attention to faces, are able to encode the differences between facial expressions, and can imitate facial gestures should not precipitate us into assuming that this means that faces are unique objects. As we have already pointed out, Meltzoff and Moore (1977) found evidence for imitation of finger gestures in their infant sample, suggesting that hands may be equally important objects. One might expect breasts to occupy a similar place of significance in the neonate's world and there may be other stimuli that also merit consideration.

So where does all this leave us in relation to the theme of this chapter? The studies of neonatal interest in facial stimuli are consistent with the idea that faces are special, but they do not support any notion that faces are unique in this respect. What evidence exists is consistent with the idea that faces are so biologically significant that some degree of hard-wiring may be evident at birth. To demonstrate that soon afterwards babies learn to distinguish one face from another (Melhuish 1982) adds some weight to the specialness argument but only in so far as faces occupy a very prominent position in the visual experience of the young child and therefore offer ample opportunity for visual learning. It may be tempting to speculate that learning to discriminate among and remember faces is also special in the sense that these cognitive skills proceed at an unusually fast pace, but we have no direct evidence either to support or refute such an hypothesis. In fact as far as the recognition of other people is concerned there is evidence that young infants may rely primarily on the voice rather than the face, since recognition of caretakers' voices is possible at ages at which face recognition has not been found to occur (Mills and Melhuish 1974; De Casper and Fifer 1980).

An intriguing possibility is that the infant's interest in and ability to imitate facial gestures may be linked to language acquisition (Studdert-Kennedy 1983). It is now known that even in adulthood people make a remarkable use of information derived from watching people's mouths and lips whilst they are speaking (Campbell 1989). McGurk and MacDonald (1976) demonstrated this phenomenon with an illusion in which a mismatch between heard and seen (mouthed) phonemes can result in the perceiver 'blending' the two. If, for instance, the sound 'ba' is superimposed on a film of the face of a person saying 'pa', most normal adults watching the resulting film find that they hear the sound as 'da'.

Like adults, infants recognize the correspondence between facial movements and speech sounds (Dodd 1979; Kuhl and Meltzoff 1982; Mackain *et al.* 1983). Dodd (1979), for instance, demonstrated this by showing that infants paid less attention to nursery rhymes when the speech sounds and lip movements were out of synchrony than when they were in synchrony. Thus the innate interest in faces and ability to discriminate and imitate facial expressions may promote the acquisition of linguistic as well as more general social skills.

At a much later stage in the child's life the ability to recognize faces undergoes a curious inflection at around the onset of puberty such that performance on face recognition tasks temporarily declines before the developmental improvement reasserts itself (Carey 1981; Carey *et al* 1980; Flin 1980, 1985). This pattern of development is found in tasks that require the encoding of sizeable numbers of unfamiliar faces for subsequent recognition; no such decline is found for the recognition of familiar faces (Carey 1981, 1982).

Carey *et al.* (1980) have used the adolescent developmental dip to argue that there are maturational changes in face recognition skills. They have demonstrated that the finding does not simply reflect changes in subject strategies by showing that the dip in performance is found even when subjects are all using the same strategy. Moreover, Diamond *et al.* (1983) produced compelling evidence in favour of a maturational explanation by demonstrating that girls undergoing the physical changes associated with puberty performed less well on recognition of unfamiliar faces than prepubescent or postpubescent girls of the same age.

This developmental dip, however, is not confined to facial recognition. Carey (1981) points out that voice recognition and tonal memory tests reveal a similar inflection or plateau around ages 10–14 years. Flin (1986) also observed clear inflection in the performances of 12–13 year olds asked to recognize pictures of flags and houses that had been presented earlier. In other words, although for a time it looked as if the developmental dip in recognition memory might be specific to faces, the effect is clearly of a more generalized nature (Young 1986).

Therefore we cannot use this line of developmental evidence for deciding on the question of the specialness of faces. It is only in the infant literature that it is possible to discern developmental phenomena that can be used to argue for the position that faces are a very special class of object. Our next area of enquiry concerns the evidence that exists in the now quite vast literature on normal adults' ability to recognize faces. In particular we will concentrate on the influential work of Robert Yin (1969, 1970).

Yin's studies

Yin, who was a student of Teuber, set about examining the possible uniqueness of face recognition by looking for differences in its salient characteristics compared with the perception and retention of other visual objects.

Yin (1969) began by comparing face recognition with recognition of other objects normally seen in one orientation (aeroplanes, houses, stick figures). Not surprisingly faces proved easier to recognize which, Yin realized, did not tell us anything very profound. Faces may be well remembered simply because of greater task familiarity or even because the particular set of faces used may have been especially easy to remember. For this reason Yin included a second condition in which the stimuli were inverted both at study and test. This condition produced a reversal in rank order, with faces now proving hardest to recognize.

Scapinello and Yarmey (1970), using pictures of dogs, houses, familiar faces, and unfamiliar faces found similar results, which Yin (1978) took as evidence to support his hypothesis that the perception of faces involves processes that are different from those employed when dealing with other classes of object. His contention is that face processing requires a different strategy in which wholistic as opposed to discrete features are extracted. When the normal strategy is disrupted, as by inversion, face recognition is more disadvantaged than is the general system required for perceiving other objects (where, presumably, a discrete-feature strategy is useful for both upright and inverted stimuli).

Two problems are immediately apparent with this argument. One is that no evidence is provided to substantiate the claim for there being a major difference in perceptual strategy between face perception and the processing of other objects. Second, it is not clear how these two putative strategies can operate in isolation. In other words, it seems *a priori* highly likely that the perception of any object involves both wholistic and discrete feature analyses. Indeed, Matthews (1978) has presented evidence that face perception itself requires an initial overall examination of external features followed by a sequential analysis of internal features. Fraser and Parker (1986) have extended this observation to show that face perception may be unusually sensitive to the order in which features are processed. They used schematic faces which were rapidly presented to subjects as a series of isolated features, the order varying from trial to trial. Overall the results indicated that subjects found the order outline, eyes, nose, mouth, easiest to perceive and discriminate. Fraser (1986) did not observe the same sensitivity to feature order when the stimuli were schematic houses rather than faces, however, which may give some support to Yin's specificity hypothesis but, of course, does not necessarily mean that houses and other stimulus objects are not perceived wholistically.

The suggestion that face perception is subserved by a possibly unique strategy has some bearing on the issue in question. Presumably, we learn to process faces in a top-down sequence because the upper half of Caucasian faces is more informative than the lower half (Shepherd et al. 1981). This is not necessarily true of Negroid faces, however, and, not surprisingly, African observers do not show the same perceptual strategy, at least when describing faces (Ellis et al. 1975). It would be difficult, if not impossible, to prove that the encoding strategy in face perception is unique.

Moreover, a series of experiments by Diamond and Carey (1986) case even further doubt on Yin's hypothesis concerning facial uniqueness. For their first experiment Diamond and Carey chose landscape pictures to compare with facial stimuli. They argued that, like faces, landscapes are highly familiar, difficult to encode verbally, and involve both an analysis of features and an examination of their spatial arrangements. Subjects were therefore required to recognize upright and inverted faces and upright and inverted landscapes. By judicious selection of stimuli Diamond and Carey were able to equate performance on the two classes of stimuli in the upright condition at almost 90 per cent accuracy. The effect of inversion on landscapes, however, was significantly less than for faces (79 per cent accuracy against 71 per cent accuracy), which then prompted Diamond and Carey to consider in what ways facial stimuli differed from their landscapes. They then acknowledged that faces are considerably more homogeneous. The features of a face and their spatial arrangements are common to all faces, whereas landscapes have different features and an almost infinite number of configurational possibilities. They decided that the acid test for homogeneity is how meaningful it would be to photographically superimpose exemplars drawn from within a class. This is possible with faces; Galton (1879) first demonstrated how easy it is to superimpose facial images to produce a 'generic image'. Diamond and Carey argue that one could not do the same thing with landscape pictures because they are insufficiently constrained; the result would be unrecognizable.

In their search for an object class that does display configurational constraints equivalent to those operating in faces Diamond and Carey hit upon the idea of using pictures of dogs. As it happens Scapinello and Yarmey (1970) did use dog pictures and found a smaller inversion effect than for faces, but Diamond and Carey argued that for true equivalence it would be necessary to employ subjects who might reasonably be expected to be highly experienced dog watchers. They predicted that dog experts would be as vulnerable to an inversion of dog pictures as recognition of human faces is for everyone else. Novices, on the other hand, should not be so affected.

By restricting the choice of dog breeds to those in which their experts were truly experienced Diamond and Carey were able to obtain the predicted three-way interaction among expertise, stimuli, and orientation. Whereas both novices and experts revealed a significant advantage in recognizing upright over inverted faces, only the experts showed a difference between the upright and the inverted dog conditions.

Unfortunately, (i) the experts were no better than the novices in the upright condition and (ii) the novices showed no difference between upright and inverted dog pictures. These factors make us a little cautious in unreservedly accepting these data, but we are none the less very sympathetic to Diamond and Carey's explanation of them. They argue that for people used to discriminating among highly similar objects from the same class an ability to extract 'second-order relational features' is essential (i.e. making use of smaller differences between the same features and of their configurational arrangements).

Diamond and Carey unequivocally conclude that faces are not special in the sense employed by Yin (1969). They further assert that face recognition is unlikely to be supported by any neural substrate devoted to face encoding. We now turn to consider this line of enquiry in some detail, examining in turn the specificity of right hemisphere involvement, prosopagnosia, and neurophysiological studies.

Specificity of right hemisphere involvement

Yin (1970) followed up his work with normal subjects by studying the responses of unilaterally and bilaterally brain-damaged patients who were asked to recognize upright and inverted faces and houses. The right posterior hemisphere damaged group were particularly impaired on the upright faces test compared both with control subjects and with left hemisphere damaged patients. There was no such difference on the upright houses recognition test. With inverted stimuli, however, the results looked rather different; here the right posterior group scored just as well as the controls and these two groups scored significantly better than all other unilaterally damaged groups (including right frontal) and bilaterally damaged patients.

The left posterior damaged group's performance on inverted faces was particularly poor. This is an important point to bear in mind because Yin (1970) argued that the relatively low score on upright faces by the right posterior damaged group coupled with their good performance on inverted faces was evidence of a double dissociation and implied that upright faces contained special characteristics which made them different from other stimuli. He did not apply the same argument to inverted faces, however, where he might have noted the egregious performance of the left posterior damaged group. Yin's data have been taken to indicate the specificity of a face recognition mechanism and its likely siting in the right posterior cerebral hemisphere. They are equally consistent with the idea of a special inverted face analyser situated in the left posterior region – admittedly an unlikely proposition but just as legitimate an inference from the data.

Yin's findings are supported, however, by studies of normal subjects. Performance for faces presented in the left visual hemifield (LVF), for which the optic nerves project to the visual cortex of the right cerebral hemisphere, is more affected by inversion than is right visual hemifield (RVF) performance (stimuli falling in the RVF are projected to the visual cortex of the left cerebral hemisphere). This effect has been found in studies by Leehey et al. (1978), Rapaczynski and Ehrlichman (1979), Young and Bion (1980, 1981) and Young (1984). The conclusion that the right cerebral hemisphere is more sensitive than the left cerebral hemisphere to face inversion is thus reasonably well established. Discrepant findings by Ellis and Shepherd (1975) and by Bradshaw et al. (1980) involved the use of very brief stimulus presentations or schematic face stimuli, each of which may have induced atypical processing strategies.

Yin's (1970) study involved a recognition memory test for faces and houses that were previously unfamiliar to the subjects concerned. Defective ability to match or remember unfamiliar faces has been found in several studies of patients with right hemisphere injuries (e.g. De Renzi & Spinnler 1966; Warrington and James 1967; Benton and Van Allen 1968). A number of investigations have been carried out to try to determine whether or not such deficits are face-specific, with rather mixed results. De Renzi *et al.* (1969) noted that patients with right cerebral injuries often showed other visual recognition problems. In contrast, Tzavaras *et al.* (1970) emphasized that problems in face processing persisted across different presentation materials (photographs or drawings), and dissociated from at least some other problems of visual recognition. Bruyer and Velge (1981) also found some evidence in favour of specificity of the right hemisphere deficit to faces in their study involving the discrimination of human faces, dog faces, cars, and houses. In this case, though, the 'face' deficit included both canine and human faces.

Mixed results also characterize equivalent investigations using visual hemifield stimulus presentations to normal subjects. Hines (1978) showed that visual hemifield asymmetries differed across word, face, and random shape stimuli. Similarly, St John (1981) found a LVF (and hence right hemisphere) advantage for face matching but not for shoe matching tasks. Anderson and Parkin (1985), however, disputed the comparability of the tasks used in such studies and themselves demonstrated LVF superiority both for matching photographs of faces and for matching photographs of people's hands.

Kolb *et al.* (1983) examined Yin's conclusions using a rather unusual procedure derived from Gilbert and Bakan (1973). This method is illustrated by the pictures in Fig. 2.2. Here (a) is the normal photograph of a person's face; (b) and (c) are made by taking the left and right halves of the face and combining each with its own mirror reversal.

Normally, when asked whether (b) or (c) looks the more like the person, right-handed people choose (b). The explanation usually offered for this phenomenon is that there is a perceptual preference for the half of the face that falls in the left visual field (LVF), which projects immediately to the right hemisphere. This explanation can, of course, only be correct if it is assumed that subjects' eye fixation positions are, on average, located near the midline of each face.

When Kolb *et al.* (1983) presented such stimuli to normal subjects they found that the phenomenon held not only for upright faces but also for inverted faces. They argue that the latter finding is inconsistent with Yin's hypothesis that the right hemisphere is adapted to perceive faces only when in an upright orientation. However, patients with damage confined to the right temporal or right parietal areas failed to make reliable choices of the (b) figure in either the upright or inverted conditions. This, perhaps, is more in line with Yin's (1970) observations on the influence of the posterior right hemisphere in normal face perception.

The studies reviewed in this section, then, have clearly established the importance of the right hemisphere to face perception, but they have not

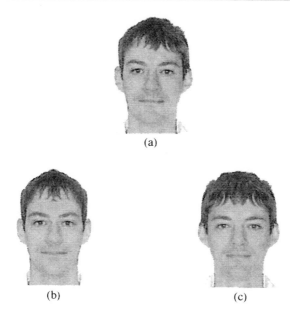

(a)

(b)   (c)

Fig. 2.2 An example of the kinds of stimuli employed by Kolb *et al.* (1983): (a) normal photograph of a face; (b), (c) left and right halves of the face, each combined with its own mirror image.

produced completely convincing evidence as regards specificity. We will now examine the evidence from patients with brain damage that has left them with not just an impairment in face perception but with a profound inability to recognize familiar people by their faces.

Prosopagnosia

Prosopagnosia was first labelled as such by Bodamer (1947) though a few cases were reported prior to that (Hécaen and Angelergues 1962). Since the topic has been examined elsewhere we will confine ourselves to discussing the implications of prosopagnosia to our question concerning the specialness of faces.

Prosopagnosia refers to an inability to recognize familiar faces following cerebral injury. Prosopagnosic patients are often unable to identify any familiar faces including famous faces, friends, family, and their own faces when seen in a mirror (Hécaen and Angelergues 1962). They can distinguish faces as a category quite easily from other visual objects (Bodamer 1947; Bruyer *et al.* 1983), but have no idea to which individual a specific face belongs. Semantic knowledge of other people is not impaired, however, and recognition is usually achieved by relying on voice, gait, clothing or context.

Despite the inability to recognize familiar faces experienced by prosopagnosic patients, recognition of other visual objects and words remains relatively intact. There is also evidence of a double dissociation between face and object agnosias, since some patients show object agnosia without prosopagnosia (Hécaen 1974; Albert *et al.* 1975) or experience more severe object than face recognition difficulties (McCarthy and Warrington 1986).

It would be easy immediately to fall into the trap of inferring specificity from the very existence of prosopagnosic patients. After all, the fact that some patients cannot recognize any faces yet are otherwise not generally agnosic surely implies the existence of a specific face recognition system? Moreover, earlier studies could be taken to indicate that not only was the dysfunction specific to faces but that there may not exist other patient groups with impairment equally circumscribed to the recognition of specific object groups. As we shall show, however, some caution is required before invoking observations on prosopagnosic patients to support the face specialness argument.

The very term 'prosopagnosia', deriving as it does from the Greek *prosopon* = face and *agnosia* = not knowing, itself implies specificity (Bodamer 1947). Yet one of Bodamer's (1947) own patients revealed deficits beyond agnosia for people. In addition to having problems with faces, this patient could not recognize a rabbit, a dog, or a chicken; nor could he recognize a wellington boot from a picture.

Further examination of the literature on prosopagnosia reveals many similar instances where prosopagnosia is accompanied by problems either in recognizing or distinguishing other classes of objects (Ellis 1975). Some examples are as follows: the patient described by Pallis (1955), apart from his inability to recognize faces, had trouble distinguishing among both foods and animals; Macrae and Trolle's (1956) patient, who also found difficulties in telling one animal species from another, in addition, complained that he could not distinguish different types of cars; Damasio *et al* (1982) reported tests on two prosopagnosic patients which revealed their difficulties in identifying animals, abstract symbols (e.g. dollar sign, swastika), and motor vehicles – particularly when there were clusters of items that were similar in form; and Bornstein (1963) discovered a prosopagnosic patient who complained that not only could she not recognize faces but that she used to enjoy ornithology but was now incapable of identifying different birds.

In addition to these other agnosic symptoms prosopagnosics have been reported as having difficulties in colour perception (e.g. Bay 1953; Beyn and Knyazeva 1962; Cole and Perez-Cruet 1964); and with topographical memory (e.g. Beyn & Knyazeva 1962; Pallis 1955).

What do these clinical observations tell us about the nature of prosopagnosia? On the basis of such evidence, Damasio *et al.* (1982) are unequivocal; they contend that 'prosopagnosia is not specific to human faces' (p. 339), and 'that the emphasis on the dissociation between facial recognition and object recognition is misleading' (p. 337).

Damasio *et al.* (1982) consider that prosopagnosia is not a cognitive deficit specific to faces. Rather they see it as one aspect of a more general problem 'to evoke the specific historic context of a given visual stimulus' (p. 339) – by which they mean that it is essentially a memory malfunction in which percepts fail to trigger their appropriate stored representations. (There are other interpretations of the cause of prosopagnosia: Hécaen 1981; Ellis 1986; but we shall ignore these for the moment.) What causes the emphasis on faces in prosopagnosic symptomatology, according to Damasio *et al.*, is that faces are peculiarly 'ambiguous' stimuli. Here they are referring to the quality of faces noted by others, including Galton (1883) and Diamond and Carey (1986), namely their inherently similar structure. Damasio *et al.* argue that most classes of object are not so well differentiated as faces and therefore may be usefully recognized following a more gross level of recognition, which they term 'generic'. In other words, while prosopagnosics may be able to identify an object as a book or a chair, if they were asked 'whose book?' or 'whose chair?' they would reveal problems similar to those experienced with faces. The difference between recognizing a generic class of object, face, book, chair, and so on is different from that involved in recognizing its 'historic context'. This is reminiscent of distinctions drawn by Tulving (1972) and others between semantic memory (i.e. knowledge of the abstract meaning of words, objects, etc.) and episodic memory (memory for specific experience), although, it must be swiftly pointed out, there is no suggestion that prosopagnosic patients display a generalized loss of episodic memory in the ways observed with amnesic patients.

The crucial question is whether there exist any prosopagnosic patients who manifest a 'pure' syndrome in which their only deficit lies in face recognition? This question is probably unanswerable because it requires one to accept proof of the null hypothesis and, of course, this is not acceptable – at least statistically. Bruyer *et al.* (1983), however, did describe a Belgian farmer, who became prosopagnosic, as a relatively 'pure' case. He complained of severe problems in recognizing faces of family and friends, yet unlike the patient of Assal *et al.* (1984) was able to identify his cows and performed adequately on a variety of tasks given to him by Bruyer *et al.* (1983). For example, he was able to identify famous buildings and flowers as well as successfully carrying out a number of face-related tasks, provided they did not require him to identify people from their faces. But this patient also had some difficulties in distinguishing within classes; he displayed problems with cars, coins, and playing cards.

However, a case of prosopagnosia apparently not accompanied by any other agnosic difficulties has been reported; this was described by De Renzi (1986). One of his four patients, a 72 year old lawyer, appeared to find difficulty only in identifying people by their face. He was able to identify his own personal belongings mixed with 6–10 similar items from the same category (i.e. razor, wallet, ties, glasses). He could also identify his own handwriting from others, he could pick out a Siamese cat from photographs of different cats, and he was able to sort out 20 Italian coins from 20 foreign coins. According to both the patient and wife he was only agnosic for faces.

De Renzi's (1986) patient shows clearly that prosopagnosia is not invariably accompanied by problems in making other within-category discriminations. If we ignore our earlier caveat and accept that this patient is indeed suffering from a disorder confined to face identification then it is legitimate to consider why pure cases are so rare. The answer to this question may lie in the fact that the majority of prosopagnosias result from infarctions and tumours which, by their very nature, are likely to involve comparatively large areas of brain tissue that may support a number of different gnostic fields. One might therefore expect that normally a deficit in face processing will occur alongside other deficits. Moreover, one would expect these accompanying problems to vary somewhat from patient to patient – which, in fact, does seem to be the case. Admittedly there are certain common themes – animals, cars, clothing – but not every prosopagnosic patient reveals all, or indeed necessarily any, of these particular additional agnosias. So, for the moment we are inclined to accept that prosopagnosia can occur in a form undiluted enough to warrant the view that it is a distinct cognitive deficit which could only arise from the existence of a system containing functional components specific to face recognition. In other words, we reject the view expressed by a number of theorists, including Damasio *et al.* (1982), that prosopagnosia is a manifestation of a more general dysfunction affecting the visual identification of objects, particularly when discrimination among exemplars is difficult.

We next briefly turn to a final line of evidence that may have a bearing on the issue of specificity in face recognition. This involves the work of Perrett and others who have been investigating the responses of single neurones in the monkey's cortex when the animal looks at faces.

Neurophysiological studies

A review of this work is given by Perrett *et al.* (1986). They report that they have located five different types of cell within the temporal cortex of the macaque, each of which responds maximally to different facial characteristics (full face, profile, back of head, head up, and head down). Other cells respond selectively to one particular individual, regardless of pose, lighting, expression, and so on and these may operate by pooling outputs of cells that are identity and pose specific.

These observations are consistent with some of the work on humans and offer some support for the specificity argument. But there are a few worrying discrepancies. For instance, the cells studied by Perrett *et al.* are situated in the superior temporal sulcus which does not exactly correspond with the regions around the inferior longitudinal fasciculus which, when damaged, can produce symptoms of prosopagnosia. Another possible problem lies in the fact that the face-specific cells are mixed in with cells responsive to other classes of object.

Unfortunately, as yet there are no data available on the time-course for the firing of the different types of cells. As we shall see in the next section, one approach to understanding human face recognition is to hypothesize a set of sub-processes, some of which precede others. It would be reassuring to know from single-cell observations that there is agreement between the neurophysiological evidence and the cognitive psychological theorizing.

We now turn to the final section of this review where we shall examine the general form that this face-specific module or gnostic area may take. Here our intention is to provide no more than a general framework for subsequent discussion, some of which will fill out the substance of the processes underlying face recognition in much greater detail.

Outline of a face-processing module

As we mentioned in the introduction to this chapter there are a number of theoretical approaches to understanding how people recognize faces and read other information from them. It is not our intention to review these here, instead all we wish to do is to demonstrate just how a face-processing module may operate by outlining some of the principal functional components necessary to support such a system.

Figure 2.3 provides a useful working plan for our present purposes. It is the model proposed by Bruce and Young (1986). It is apparent from

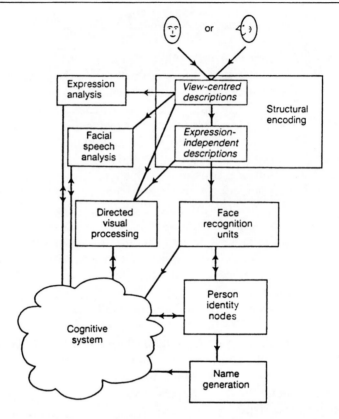

Fig. 2.3 Bruce and Young's (1986) model of face recognition.

the model that what we have termed the face-processing module is rather more like Konorski's (1967) notion of a gnostic field – that is, a set of related modules that normally act in an orchestrated way but that may sometimes operate in solo fashion. What is also clear from the model is that surrounding the core identification system are a number of satellite systems designed to process different kinds of facial information. In addition the model assumes that the semantic information stored about people can be accessed in ways other than by the face. In the following discussion we shall describe separately the three conceptual areas of the model. Before doing so, however, it is timely to repeat the warnings usually given with information processing models such as this one, namely

(1) that it is a gross simplification of the likely system, indicating only some of the possible pathways involved;

(2) that no detailed links to other parts of the cognitive system are shown (including those that may exert contextual influence); and

(3) that the system is shown largely as a bottom-up process and ignores the fact that there are, undoubtedly, top-down influences.

Identification

Identification is depicted in Fig. 2.3 as a three-stage process in which the raw image first undergoes whatever computational processes are necessary for later perceptual processing. There are a number of ways by which this may be achieved but one favoured theory has been that proposed by Marr (1982) whereby first a raw primal sketch is derived, then a viewer-centred (two-and-a-half-dimensional) image is computed, followed by an object-centred (or three-dimensional) image.

This stage is fast and displays the quality of encapsulation that Fodor (1983) identified as a feature of modular systems (i.e. it is automatic and cannot be influenced by top-down processes). One further feature of the structural encoding stage may be its selective tuning to encode face-like stimuli. It is a common observation that ambiguous natural stimuli such as those provided by flames or clouds are often 'resolved' as being faces. This classification is not exclusive but it may be that any pattern that in the least corresponds to the basic facial structure is perceived as such – that is, it has an unusually lax criterion for including patterns into the face-processing module.

Ellis (1981a,b, 1983) has suggested that the face-processing system may only be activated following an initial classification of patterned input as a face. If any such active selection does occur then early detection would be a prerequisite. One measure of the significance of faces, in fact, may be the relative breadth of criterion tolerance at the structural encoding stage which allows fast routing of information to the face-processing system.

It is not necessary to postulate such an early selection or switching mechanism; it is equally possible to suggest that no preprocessing is necessary, but if an active categorization process does precede detailed analysis it may take place at the structural encoding stage. This means, of course, that this stage is either not exclusive to faces, because it has to cope with other classes of input, or that some part of the computational processes within it is shared with these other categories of objects.

The structural encoding provides data for the next stage, the face recognition units, in which 'descriptions' of known faces are contained. When a facial input makes contact with its representation at this stage the output is of two kinds:

(1) a signal of familiarity is given and
(2) there is a signal given to the corresponding person node within semantic memory.

There is a controversy concerning the nature of these units. Do they operate like the word units, logogens, proposed by Morton (1969), as though they each possess a variable threshold? Or, instead, do they work by giving out a graded response depending on the degree of similarity between the stored representation and current percept? (Ellis *et al.* 1987). It is known that the greater the familiarity of a face the more likely it is to be recognized despite masking, distortion, and so on, consistent with a variable threshold mode of operation (Ellis 1981*b*). But we also know that we are sometimes aware that one face resembles another yet is not the same. This is difficult to reconcile with a threshold mechanism, but it may be possible to do so by suggesting a further decision-making stage in which other knowledge may be brought to bear (e.g. 'It looks like Paul Newman's face but he is unlikely to visit this particular pub therefore it's someone else').

Following the establishment of a face's familiarity the next stage is to identify who the person is. Information about the person including his or her occupation, status, and so on is thought to be held in a separate store that may form part of semantic memory in general.

These 'person-identity nodes' (Hay and Young 1982) may also be accessed via other routes not specifically shown in the model such as name, voice, and gait and so are not exclusive to the facial route. If the latter should fail, as it does in cases of prosopagnosia, then these alternative routes may be used, often quite successfully.

At this point it is worthwhile pointing out that prosopagnosia may arise from damage at any point in the system (Hécaen 1981; De Renzi 1986; Ellis 1986). Indeed the fact that some prosopagnosics cannot form a good structural representation of a face while others have problems either extracting general facial characteristics (sex, age, etc.) or in reading emotional expressions and others still can do all of these yet fail to achieve a sense of familiarity when confronted by someone they know supports the functional architecture shown in Fig. 2.3.

Other support comes from the everyday errors recorded by Young *et al.*'s (1985) subjects; sometimes they saw someone they knew to be familiar yet whose full identity eluded them for some time.

Associated facial analyses

Figure 2.3 shows three structures associated with face identification yet possibly distinct from it. These are modules concerned with interpreting emotional expression, facial speech analysis, and directed visual processing. The existence of these is supported by neuropsychological evidence in which patients have been described who can process one or

other type of information but not the remaining one. Not all prosopagnosics, for instance, report difficulties in interpreting emotional
expressions displayed in faces. Some do, however, and the ability to
recognize faces has been known to recover before the ability to identify
their emotional state (Bornstein 1963). Malone *et al.* (1982) describe a
double dissociation between impairments affecting recognition of
familiar faces and ability to match views of unfamiliar faces (which
would, in our terms, depend on directed visual processing).

Campbell (1989) reports the double dissociation of prosopagnosia
and the ability to lip-read, suggesting that these skills are governed by
separate systems.

Alternative routes to recognition

The final area of the schematic face-processing model we wish briefly to
discuss concerns the obvious fact that the person-identity nodes may be
accessed by routes other than the facial one. As we mentioned earlier, it
is a common observation that prosopagnosic patients rely heavily on
voices for identification, sometimes using gait or clothing as additional
cues.

Voice identification, though on occasion useful to normal individuals,
appears to be a less reliable means of establishing identity. Instead, what
seems to us to happen quite often is that familiar voices are easily
classified as known or unknown but that the actual identity of the
speaker may elude one for some time. Advertising agencies, well aware
of this phenomenon, frequently employ well-known actors to perform
voice-overs on TV commercials. They have realized how reassuring it is
for the voice to seem comfortingly familiar without full identification
taking place.

Conclusions

We began by posing once again the question 'Are faces special?'. Our
conclusion is that they are special but that they are not unique. The model
of face recognition proposed by Bruce and Young (1986) outlines the
likely stages leading up to identification but it does not, of course, identify
which one, if any may be specific to faces. Many object classes may be
analysed in similar parallel ways (cf. Konorski 1967), but faces may be
special simply because we all experience them so extensively and are
continually required to make fine discriminations among them.
Moreover, faces provide an unusually rich source of information that

covers not only identification but emotional expression as well as verbal and non-verbal communication. These factors may mean that the face recognition module is rather more elaborate than is usually the case for other classes of object. However, in our opinion, provided there is a need for it, any other class could develop such a system of its own, displaying a similar architecture as that shown in Fig. 2.3. Faces are special but not unique objects. Therefore their study is of interest not only to those interested in physiognomic processing, but also to those interested in the way any objects or patterns, including words, are recognized by the brain. Indeed, A. Ellis *et al.* (1987) have argued that the face recognition module could have provided the original model for a visual recognition system and that evolutionarily subsequent needs, such as reading, may have employed the existing system such as that used for faces.

References

Albert, M. L., Reches, A., and Silverberg, R. (1975). Associative visual agnosia without alexia. *Neurology*, **25**, 322–6.

Anderson, E. and Parkin, A. (1985). On the nature of the left visual field advantage for faces. *Cortex*, **21**, 453–9.

Assal, G., Favre, C., and Anderes, J. P. (1984). Non-reconnaissance d'animaux familiers chez un paysan. *Revue Neurologique*, **140**, 580–4.

Baron, R. J. (1981). Mechanisms of human facial recognition. *International Journal of Man–Machine Studies*, **15**, 137–78.

Bateson, P. P. G. (1977). Testing an observer's ability to identify individual animals. *Animal Behaviour*, **25**, 247–8.

Bay, E. (1953). Disturbances of visual perception and their examination. *Brain*, **76**, 515–51.

Benton, A. L. and Van Allen, M. W. (1968). Impairment in facial recognition in patients with cerebral disease. *Cortex*, **4**, 344–58.

Beyn, E. S. and Knyazeva, G. R. (1962). The problem of prosopagnosia. *Journal of Neurology, Neurosurgery, and Psychiatry*, **25**, 154–9.

Blanc-Garin, J. (1984). Perception des visages et reconnaissance de la physionomie dans l'agnosie des visages. *L'Année Psychologique*, **84**, 573–98.

Bodamer, J. (1947). Die Prosopagnosie. *Archiv Für Psychiatrie und Nervenkrankheiten*, **179**, 6–53.

Bornstein, B. (1963). Prosopagnosia. In *Problems of dynamic neurology*, (ed. L. Halpern), pp. 283–318. Hadassah Medical Organization, Jerusalem.

Bradshaw, J. L., Taylor, M. J., Patterson, J. and Nettleton, N. C. (1980). Upright and inverted faces, and housefronts, in the two visual fields: a right and a left hemisphere contribution. *Journal of Clinical Neuropsychology*, **2**, 245–57.

Broadbent, D. (1985). A question of levels: comment on McClelland and Rumelhart. *Journal of Experimental Psychology: General*, **14**, 189–92.

Bronson, G. W. (1974). The postnatal growth of visual capacity. *Child Development*, **45**, 873–90.

Bruce, V. and Young, A. (1986). Understanding face recognition. *British Journal of Psychology*, **77**, 305–27.

Bruyer, R. and Velge, V. (1981). Lésion unilatérale et trouble de la perception de visages: specificité du déficit? *Acta Neurologica Belgica*, **81**, 321–32.

Bruyer, R., Laterre, C., Seron, X., Feyereisen, P., Strypstein, E., Pierrard, E. and Rectem, D. (1983). A case of prosopagnosia with some preserved covert remembrance of familiar faces. *Brain and Cognition*, **2**, 257–84.

Campbell, R. (1989). Lipreading. In *Handbook of research on face processing*, (ed. A. W. Young and H. D. Ellis), pp. 187–205. North Holland, Amsterdam.

Carey, S. (1981). The development of face perception. In *Perceiving and remembering faces*, (ed. G. Davies, H. Ellis, and J. Shepherd), pp. 9–38. Academic Press, London.

Carey, S. (1982). Face perception: anomalies of development. In *U-Shaped behavioral growth*, (ed. S. Strauss and R. Stavy), pp. 169–91. Academic Press, New York.

Carey, S., Diamond, R. and Woods, B. (1980). Development of face recognition – a maturational component? *Developmental Psychology*, **16**, 257–69.

Cole, M. and Perez-Cruet, J. (1964). Prosopagnosia. *Neuropsychologia*, **2**, 237–46.

Conrad, V. K. (1947). Uber den begriff der Vorgestalt und seine Bedeutung für die Hirnpathologie. *Der Nervenarzt*, **38**, 289–93.

Damasio, A. R., Damasio, H., and Van Hoesen, G. W. (1982). Prosopagnosia: anatomical basis and behavioral mechanisms. *Neurology*, **32**, 331–41.

De Casper, A. J. and Fifer, W. P. (1980). Of human bonding: Newborns prefer their mothers' voices. *Science*, **209**, 1174–7.

De Renzi, E. (1986). Current issues on prosopagnosia. In *Aspects of face processing*, (ed. H. D. Ellis *et al.*), pp. 243–52. Nijhoff, Dordrecht.

De Renzi, E. and Spinnler, H. (1966). Facial recognition in brain-damaged patients. *Neurology*, **16**, 145–52.

De Renzi, E., Scotti, G. and Spinnler, H. (1969). Perceptual and associative disorders of visual recognition: relationship to the side of the cerebral lesion. *Neurology*, **19**, 634–42.

Diamond, R. and Carey, S. (1986). Why faces are and are not special: an effect of expertise (1986). *Journal of Experimental Psychology: General*, **115**, 107–17.

Diamond, R., Carey, S., and Back, K. J. (1983). Genetic influences on the development of spatial skills during early adolescence. *Cognition*, **13**, 167–85.

Dickinson, A. and Boakes, R. (1979). *Mechanisms of learning and motivation: a memorial to Jerzy Konorski*. Lawrence Erlbaum, Hillsdale, NJ.

Dodd, B. (1979). Lip reading in infants: attention to speech presented in- and out-of-synchrony. *Cognitive Psychology*, **11**, 478–84.

Ellis, H. D. (1975). Recognizing faces. *British Journal of Psychology*, **66**, 409–26.

Ellis, H. D. (1981a). Introduction. In *Perceiving and remembering faces*, (ed. G. Davies, H. Ellis, and J. Shepherd), pp. 1–5. Academic Press, London.

Ellis, H. D. (1981b). Theoretical aspects of face recognition. In *Perceiving and remembering faces*, (ed. G. Davies, H. Ellis, J. Shepherd), pp. 171–97. Academic Press, London.

Ellis, H. D. (1983). The role of the right hemisphere in face perception. In *Functions of the right hemisphere*, (ed. A. W. Young), pp. 33–64. Academic Press, London.

Ellis, H. D. (1986). Processes underlying face recognition. In *The neuropsychology of face perception and facial expression*, (ed. R. Bruyer), pp. 1–27. Lawrence Erlbaum, Hillsdale, NJ.

Ellis, H. D. (1986). Disorders of face recognition. In *Neurology*, (ed. K. Poeck *et al.*), pp. 179–87. Springer, Heidelberg.

Ellis, H. D. and Shepherd, J. W. (1975). Recognition of upright and inverted faces presented in the left and right visual fields. *Cortex*, **11**, 3–7.

Ellis, H. D., Deregowski, J. B. and Shepherd, J. W. (1975). Descriptions of white and black faces by white and black subjects. *International Journal of Psychology*, **10**, 119–23.

Ellis, A. W., Young, A. W. and Hay, D. C. (1987). Modelling the recognition of faces and words. In *Modelling cognition* (ed. P. E. Morris), pp. 269–97. Wiley, Chichester.

Field, T. M. Woodson, R., Greenberg, R. and Cohen, D. (1982). Discrimination and imitation of facial expressions by neonates. *Science*, **281**, 179–81.

Flin, R. H. (1980). Age effects in children's memory for unfamiliar faces. *Developmental Psychology*, **16**, 373–4.

Flin, R. H. (1985). Development of face recognition: an encoding switch? *British Journal of Psychology*, **76**, 123–34.

Flin, R. H. (1986). Development of visual memory: an early adolescent regression. *Journal of Early Adolescence*.

Fodor, J. A. (1983). *The modularity of mind*. MIT Press, Cambridge, MA.

Fraser, I. H. (1986). Temporal discrimination and integration in visual pattern perception. PhD thesis, University of Aberdeen.

Fraser, I. H. and Parker, D. M. (1986). Reaction time measures of feature saliency in a perceptual integration task. In *Aspects of face processing*, (ed. H. D. Ellis *et al.*), pp. 45–52. Nijhoff, Dordrecht.

Galton, F. (1879). Generic images. *Proceedings of the Royal Institution*, **9**, 161–70.

Galton, F. (1883). *Inquiries into human faculty and development*. Macmillan, New York.

Gilbert, C. and Bakan, P. (1973). Visual asymmetry in perception of faces. *Neuropsychologia*, **11**, 355–62.

Goren, C. C., Sarty, M. and Wu, R. W. K. (1975). Visual following and pattern discrimination of face-like stimuli by newborn infants. *Pediatrics*, **56**, 544–9.

Hay, D. C. and Young, A. W. (1982). The human face. In *Normality and pathology in cognitive functions*, (ed. A. W. Ellis), pp. 173–202. Academic Press, New York.

Hayes, L. A. and Watson, J. S. (1981). Neonatal imitation: fact or artifact? *Developmental Psychology*, **17**, 655–60.

Hécaen, H. (1981). The neuropsychology of face recognition. In *Perceiving and remembering faces*, (ed. G. Davies, H. Ellis, and J. Shepherd), pp. 39–54. Academic Press, London.

Hécaen, H. and Angelergues, R. (1962). Agnosia for faces (prosopagnosia). *Archives of Neurology*, **7**, 92–100.

Hécaen, H., Goldblum, M. C., Masure, M. C. and Ramier, A. M. (1974). Une nouvelle observation d'agnosie d'objet. Deficit de l'association ou de la categorisation specifique de la modalité visuelle? *Neuropsychologia*, **12**, 447–64.

Hines, D. (1978). Visual information processing in the left and right hemispheres. *Neuropsychologia*, **16**, 593–600.

Hinton, G. E. and Anderson, J. A. (1981). *Parallel models of associative memory*. Lawrence Erlbaum, Hillsdale, NJ.

Jacobson, S. W. (1979). Matching behavior in the young infant. *Child Development*, **50**, 425–30.

Johnson, M., Dziurawiec, S., Ellis, H. and Morton, J. (1991). Newborns' preferential tracking of face-like stimuli and its subsequent decline. *Cognition*, **40**, 1–19.

Koepke, J. E., Hamm, M., Legerstee, M. and Russell, M. (1983). Neonatal imitation: two failures to replicate. *Infant Behavior and Development*, **6**, 97–102.

Kohonen, T., Oja, E. and Lehtio, P. (1981). Storage and processing of information in distributed associative memory systems. In *Parallel models of associative memory*, (ed. G. E. Hinton and J. A. Anderson). Lawrence Erlbaum, Hillsdale, NJ.

Kolb, B., Milner, B. and Taylor, L. (1983). Perception of faces by patients with localized cortical excisions. *Canadian Journal of Psychology*, **37**, 8–18.

Konorski, J. (1967). *Integrative activity of the brain. An interdisciplinary approach*. University of Chicago Press.

Kuhl, P. K. and Meltzoff, A. N. (1982). The bimodal perception of speech in infancy. *Science*, **218**, 1138–41.

Leehey, S. C., Carey, S., Diamond, R. and Cahn, A. (1978). Upright and inverted faces: the right hemisphere knows the difference. *Cortex*, **14**, 411–19.

Light, L. L., Kayra-Stuart, F. and Hollander, S. (1979). Recognition memory for typical and unusual faces. *Journal of Experimental Psychology: Human Learning and Memory*, **5**, 212–28.

McCarthy, R. and Warrington, E. K. (1986). Visual associative agnosia: a clinico-anatomical study of a single case. *Journal of Neurology, Neurosurgery, and Psychiatry*, **49**, 1233–40.

Macrae, D. and Trolle, E. (1956). The defect of function in visual agnosia. *Brain*, **79**, 94–110.

McGurk, H. and Macdonald, J. (1976). Hearing lips and seeing voices. *Nature*, **264**, 746–8.

Mackain, K. S. Studdert-Kennedy, M., Spieker, S. and Stern, D. (1983). Infant intermodal speech perception is a left hemisphere function. *Science*, **219**, 1347–9.

McKenzie, B. and Over, R. (1983). Young infants fail to replicate facial and manual gestures. *Infant Behavior and Development*, **6**, 85–9.

Malone, D. R., Morris, H. H., Kay, M. C. and Levin, H. S. (1982). Prosopagnosia: a double dissociation between the recognition of familiar and unfamiliar faces. *Journal of Neurology, Neurosurgery, and Psychiatry*, **45**, 820–2.

Marr, D. (1982). *Vision*. W. H. Freeman, San Francisco.

Martindale, C. (1981). *Cognition and consciousness*. Dorsey, Homewood, Ill.

Matthews, M. L. (1978). Discrimination of Identikit constructions of faces: evidence for a dual processing strategy. *Perception and Psychophysics*, **23**, 153–61.

Melhuish, E. C. (1982). Visual attention to mother's and stranger's faces and facial contrast in 1-month-old infants. *Developmental Psychology*, **18**, 229–31.

Meltzoff, A. N. (1981). Imitation, intermodal co-ordination and representation in early infancy. In *Infancy and Epistemology*, (ed. G. Butterworth), pp. 85–114. Harvester Press, Brighton.

Meltzoff, A. N. and Moore, M. K. (1977). Imitation of facial and manual gestures by human neonates. *Science*, **198**, 75–8.

Meltzoff, A. N. and Moore, M. K. (1983a). Newborn infants imitate adult facial gestures. *Child Development*, **54**, 702–9.

Meltzoff, A. N. and Moore, M. K. (1983b). The origins of imitation in infancy: paradigm, phenomena, and theories. In *Advances in infancy research*, vol. 2, (ed. L. P. Lipsitt and C. K. Rovee-Collier), pp. 265–301. Ablex, New Jersey.

Meltzoff, A. N. and Moore, M. K. (1983c). Methodological issues in studies of imitation: comments on McKenzie and Over and Koepke *et al*. *Infant Behavior and Development*, **6**, 103–8.

Mills, M. and Melhuish, E. (1974). Recognition of mother's voice in early infancy. *Nature*, **252**, 123–4.

Morton, J. (1969). Interaction of information in word recognition. *Psychological Review*, **76**, 165–78.

Pallis, C. A. (1955). Impaired identification of faces and places with agnosia for colours. Report of a case due to cerebral embolism. *Journal of Neurology, Neurosurgery, and Psychiatry*, **18**, 218–24.

Perrett, D. I., Mistlin, A. J. Potter, D. D., Smith, P. A. J., Head, A. S., Chitty, A. J., *et al.* (1986). Functional organisation of visual neurones processing face identity. In *Aspects of face processing*, (ed. H. D. Ellis *et al*), pp. 187–98. Nijhoff, Dordrecht.

Rapaczynski, W. and Ehrlichman, H. (1979). Opposite visual hemifield superiorities in face recognition as a function of cognitive style. *Neuropsychologia*, **17**, 645–52.

Rhodes, G. (1985). Lateralized processes in face recognition. *British Journal of Psychology*, **76**, 249–71.

St John, R. C. (1981). Lateral asymmetry in face perception. *Canadian Journal of Psychology*, **35**, 213–23.

Scapinello, K. F. and Yarmey, A. D. (1970). The role of familiarity and orientation in immediate and delayed recognition of pictorial stimuli. *Psychonomic Science*, **21**, 329–31.

Seymour, P. H. K. (1979). *Human visual cognition.* Collier-McMillan, London.

Shepherd, J. W., Davies, G. M. and Ellis, H. D. (1981). Studies of cue saliency. In *Perceiving and remembering faces*, (ed. G. Davies, H. Ellis and J. Shepherd), pp. 105–31. Academic Press, London.

Souther, A. F. and Banks, M. S. (1979). The human face: a view from the infant's eye. Paper presented at the meetings of the Society for the Research in Child Development, San Francisco, California.

Studdert-Kennedy, M. (1983). On learning to speak. *Human Neurobiology*, **2**, 191–5.

Teuber, H. L. (1978). The brain and human behaviour. In *Handbook of sensory psychology*, Vol. 8, (ed. R. Held *et al.*). Springer, Berlin.

Tulving, E. (1972). Episodic and semantic memory. In *Organization and memory*, (ed. E. Tulving and W. Donaldson). Academic Press, London.

Tzavaras, A., Hécaen, H. and Lebras, H. (1970). Le problème de la specificité du deficit de la reconnaissance du visage humain lors des lésions hémisphériques unilatérales. *Neuropsychologia*, **8**, 403–16.

Vinter, A. (1985). La capacité d'imitation à la naissance: elle existe, mais que signifie-t-elle? *Canadian Journal of Psychology*, **39**, 16–33.

Warrington, E. K. and James, M. (1967). An experimental investigation of facial recognition in patients with unilateral cerebral lesions. *Cortex*, **3**, 317–26.

Yin, R. K. (1969). Looking at upside-down faces. *Journal of Experimental Psychology*, **81**, 141–5.

Yin, R. K. (1970). Face recognition by brain-injured patients: a dissociable ability? *Neuropsychologia*, **8**, 395–402.

Yin, R. K. (1978). Face perception: a review of experiments with infants, normal adults and brain-injured persons. in *Handbook of Sensory Physiology, Vol VIII* (ed. R. Held *et al.*), pp. 593–608. Springer-Verlag, Berlin.

Young, A. W. (1984). Right cerebral hemisphere superiority for recognising the internal and external features of famous faces. *British Journal of Psychology*, **75**, 161–9.

Young. A. W. (1986). Subject characteristics in lateral differences for face processing by normals: age. In *The Neuropsychology of face perception and facial expression*, (ed. R. Bruyer), pp. 167–200. Erlbaum, New Jersey.

Young, A. W. and Bion, P. J. (1980). Absence of any developmental trend in right hemisphere superiority for face recognition. *Cortex*, **16**, 213–21.

Young, A. W. and Bion, P. J. (1981). Accuracy of naming laterally presented known faces by children and adults. *Cortex*, **17**, 97–106.

Young, A. W., Hay, D. C. and Ellis, A. W. (1985). The faces that launched a thousand slips: everyday difficulties and errors in recognizing people. *British Journal of Psychology*, **76**, 495–523.

3

A theoretical perspective for understanding face recognition

Reprinted in slightly modified form from Bruce, V. and Young, A. W. (1986), Understanding face recognition, *British Journal of Psychology*, **77**, 305–27. With kind permission of Professor V. Bruce and the British Psychological Society.

Summary

The aim of this paper is to develop a theoretical model and a set of terms for understanding and discussing how we recognize familiar faces, and the relationship between recognition and other aspects of face processing. It is suggested that there are seven distinct types of information that we derive from seen faces; these are labelled pictorial, structural, visually derived semantic, identity-specific semantic, name, expression, and facial speech codes. A functional model is proposed in which structural encoding processes provide descriptions suitable for the analysis of facial speech, for analysis of expression, and for face recognition units. Recognition of familiar faces involves a match between the products of structural encoding and previously stored structural codes describing the appearance of familiar faces, held in face recognition units. Identity-specific semantic codes are then accessed from person identity nodes, and subsequently name codes are retrieved. It is also proposed that the cognitive system plays an active role in deciding whether or not the initial match is sufficiently close to indicate true recognition or merely a 'resemblance'; several factors are seen as influencing such decisions.

This functional model is used to draw together data from diverse sources including laboratory experiments, studies of everyday errors, and studies of patients with different types of cerebral injury. It is also used to clarify similarities and differences between processes responsible for object, word, and face recognition.

Introduction

A human face reveals a great deal of information to a perceiver. It can tell about mood and intention and attentiveness, but it can also serve to identify a person. Of course, a person can be identified by other means than the face. Voice, body shape, gait, or even clothing may all establish identity in circumstances where facial detail may not be available. Nevertheless, a face is the most distinctive and widely used key to a person's identity, and the loss of ability to recognize faces experienced by some neurological (prosopagnosic) patients has a profound effect on their lives.

Many studies of face recognition have been carried out; the bibliography compiled by Baron (1979) lists over 200. However, as H. Ellis (1975, 1981) pointed out, this considerable empirical activity was not initially accompanied by developments in theoretical understanding of the processes underlying face recognition. It is only comparatively recently that serious theoretical models have been put forward (Bruce 1979, 1983; Baron 1981; H. Ellis 1981, 1983, 1986a; Hay and Young 1982; Rhodes 1985; A. Ellis *et al.* 1987).

Here, we present a theoretical framework for face recognition which draws together and extends these models. This framework is used to clarify what we now understand about face recognition, and also to point to where the gaps in our knowledge lie. It is also used to compare and contrast the recognition of people's faces with the recognition of other types of visual stimuli, and to explore ways in which mechanisms involved in human facial recognition relate to other types of face processing, such as the analysis of expressions or the interpretation of lip and tongue movements in speech comprehension.

Our principal concern is to present a functional model to account for the perceptual and cognitive processes involved when people recognize faces. We use the term recognition here in a broad sense, covering the derivation of any type of stored information from faces. Thus we are also using face recognition to include what might well be called identification or retrieval of personal information. We develop the view that recognition in this sense is not a unitary event, and that it involves the interaction of a number of different functional components.

In the present paper we are concerned almost exclusively with evidence in favour of *functional* components in the human face processing system, without regard to whether or not these are localized to specific areas of the brain. The evidence of localization (and especially cerebral lateralization) of the component processes has been reviewed by H. Ellis (1983) and Rhodes (1985). Although we do not discuss the evi-

dence for localization of function, we do, however, pay close attention
to the functional deficits which can result from certain kinds of cerebral
injury. Different patterns of breakdown can yield important information about what the functional components of the system are, and how
they are organized. For this reason we pay attention not only to
conventional experimental studies of face processing, but also to studies
of the disorders of face processing caused by different types of cerebral
injury. Temporary breakdowns of face processing also occur in everyone from time to time, and here too the patterns of breakdown yield
important evidence. Therefore we also discuss studies of errors of
recognition made by normal people both in everyday life and under
laboratory conditions.

In understanding face processing a crucial problem is to determine
what uses people need to make of the information they derive from
faces. We argue here that there are at least seven distinct types of
information that can be derived from faces; we describe these as
different types of information *code*. We distinguish pictorial, structural,
visually derived semantic, identity-specific semantic, name, expression,
and facial speech codes; this list can cover all of the uses of facial
information of which we are at present aware. We assume that these
codes are not themselves the functional components of the face processing system, but rather that they are the products of the operation of
the functional components.

The idea of different ways of coding facial information provides a
convenient set of terms for talking about face processing, particularly in
the context of typical laboratory experiments n face recognition, where
it is important to distinguish different sources of information which
could mediate decisions about the earlier occurrence of faces (cf. Bruce
1982). More importantly, though, it also makes clear what we need to
understand about the human face processing system. It is clear that
there are two major questions that we must address:

1. What different information codes are used in facial processing?
2. What functional components are responsible for the generation and
   access of these different codes?

An additional question of importance to the present discussion concerns which of the types of facial information are used in recognizing a
familiar person in everyday life. As will become clear, our view is that
recognition of familiar faces mainly involves structural, identity-specific
semantic, and name codes, and that pictorial, expression, and facial
speech codes usually play no more than a minor role in recognition.

We deal in turn with each of the questions, before turning to compare our framework for face recognition with contemporary models of object and word recognition. We then consider some of the unresolved issues deriving from our functional model.

What different codes are involved in face processing?

A photograph or other picture of a face will lead to the generation of a *pictorial code*. A pictorial code is a description of a *picture*. It should not be equated with view-specific information derived, and continuously updated, during early visual processing of moving faces (see later). Nor is it simply equivalent to the viewer-centred information derived when a picture is viewed, since what we term a 'pictorial' code is at a more abstract level, at which information from successive fixations has been integrated. The pictorial code may contain details of the lighting, grain, and flaws in a photograph, as well as capturing the static pose and expression portrayed. A match at the level of the pictorial code can be used to mediate yes/no recognition memory decisions in many laboratory studies of episodic memory for faces, where the same pictures of previously unfamiliar faces are used as targets at presentation and test (Bruce 1982; Hay and Young 1982).

Even if our experience of faces were confined entirely to pictures of them, a pictorial coding system could not alone subserve the task of recognizing faces *despite* changes in head angle, expression, lighting, age, or hairstyle. Yet we can readily cope with such transformations, at least across a certain range. Thus from a picture of a face, as well as from a live face, some yet more abstract visual representation must be established which can mediate recognition, despite the fact that in real life the same face will hardly ever form an identical image on successive occasions. Our ability to do this shows that we can derive *structural codes* for faces, which capture those aspects of the structure of a face essential to distinguish it from other faces.

The distinction between structural and pictorial codes is easily demonstrated in laboratory experiments. Bruce (1982), for instance, showed that episodic recognition memory for unfamiliar faces was impaired if views of faces were changed between presentation and test, with more impairment if both head angle and expression were changed than if only one change was made. More importantly, Bruce also showed that there was an effect of changing view even for episodic recognition of *familiar* faces, where recognition was significantly slower for changed compared with same views. Since structural codes must already be established for familiar faces, to allow their familiarity to be recognized, the effect of changing the view of familiar faces gives strong evidence for the additional retention of characteristics of a particular picture of a face in laboratory episodes. Further evidence for pictorial coding comes from the observation that subjects are better than chance at deciding whether a test picture is the same as, or different from, the picture of the person shown at presentation (Bruce 1977).

We regard the pictorial code as a general code formed for any visual pattern or picture. It is a record of a particular, static, visual event. Studies of face memory which use the same pictures at presentation and test may tell us as much about picture memory generally as about face recognition. Pictorial coding is probably of little importance in everyday life, where faces are seldom encountered under identical conditions. The importance of pictorial coding lies in the interpretation of much of the research literature on face recognition, and in the design of future experiments.

It is the more abstract, structural codes which mediate everyday recognition of familiar faces. What can be said about the nature of such codes? Many studies (reviewed extensively by H. Ellis 1975; Davies et al. 1981) have shown that some areas of the face provide more information about a person's identity than other areas, and have led to the widespread view that face recognition is dependent on the arrangement of features with respect to each other (configuration) as much as the features themselves (e.g. Matthews 1978; Sergent 1984). While it is difficult to make a very clear-cut distinction between features and 'configuration', an emphasis on configural aspects of face processing may explain how we are able to identify celebrities' faces both from low spatial frequencies (blurred pictures in which all fine detail of features has been removed, see Harmon 1973) and from caricatures, where individual features may be grossly distorted.

One important finding is that structural codes for familiar faces differ from those formed to unfamiliar faces. This is perhaps not too surprising as the formation of structural codes for unfamiliar faces will be limited by the conditions of initial exposure – whether the face is seen in one or many views, whether different expressions are seen, and so on. H. Ellis et al. (1979) have shown that the internal features of familiar faces are differentially important for recognition, while internal and external features are equally important in the recognition of unfamiliar faces. This shows that structural codes for familiar faces emphasize the more informative and less changeable (cf. hairstyles) regions of the face. The finding has been replicated with Japanese subjects and Japanese faces (Endo et al. 1984), and the differential salience of the internal features of familiar faces has also been demonstrated in a recognition task by

Young (1984) and in a matching task by Young *et al.* (1985*a*). Young *et al.* (1985*a*) were able to demonstrate that the finding only arises when people match structural rather than pictorial codes.

There is evidence, then, demonstrating differences between the structural coding of familiar and unfamiliar faces. We will argue later that these differences probably arise because stored structural codes for known faces have become elaborated through frequent exposure, and represented within recognition units which are not present for unfamiliar faces. The precise nature of the structural codes used to recognize familiar faces remains, however, unknown. In thinking what form they might take it is probably useful to consider the idea of different levels of visual representation used by Marr (1982).

Marr distinguished three representational stages beyond the retinal image. The *primal sketch* makes explicit the intensity changes present in the image and groups these into larger structures. The *viewer-centred representation* (which Marr called the 2½D sketch) describes the surface layout of a viewed scene relative to the viewer. Finally there is an *object-centred representation* (which Marr called the 3D model) allowing the recognition of objects from any viewpoint.

We assume that when a face is perceived, primal sketch and viewer-centred descriptions are constructed which describe, respectively, the layout of the image of the face, and the layout of the surfaces which gave rise to this image. What is less clear at the moment is what description, or set of descriptions, of the face is necessary before recognition can occur. Marr and Nishihara (1978) and Marr (1982) argued persuasively that the representational system used for recognizing objects must be based on an interlinked set of descriptions at different levels of detail. The description needed to recognize the shape of a human body cannot be sensitive enough to recognize the shape of a human hand simultaneously. Clearly different descriptions are needed, but these must be connected, so that recognizing a part of a body can facilitate recognition of the whole, and vice versa. In a similar way we argue that a familiar face is represented by an interconnected set of descriptions – some describing the configuration of the whole face, and some describing the details of particular features. Such a representational format could allow us to recognize a person's face both from distinctive features in isolation (e.g. Margaret Thatcher's eyes) and in situations where certain features are concealed (e.g. Margaret Thatcher wearing sunglasses). Therefore we propose that a familiar face is not represented by a single structural code, but by a set of codes. Can we say more about the nature of these descriptions?

While Marr and Nishihara (1978) and Marr (1982) argued that

object-centred descriptions should form the basis of recognition, the specific (axis-based) representation which they proposed is not suitable to cope with the fine discriminations needed in face recognition, where similar three-dimensional structures hold for all members of the class of stimuli (i.e. for all faces). Moreover, the range of transformations of viewpoint across which we need to recognize faces in everyday life is considerably smaller than the range of transformations involved in object recognition, so that it is conceivable that object-centred descriptions are less important to face recognition. People usually stand with their heads more or less upright, and indeed face recognition is particularly prone to disruption when faces are inverted (Yin 1969; Valentine and Bruce 1986). In addition, people will often look toward you, though recognition of profiles is of course quite possible. However, there are also transformations such as expression and hairstyle which apply only in the case of face (as opposed to object) recognition. While it seems unlikely that recognition of familiar faces is based on 'raw' viewer-centred descriptions, we think it possible that the face recognition system might make use of separate representations of discrete head angles, each in an expression-independent form. Our thinking here has been influenced by the work of Perrett and his colleagues (Perrett *et al.* 1982, 1984, 1985) who have argued on the basis of properties of single cells in monkey infero-temporal cortex that the sensitivity of these cells to facial identity arises at the level of specific views of the individual. Further experimental and computational investigations are clearly needed to clarify these ideas, but for the moment we propose that a familiar face is represented via an interlinked set of expression-independent structural codes for distinct head angles, with some codes reflecting the global configuration at each angle and others representing particular distinctive features.

A face can be recognized as familiar when there is a match between its encoded representation and a stored structural code. However, we are generally not satisfied that we know a face until more than a sense of familiarity is achieved. We need to know to whom a face belongs.

Some information about the face's owner can be obtained even for unfamiliar faces. We can judge age and sex reasonably accurately, we can give to unfamiliar faces attributions like honesty or intelligence, and we can think of known individuals that faces remind us of. We will refer to this type of information as a *visually derived semantic code.*

Visually derived semantic codes are readily formed, and can be useful in remembering unfamiliar faces (Klatzky *et al.* 1982a,b). Indeed attempts to apply the 'levels of processing' framework to face recognition can be described as attempts to influence the kind of visually derived semantic codes formed by subjects viewing unfamiliar faces (e.g. Bower and Karlin 1974; Patterson and Baddeley 1977). We contrast visually derived semantic codes with information in the form of an *identity-specific semantic code*. Identity-specific semantic codes might describe a familiar person's occupation, where he or she is usually encountered, who his or her friends are, and so on.

Not everyone makes this distinction between visually derived and identity-specific semantics. Rhodes (1985), for instance, suggests that there is a continuum of meaningfulness ranging from the once-viewed, unfamiliar face to the extremely familiar face of a friend or public figure, reflected in a continuum of strength of the semantic code. However, we prefer to think of qualitatively distinct kinds of associative coding, only some of which are available for the unfamiliar face.

One reason for this preference is the different relationships which hold between the physical form of a face and different aspects of its meaning. Judgements about sex, age, expression, and so on are dependent upon physical 'features' (used neutrally here) of the perceived face. But the identity-specific semantics are not dependent upon surface form except in the loosest of ways. Although pop stars are likely to look different from politicians, in general the shape of a person's nose, mouth, or hairstyle cannot tell you whether they are a politician, actor, or secret agent. Thus identity-specific semantics bear a largely arbitrary relationship with the physical form of the face, rather like the relationship which holds between the semantics of a word in relation to its spelling. Other aspects of facial meaning are dependent on surface form, and may thus be more analogous to the relationship between an object's structure and its meaning. For objects, appearance alone would be sufficient to determine membership of many categories (Rosch *et al.* 1976; Sperber *et al.* 1979). For example, it would be possible to discriminate animals from items of furniture even in the case of unfamiliar members of each category, whereas reliable discrimination of unfamiliar politicians from unfamiliar stockbrokers could not be achieved on a purely visual basis.

A further reason for our distinction between different kinds of semantic code is that, for a familiar face, it is access of identity-specific semantic codes which gives the feeling that the person has been successfully recognized. A familiar face that we are struggling to 'place' nevertheless has meaning in terms of expression, resemblance to other faces, age, sex, and so forth. But it is recovery of identity-specific semantic codes which resolves the 'feeling of knowing'.

In addition to the identity-specific semantic codes we also postulate a separate *name code*, holding the information that the person's name is

Colin Smith, or whatever. We all have acquaintances who we know well enough to talk to, and to talk about to others, but whose names we may never have heard. Thus it is clearly possible to have an identity-specific semantic code for a person with no name code.

Name codes as here conceived are output codes which allow a name to be generated. It is thus important that they are distinguished from input codes used in recognizing written or spoken names. [See Morton (1979, 1984) for detailed reasons for distinguishing input from output codes.]

It would, of course, be possible simply to view names as a particular type of identity-specific semantic code, with rather different properties from other aspects of a person's identity. Someone's name is an essentially arbitrary label, and is relatively unimportant for guiding social interaction compared with other aspects of their identity. This alone might explain why names are particularly hard to remember (see below). However, we feel there are good empirical grounds for distinguishing names as a separate class of code. The experience of knowing who a person is without being able to recall their name is common in both everyday (Reason and Mycielska 1982; Reason and Lucas 1984; Young et al. 1985b) and laboratory (Yarmey 1973; Williams and Hollan 1981; Read and Bruce 1982) studies of problems in recognizing people. Moreover, disorders of name retrieval (anomias) are also often seen in patients with cerebral injuries (Caramazza and Berndt 1978; Goodglass 1980; Ratcliff and Newcombe 1982). Anomic disorders affect face naming (Warrington and James 1967) and in some cases the anomia has even been reported as being restricted to proper names (McKenna and Warrington 1980).

For both familiar and unfamiliar faces we are not only able to derive information concerning the person's likely age, sex, and so on, but we are also able to interpret the meaning of their facial expressions. By analysing the relative shapes or postures of facial features we are able to categorize a person as looking 'happy', 'sad', 'angry', 'worried', and so on (Ekman and Oster 1979). We will refer to this as the formation of an *expression* code. More recently, it has also been established that observation of a person's lip movements while speaking can affect speech perception of adults (McGurk and MacDonald 1976; Campbell and Dodd 1980) and infants (Dodd 1979; Kuhl and Meltzoff 1982; Mackain et al. 1983). It seems that movements of the lips and tongue are used to derive a representation that shares at least some properties with representations derived from heard speech. We will describe the output of such analysis as a *facial speech code*.

At present, there is no evidence to suggest that expression codes (except, perhaps, for *characteristic* expressions) and facial speech codes are important in recognizing faces, which is our principal concern in this paper. Thus we largely restrict ourselves to briefly discussing how these codes might relate to the codes involved in recognition. As will be seen, we take the view that distinct functional components are involved in the generation of expression and facial speech codes. This is not surprising when thought is given to how heavily dependent they may be on analysis of *changes* in the shape and position of facial features across time.

Functional components in the human face processing system

We can account for several aspects of face processing simply in terms of the different codes we have already outlined. Recognition memory experiments can be interpreted in terms of the formation and recovery of codes of different kinds (Bruce 1982; Memon and Bruce 1985), with performance better if many codes at test match those formed at presentation. To a certain extent, everyday recognition of familiar faces can be described in terms of the sequential access of different codes. However, there is a distinction to be drawn between the *products* of a process, or set of processes, and the processes themselves. To take Marr's work again as an example, his primal sketch is the product of a number of procedures which analyse the intensity changes in an image, while his 2½D sketch results from the analysis of contours, depth, motion, and shading.

Having emphasized the products of facial processing, we now turn to offer a suggestion about some of the procedures which generate and access the codes we have described. We here focus on the interrelationship of a number of broad functional components, though we also offer some more tentative suggestions about the fine-grained structure of these components. Our model is compatible with existing evidence derived from normal people's errors, descriptions of clinical conditions, and experiments involving normal and clinical subject populations.

The model is shown in the form of a box diagram in Fig. 3.1, which is a convenient way of representing what we consider to be involved in face processing, and how the different components are thought to relate to each other. In constructing this box diagram, we have adhered to the convention of similar models used in the related areas of word and object recognition. A 'box' represents any processing module, or store, which plays a distinct functional role, and whose operation can be eliminated, isolated, or independently manipulated through experiment or as a consequence of brain damage. (The 'cognitive system', by

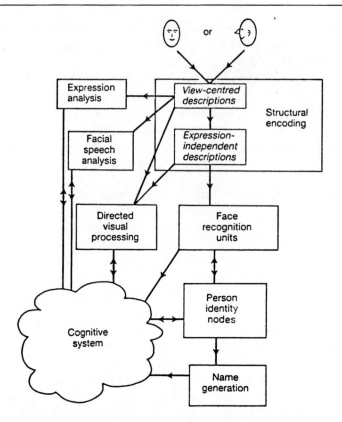

Fig. 3.1 Bruce and Young's (1986) model of face recognition.

convention, is somewhat cloudy.) Arrows between boxes variously denote the access of information, the conversion or recoding of information, and the activation of one component by another. We recognize that the differences in the statuses of the arrows and the boxes used in models of this type are problematic. However, the heuristic value of such models has been more than adequately demonstrated in other areas of research. In addition, use of a familiar format will allow us (see later) to draw explicit comparisons between the recognition of faces, objects, and words.

Structural encoding produces a set of descriptions of the presented face, which include view-centred descriptions as well as more abstract descriptions both of the global configuration and of features. View-centred descriptions provide information for the *analysis of facial speech*, and for the *analysis of expression*. The more abstract, expression-independent descriptions provide information for the *face recognition units*. Each of these three components (analysis of facial speech, analysis of expression, and face recognition units) serves a different kind of perceptual classification function. The visible movements of the mouth and tongue are categorized in the analysis of facial speech, while the configuration of various features leads to categorization of expression. Facial speech codes and expression codes result, respectively, from these categorization processes. Beyond this, however, we will not speculate about the details of how such categorization is achieved. It is the third perceptual classification system – the face recognition units – which holds most interest here. Each face recognition unit contains stored structural codes describing one of the faces known to a person. When a face is seen, the strength of the recognition unit's signal to the cognitive system will be at a level dependent on the degree of resemblance between its stored description and the input provided by structural encoding. The basic level of activation of the recognition unit can also, however, be raised (primed) indirectly from the person identity node when we are expecting to see a particular person, or directly raised because that face has been recently seen (primed by recent use).

The face recognition units can access identity-specific semantic codes held in a portion of the associative memory which we term *person identity nodes*. The idea is that there is one person identity node for each person known, and that this contains the identity-specific semantic codes that allow us to feel we have successfully identified the person concerned. *Names* are accessed only via the person identity nodes. The distinction between face recognition units and person identity nodes is made clear when we consider the different inputs which each will respond to. A face recognition unit will respond when any view of the appropriate person's *face* is seen, but will not respond at all to his or her voice or name. The person identity node, in contrast, can be accessed via the face, the voice, the name or even a particular piece of clothing (only access via the face is shown in Fig. 3.1). It is the point at which *person* recognition, as opposed to face recognition, is achieved. It is clear that face recognition can break down whilst person recognition via other visual cues remains intact, since prosopagnosics become adept at using other visual cues (Hécaen 1981). Moreover, disorders of visual and auditory recognition of people are dissociable, though they do co-occur in some cases (Assal *et al.* 1981; Van Lancker and Canter 1982).

The associative memory, to which the person identity nodes form an entry point, forms one component of the box we have labelled the 'cognitive system'. In Fig. 3.1 we have taken the person identity nodes 'outside' the rest of the cognitive system, in order to emphasize the logically distinct role that they play in person recognition. However, we must stress that person identity nodes are not seen as fundamentally different from other 'nodes' in semantic memory – they just serve a key role in the identification of people. The cognitive system includes or accesses all other associative and episodic information which falls outside the scope of our 'person identity nodes'. For example, occasionally people who had been asked to keep records of difficulties in person recognition (Young *et al.* 1985*b*) reported that they had experienced difficulty retrieving some 'identity-specific' semantic information even after a face had been successfully named, though there was never any doubt that the person had been successfully identified. Invariably, the information sought concerned some precise detail, such as some of the films that a named actor had appeared in. It seems to us that there is a distinction to be drawn between such peripheral details, which blend imperceptibly into general knowledge about the film industry, literature, and so on, and information which is essential to specify a person's identity. The latter we see as being accessed directly from the 'person identity nodes'; all other information lies within the rest of associative memory.

A further function of the cognitive system is to direct attention to other components of the system. Just as we have taken the person identity nodes 'outside' the cognitive system, so too have we taken out a component which we label 'directed visual processing', since selective attention to the visual form of a face may play an important role in certain tasks. As well as 'passively' recognizing expressions, identities, and so forth from faces, we also encode certain kinds of information selectively and strategically. For example, if we are going to meet a friend at the station, we will actively look out for faces sharing particular critical features with the friend. Alternatively, we may scrutinize a stranger's face to try to ensure we remember it in the future – carefully looking for distinctive features. We may make considerable use of such processes when asked to compare unfamiliar faces or to remember sets of unfamiliar faces in laboratory experiments. We thus contrast the processes used to compare and remember unfamiliar faces (via structural encoding and directed visual processing) from those which are used to identify familiar faces (via face recognition units). We assume that visual processing can be directed to any of the different representations produced by the structural encoding processes.

The analysis of facial speech, expression analysis, face recognition units, directed visual processes, and person identity nodes all provide information to the rest of the cognitive system, which is in turn able to influence all these functional components. The cognitive system is also responsible for various decision processes, which we describe below.

In describing the functional model, we have mentioned components which generate structural, expression, facial speech, identity-specific semantic, and name codes. The relationship between the functional model and the other two codes we described – pictorial and visually derived semantic – is not so clear-cut. Pictorial codes are by-products of some of the processes which we have housed within the 'structural encoding' component, but may also be enhanced by directed visual processing – for example when subjects in a face memory experiment pay attention to flaws in the photographs in an effort to remember them. We propose that the cognitive system is responsible for the generation of visually derived semantic codes, using information from the analysis of expression, structural encoding, directed visual processing, and the face recognition units. However, we note that future studies may allow the separation of 'visually derived semantic codes' into distinct types, produced by different routes. The classification of the sex and approximate age of a face, for example, may involve different processes from those involved in judging that a face appears honest, or resembles that of a particular relative (cf. H. Ellis 1986a, who suggests that categorization of age and sex occurs very early in the processing sequence).

This functional model is clearly related to those proposed by Hay and Young (1982) and H. Ellis (1986a), and we will not go through all of the evidence discussed in those papers. We will, however, look at some of the main lines of evidence in support of this type of model, and the principal unresolved issues that arise.

Consider first everyday difficulties in recognizing people that we all experience from time to time. These can be studied either by asking people to keep records of problems that they experience (Reason and Mycielska 1982; Reason and Lucas 1984; Young et al. 1985b), or by examining errors and difficulties that arise when people are asked to identify a set of faces (Yarmey 1973). These difficulties and errors can take a number of different forms, but two that are quite commonly reported are of particular interest here. The first involves knowing that a face is familiar, but being unable to recall any information about the person. In this case the face recognition unit has failed to access either the person identity node, and thereby the identity-specific semantic code or a name code for the person seen.

The second type of difficulty involves the well known 'tip-of-the-tongue' state in which we can identify the face's owner but cannot recall his or her name. This shows that identity-specific semantic codes can be accessed from structural codes without any need to proceed through an intervening name. Closer examination of tip-of-the-tongue states also suggests that the name code can only be accessed via an identity-specific semantic code, since one of the strategies that people use to guide their search for the name is to concentrate on the things that they know about the person (i.e. on the identity-specific semantic codes); they do not report trying to find the name by concentrating on the appearance of the face (which would be an appropriate strategy if name codes were accessed directly from structural codes).

Also of interest are types of error and difficulty that do *not* occur. In particular, if name codes could be accessed directly from the structural codes then it would be expected that there would be occasions on which people were able to put a name to a seen face but had no idea who the person was. In the studies of McWeeny (1985) and Young *et al.* (1985*b*), which between them involve a large corpus of errors and difficulties, this never happened. The only examples of such errors that we have been able to find are briefly mentioned in a report of cases of tuberculous meningitis by Williams and Smith (1954). One patient was able to name people from a photograph of the men on one of his former military training courses, but could give no indication as to when or where he had met them. However, such patients are in any case amnesic and often confused, so that it is difficult to know exactly how to interpret this error. In addition, the fact that all the pictured men share the same identity-specific semantics makes the task particularly tricky to interpret. We would wish to know whether such a patient was able to pick out his ex-colleagues from an array containing other familiar faces (e.g. politicians) before being persuaded of the lack of identity-specific semantic information.

Neuropsychological evidence is also consistent with our model (see also H. Ellis 1986*b*). The most relevant neuropsychological findings are the dissociation between disorders of familiar and unfamiliar face recognition, the dissociation between disorders of face recognition and analysis of facial expressions, and the dissociation between facial speech analysis and other aspects of facial processing.

The dissociation between disorders of familiar and unfamiliar face recognition was shown by Warrington and James (1967), who observed no correlation between these deficits for a group of patients with right cerebral hemisphere injuries. A number of findings consistent with the view of a dissociation between deficits of recognition of familiar and unfamiliar faces were subsequently obtained (see Benton 1980). The strongest evidence comes from the two single case studies of proso-pagnosic patients presented by Malone *et al.* (1982) who described one patient whose ability to match unfamiliar faces recovered whilst the severe recognition deficit for familiar faces persisted, and a second patient whose ability to recognize familiar people recovered whilst problems in matching unfamiliar faces persisted. Such dissociations would be expected from our model in which the recognition units and person identity nodes used in identifying faces that are already familiar form a route quite distinct from that used temporarily to store and recognize unfamiliar faces.

Clinical disorders of analysis of facial expressions also dissociate from disorders of face recognition. Although it is not unusual to find that prosopagnosic patients can neither identify faces nor understand their expressions (Bodamer 1947), it is now known that some patients are able to interpret facial expressions correctly despite an almost complete inability to identify familiar faces (Shuttleworth et al. 1982; Bruyer et al. 1983). The opposite dissociation is seen in the work of Kurucz and Feldmar (1979) and Kurucz et al. (1979) who observed that patients diagnosed as having 'chronic organic brain syndrome' found it difficult to interpret facial emotions yet were still able to identify photographs of American Presidents. For these patients there was no correlation between performance on recognizing affect and identity from the face. Similarly, Bornstein (1963) described patients for whom there was some degree of recovery of ability to identify familiar faces whilst they remained unable to interpret facial expressions.

Neuropsychological studies of patients with impairments that severely affect the identification of familiar faces or the interpretation of facial expressions thus show that such impairments can dissociate from each other. Other neuropsychological evidence pointing to the conclusion that analyses of facial identity and facial expression proceed independently can be found in studies of patients with unilateral cerebral lesions (Cicone et al. 1980; Etcoff 1984; Bowers et al. 1985) and in studies that have used brief lateral stimulus presentations to investigate cerebral hemisphere differences for face processing in normal subjects (Suberi and McKeever 1977; Ley and Bryden 1979; Hansch and Pirozzolo 1980; Strauss and Moscovitch 1981; Pizzamiglio et al. 1983). These studies have shown that although the right cerebral hemisphere makes an important contribution to analyses both of facial identity and expression, the right hemisphere superiorities for identity and expression seem to be independent of each other. A review is given by Etcoff (1986).

Finally Campbell et al. (1986) describe a dissociation between facial speech analysis and the recognition of faces and their expressions. The dissociation was observed in two patients. One was a severely proso-pagnosic lady who failed to recognize faces or even to say what sex they were, and failed to categorize expressions correctly. She could, however, judge what phonemes were mouthed in photographs of faces and was susceptible to the McGurk and MacDonald (1976) illusion, where a mismatch between heard and seen (mouthed) phonemes results in the perceiver 'blending' the two. The second was an alexic patient who had no difficulties in recognizing faces or expressions, but who was impaired at phonemic judgements to face stimuli and was not susceptible to the McGurk and MacDonald illusion.

Support for our model also derives from laboratory experiments. Such studies support the view that structural codes lead to the access of identity-specific semantic codes before name codes. Young *et al.* (1986*a*) showed that decisions requiring access only to structural codes (deciding whether or not a face was familiar) were more quickly made than semantic decisions that required access to an identity-specific code (deciding whether or not a face was a politician). Young *et al.* (1986*a*) also showed that the use of familiar stimuli drawn from a homogeneous semantic category could speed up semantic decisions without affecting familiarity decisions. Thus semantic decisions can be affected by factors that do not influence familiarity decisions, a finding consistent with the view that a structural code is sufficient to determine familiarity whereas an identity-specific semantic code must be accessed from the structural code in order to determine category membership.

Although semantic decisions are usually made more slowly than familiarity decisions, they are made much more quickly than responses that require faces to be named, even when the set of possible faces occurring in the experiment is quite small (Young *et al.* 1986*b*). Thus access to a name code from a face takes longer than access to an identity-specific semantic code, a finding consistent with the view that name codes are accessed via the person identity nodes.

There is good evidence, then, that names are accessed via the identity-specific semantic codes available at the person identity nodes. This is by no means a trivial conclusion. As we will see later, direct links between structural codes and name codes certainly do seem to exist for visually presented words (including people's names).

Experiments have also provided some support for the 'face recognition unit' component. Bruce and Valentine (1985) found that recognition of a face as familiar was facilitated by earlier presentation of the same picture, and to a lesser extent by a different picture of the same person's face, but was not facilitated by earlier presentation of the person's name. If it is thought that seen names can access the same identity-specific semantic codes as seen faces, then this priming effect must clearly be located in an earlier component than the person identity nodes. However, Bruce and Valentine also found that the amount of priming in the different picture condition was not correlated with the rated visual similarity between the two different pictures used. Hence, though re-presenting the same picture confers additional benefit (presumably via a match at the level of the pictorial code), the results of Bruce and Valentine's (1985) experiment are not consistent simply with a visual memory effect. The effect of a different picture can instead be explained as mediated by residual activation in a face recognition unit which responds when any view of a face is seen.

In our (Fig. 3.1) model, we have suggested, like Hay and Young (1982), that face recognition units can be primed by the presence of an appropriate context, and some evidence consistent with this has also been obtained (Bruce 1983; Bruce and Valentine 1986). Bruce and Valentine found that the familiarity decisions to faces were speeded if each face was preceded by a related face (e.g. Stan Laurel followed by Oliver Hardy), compared with preceding the face by a neutral or un-related familiar face. This facilitation occurred even when the interval between onset of prime and target faces was as little as 250 ms, which rules out an explanation in terms of conscious expectancy. Thus we have an apparent example of interpriming of face recognition units for people associated with each other.

The findings of Bruce (1979) also fit well with the model. Her tasks involved searching for familiar faces (politicians) in sequences of familiar and unfamiliar faces. She showed that search for the faces of four politicians could be affected by the presence of visually or semantically similar distractor faces. Distractors rated as visually similar to the targets and distractors who were other familiar politicians took longer to reject than visually dissimilar and non-politicians' faces respectively, and these effects of visual and semantic similarity were additive. This led Bruce to argue that in visual search tasks involving faces, visual and semantic analyses can proceed in parallel, with both providing information that can be employed in making a decision. Our (Fig. 3.1) model allows semantic analysis via the person identity nodes to occur in parallel with directed visual processing, which in Bruce's task would involve a careful, feature-by-feature visual analysis of each face for remembered features of the target faces. Both components could then send outputs to decision processes set up by the cognitive system.

In a task such as Bruce's (1979), in which *particular* targets are to be found, there is an obvious need for some kind of decision mechanism. Experiments on episodic memory for familiar and unfamiliar faces can also be analysed in this way (Bruce 1982). However, we feel that decision processes may have a more general role to play in everyday face recognition. Some kind of decision-making machinery seems necessary to account for a number of rather striking errors in Young *et al.*'s (1985*b*) diary study of difficulties and errors in everyday recognition. Such errors included, for instance, uncertainty as to whether or not a seen person was a particular friend, and thinking that a seen person must be someone unfamiliar who looked remarkably like the person is actually was!

Young *et al.* (1985*b*) also found that a common experience, which is in no sense an error, is to notice that someone bears a striking resemblance to someone else. This 'resemblance' experience also illustrates the importance of decision processes since it is most readily accounted for by proposing that the recognition unit fires and accesses the appropriate person identity node and via this the name code, but a decision has been taken that this firing is not to be seen as sufficient evidence that it is that person (often because the context is wrong for such an encounter). We do not think that it would be adequate to try to account for all such experiences simply by postulating a threshold of recognition unit firing, above which the level of firing would be taken to indicate recognition and below which it would be taken to indicate resemblance, since the experience can occur even to very strong resemblances (lookalikes).

The role of decision processes in recognition would clearly repay further investigation. In our (Fig. 3.1) model, such decisions are assigned to the cognitive system component, which can be seen as evaluating the strength of activity in various components of the system.

Comparisons between face, object and word recognition

Our theoretical framework allows us to draw parallels as well as highlighting differences between the recognition of faces and the recognition of other objects and words.

In broad outline, our model shares much in common with recent functional models of word and object recognition, such as those of Nelson *et al.* (1977), Seymour (1979) and Warren and Morton (1982). In particular, our account of face recognition shares the 'recognition unit' metaphor which has previously been used in theories of word recognition (logogens) and object recognition (pictogens) (Morton 1969, 1979; Seymour 1979). The advantage of this idea is that it sidesteps the difficult issue of the nature of the structural codes used to effect recognition, and concentrates attention on to questions about the interrelationship of different coding processes – questions that are more amenable to investigation using current experimental techniques.

Hay and Young (1982) first put forward the explicit suggestion that the same idea might help in understanding face recognition. They proposed that face recognition units mediate between the establishment of a facial representation and the access of 'person information' concerning a person's identity. The same recognition unit would respond when any view of a known individual's face was seen, and a different face recognition unit would be constructed for each known person's face. Much the same conception of face recognition units has been used in the present paper, except that we have followed the emphasis placed by Young *et al.* (1985*b*) and A. Ellis *et al.* (1987) on recognition units giving a graded signal of degree of resemblance to a familiar face, rather than acting as simple triggers. Thus we have modified the original analogy with the 'logogen' concept, used by Hay and Young (1982), and the recognition units described in this paper function more like the 'cognitive demons' in a pandemonium type of system, signalling degree of resemblance by the intensity with which they shout to a decision demon (see Lindsay and Norman 1977).

Several authors have proposed a similar sequence of accessing semantic and name codes from objects to that proposed here for faces (Potter and Faulconer 1975; Nelson and Reed 1976; Warren and Morton 1982). For recognition of visually presented words, however, existing evidence favours something more complex in which recognition units are able to access name codes directly as well as via the semantic representations (Warren and Morton 1982; A. Ellis 1984). These arrangements are shown in Fig. 3.2. The diagram of visual word recognition would, of course, be more complex still if it also included the possibility of using spelling–sound correspondences.

Reasons for postulating a more complex arrangement for visual word recognition include the descriptions by Schwartz *et al.* (1979, 1980) of a patient who was able to read single words that she could not classify on a semantic basis. Moreover, this patient could correctly name irregular words such as 'leopard', which showed that she did not rely on spelling–sound correspondences. This phenomenon of correct naming without understanding has not been observed in the case of disorders of object recognition (Ratcliff and Newcombe 1982) and, we have argued, it has yet to be clearly established for disorders of face recognition.

In some types of experiment, objects and words also show different properties that can be interpreted in terms of the arrangements shown in Fig. 3.2. Objects can, for instance, often be categorized semantically more quickly than they can be named, whereas words can be named more quickly than they can be categorized (Potter and Faulconer 1975). Faces share with objects this property of being semantically categorized more quickly than they can be named (Young *et al.* 1986*b*). Moreover by using categories of faces that do not differ visually from each other,

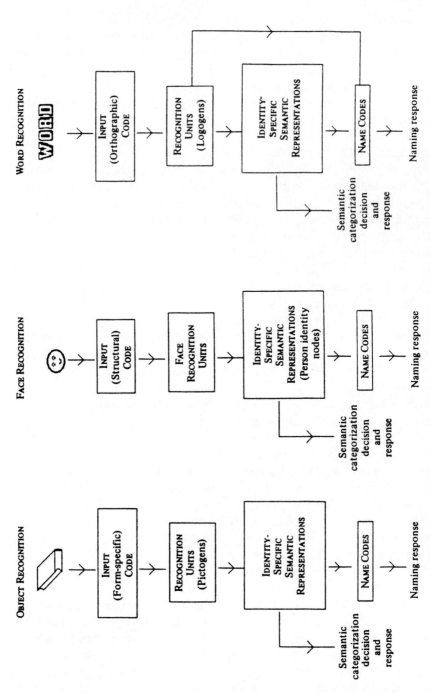

Fig. 3.2 A comparison of the routes involved in recognition and naming of objects, faces and words.

Young *et al.* (1986*b*) were able to show that the rapid categorization of faces is not entirely due to the use of visually derived semantic codes.

In interference experiments the presence of irrelevant printed words will interfere with naming depicted objects, whilst irrelevant pictures of objects do not interfere much with word naming (Rosinski *et al.* 1975; Glaser and Düngelhoff 1984). This interference effect reverses in categorization tasks, where irrelevant pictures of objects will interfere more with word categorization (Smith and Magee, 1980; Glaser and Düngelhoff, 1984). In comparisons of interference between faces and written names of familiar people, photographs of faces produce interference effects corresponding to those found for pictures of objects, and people's names produce interference effects corresponding to those found for words (Young *et al.* 1986*c*, 1987).

In semantic categorization, naming, and interference tasks, faces behave rather like objects whereas people's names and other types of word behave differently. If we shift to examining each system at a different (earlier) level, however, object, face, and word recognition findings are similar to one another. The results of Bruce and Valentine (1985, 1986), for example, supporting the hypothesis of face recognition units by identity priming and associative priming, are similar to findings that have pointed to object and word recognition units. Likewise Bruce (1981) was able to show that visual and semantic analyses involved in searches for words appeared to proceed in the same parallel fashion as those involved in searches for faces (Bruce 1979).

What these similarities and differences between object, face, and word recognition relate to is the way in which what might be considered analogous functional components in each system are arranged with respect to each other. However, when we turn to consider the *demands* placed on these functional components in each case it becomes clear that some of the apparent similarities may be only superficial.

In recognizing objects, for instance, we usually rely on analysis to a level at which objects belong to broad categories that maximize the functional and visual similarities of the objects within each category (dogs, tables, houses, etc.). Rosch (1978) and Rosch *et al.* (1976) refer to these as 'basic level' categories, and a considerable body of evidence has accumulated indicating their primacy in object recognition. However, although the members of these basic level categories may be more visually similar to each other than to members of other categories (i.e. different dogs are more like each other than they are like tables or houses), the task facing the perceptual system is none the less one of assigning different stimuli (different dogs, different tables, different houses) to the same category (dog, table, or house). For face recognition, the task is quite different. First, functional semantic categories such as actors, politicians, or television newsreaders are often not visually distinct. Indeed, we suspect that visually derived semantics may be much more important to object than to face processing. Second, with people's faces we want to identify the actual individuals. In Rosch's terms 'faces' are themselves a kind of basic level category; what we have to do is to discriminate *within* this rather homogeneous visual category to determine which of the already known exemplars a face actually is. In some cases the visual differences between different people might only be very slight.

When these requirements are taken into consideration it is clear that face recognition units are really doing a rather different job from pictogens, and the clinical observations of object agnosia without prosopagnosia and of prosopagnosia without object agnosia become less surprising (see also Hécaen 1981; Damasio *et al.* 1982; Blanc-Garin 1984; Jeeves 1984). In fact, the requirements for face recognition, of discrimination within a class of rather homogeneous stimuli on the basis of any difference in individual features or their arrangement, are more reminiscent of the requirements of word than of object recognition units. With written words, however, the range of potential distinguishing features is limited to the set of letters in the language and the crucial spatial arrangement is in the form of a sequence. Word recognition disorders can, of course, dissociate perfectly from both object agnosia and prosopagnosia.

In making our comparisons between face, word, and object recognition we have been touching on the question of whether specialized mechanisms are involved in face processing. Hay and Young (1982) suggested that this question can in turn be broken down into that of whether some components of the face-processing system are qualitatively different from those involved in the processing of other visual stimuli (the question of face uniqueness) or whether some of the components are used only for faces despite similarities to equivalent components used in processing other visual stimuli (the question of face specificity). The present paper is not directly addressed to such issues. However, the clinical dissociations mentioned clearly suggest that there are at least some face-specific components. Moreover, the preceding discussion of the requirements of object, face, and word recognition, together with our earlier comments on the particular demands made by expression codes and facial speech codes, should make it clear why we are inclined to think that some of the components are unique to faces (see also Young 1986 for evidence concerning innate specification of some components).

Unresolved issues

A reasonably detailed functional model is clearly valuable in accounting for existing findings and clarifying the issues that need to be addressed in future work. In this final section we draw attention to these issues. In doing this we hope to stimulate the research that will lead to an improvement of the model. Three main issues will be addressed. These involve the breadth of specification of functional components, the question of whether faces must first be classified *as faces*, and the roles of contextual information.

Breadth of specification of functional components

Not all of the components have been specified with the same degree of precision. Face recognition units are, for instance, more narrowly and precisely specified than structural encoding, which is in turn more narrowly and precisely specified than the cognitive system. Our view is that as more evidence is gathered this will lead to the division of some of the components shown in Fig. 3.1.

For example, while we have offered suggestions about the nature of structural codes for familiar face recognition, these ideas will become further refined through experimentation. A computational approach to face recognition is also likely to prove fruitful in this respect, and we note the possibility that it may prove feasible to account for the properties of face recognition units in terms of distributed representations (e.g. McClelland and Rumelhart 1985). In addition, careful investigation of the neuropsychological symptom of 'metamorphopsia', in which faces appear distorted to certain patients (Hécaen and Angelergues 1962; Whiteley and Warrington 1977; Hécaen 1981), may give us further clues about the nature of visual representations used in face recognition. Further experimental, computational, and neuropsychological investigations will also allow us to specify more details of the analyses of expressions and facial speech.

The broadest component in our (Fig. 3.1) model at present is the cognitive system. This serves to catch all those aspects of processing not reflected in other components of our model. Such a component is a common one in other functional models of human memory. For example, the cognitive system in Morton's (1969, 1979) logogen model of word recognition is directly analogous to the same component in our own model, and Baddeley and Hitch (1974) include a similar 'catch-all' component in the 'central executive' of their working memory model. In the future we aim to specify in more detail the finer structure of this component. As described here, the cognitive system has at least three distinct functions. The first of these functions is to house the associative memory, and the second to take decisions on the basis of information received from other components of the system. The third is to direct attention to various other components of the system, as in the directed visual processing which plays an important role in perception of unfamiliar faces. The details of each of these aspects of the cognitive system, and their interactions, should be made clearer through further experimental studies, and simulation could provide a further way of exploring this.

Is the input first classified as a face?

When we look at a face, we know that we are seeing a face rather than some other object. As we discussed above, it may be the *object* classification system which allows us to make this basic level judgement, and it is possible that such a judgement *precedes* further analysis of who the face belongs to (H. Ellis 1981, 1983). Prosopagnosic patients can, for instance, recognize faces as such even though they do not know whose face they are seeing (Bodamer 1947; Bruyer *et al.* 1983; Jeeves 1984).

H. Ellis (1981, 1983) argued that without such a classification faces could not be treated differently from any other visually presented stimulus. However, we have not included this 'classification as a face' stage as an explicit component in our model for three reasons. First, it prejudges the issue of whether faces actually do require a special type of analysis. We do not want to do this at present, even though we (like Ellis) now strongly suspect that specialized processes are involved. Second, even if face-specific analyses do occur, it is not clear to us that an explicit face 'switch' is needed. Appropriate analysers might just pick up the input to which they are attuned, thereby classifying the input implicitly. Third, we are uncertain about the level of visual information processing at which the decision to classify an input as a face is taken (see Young *et al.* 1985c). It could be that classification as a face is an essential first step that must be taken before processing is directed to other components in our system, or it might be that classification as a face is achieved on the basis of a very general global structural description simultaneous with the classification of particular faces on the basis of more detailed local information. Future studies examining which disorders of structural encoding are or are not specific to faces should help to answer such questions. In the meantime we assume that if classification of the input as a face is necessary it occurs as part of the structural encoding component.

The roles of contextual information

The semantic priming experiments of Bruce (1983) and Bruce and Valentine (1986) illustrate the way in which one kind of context can affect the recognition of familiar faces. A face is easier to recognize if accompanied by an appropriate partner (e.g. Stan Laurel with Oliver Hardy). This effect can be compared with that of facilitation of word recognition by appropriate accompanying words in lexical decision (Meyer and Schvaneveldt 1971) or facilitation of object naming by the presence of semantically related objects (Sperber *et al.* 1979).

However, contextual information might also include the place where a face is usually seen. We might expect to find the recognition of, say, Margaret Thatcher, to be more difficult if she were shown against a picture of a launderette than if she were shown along with a picture of the Houses of Parliament, although the difficulty of producing a range of distinctive visual contexts for celebrities makes it unlikely that such an experiment will be conducted. However, we note that Palmer (1975) found that appropriate scenic contexts (e.g. a kitchen) facilitated the recognition of objects appropriate to that context (e.g. loaf of bread).

The kinds of contextual effects we have described above could be explained in terms of the 'priming' of face recognition units for familiar people. However, when we turn to the episodic recognition of unfamiliar faces, for whom we assume face recognition units have not been formed, context effects also abound. Episodic recognition of unfamiliar faces is facilitated if faces are retested along with the same partners that accompanied them at presentation (Winograd and Rivers-Bulkeley 1977), or if they are retested against the same distinctive background context with which they were originally presented (Beales and Parkin 1984; Memon and Bruce 1983). There have even been claims (e.g. Wagstaff 1982) that performance on a photo-lineup task is improved if this is conducted in the same room in which a staged incident occurred.

Such contextual effects both in the recognition of familiar faces and in episodic recognition of unfamiliar faces scarcely seem surprising when we consider the relationship between identity-specific semantic codes and context. Even for familiar celebrities, part of their meaning is where they live, who their associates are, and so on. Thus we would expect the person identity node for Stan Laurel to include a strong link to that for Oliver Hardy, and we would expect the person identity node for Margaret Thatcher to be associated with '10 Downing St', however temporarily.

For less familiar, and less 'public' figures, their identity is even more bound up in the contexts with which they are associated. In Young *et al.*'s (1985*b*) diary study, for instance, a commonly reported way of trying to resolve the irritating 'I know that face' feeling was to try to think where the person was usually encountered. For many people that we know, their identity goes together with where we know them from, and the role we ourselves play when we see them. This is particularly clearly seen in Young *et al.*'s (1985*b*) example of a person who thought for a long time that one of her somewhat casual acquaintances was two different people because she met him in two different places. We have yet to examine closely the relationship between categorical aspects of a person's identity (e.g. their occupation) and aspects more closely tied to time or place of occurrence.

Our ability to link faces to a context may explain why faces are often remarkably resistant to forgetting in laboratory experiments, despite all the 'real-world' faces, which include newspaper and television photographs, seen between presentation and test. Yet striking interference can be obtained retroactively from a later set of faces (Deffenbacher *et al.* 1981) or from distractors within a test series (Laughery *et al.* 1974). Thus, much more interference seems to be obtained from faces seen in the same laboratory context than from those seen in a different context.

We suggested above that certain of these contextual effects could be seen as resulting from the priming of face recognition units via the person identity nodes, but noted that this explanation was not satisfactory for the effects in episodic memory for unfamiliar faces. The most common explanation offered in the literature is some variant of Tulving's encoding specificity theory (Tulving and Thomson, 1973). Recognition will be easier the greater the overlap between retrieval cues at test and features of the encoded trace. Although it is difficult to translate the terminology of encoding specificity into that of our own framework, which is not designed specifically to account for episodic memory, Memon and Bruce (1985) argue that by considering the different codes derived from faces, we can provide a better account of contextual effects in face recognition than that given by theories borrowed directly from the verbal memory literature.

One recent theory attempts, like us, to explain people's difficulties in remembering names, and certain contextual effects in remembering. The headed records framework (Morton *et al.* 1985) copes well with such phenomena which are difficult for traditional associative network conceptions of long-term memory. Headed records is an 'episodic' theory, in which information about a person's identity would be discovered by accessing the appropriate record via the access key contained in the heading. Headings themselves cannot be retrieved, and Morton *et al.* explain the particular difficulty in recalling names by suggesting that these often form the headings to records containing details of person information. Morton *et al.*'s model, unlike our own, does not address the relationship between perceptual classification and access of semantic information, and would have difficulty accommodating some of the clinical evidence we have discussed.

Overview and conclusions

We have presented a functional framework for face recognition, in which a number of components are distinguished. Different processes are involved in the generation and storage of different kinds of information, or 'codes'. We have described seven codes that can be distinguished in face processing, which we label pictorial, structural, identity-specific semantic, visually derived semantic, name, expression, and facial speech codes. The last two of these are not directly involved in face *recognition*, though they are clearly important for other aspects of face *perception*, and pictorial codes are probably only of major importance in laboratory experiments of a certain kind. Everyday face recognition is seen as involving use of structural codes to access identity-specific semantic information and names, where available, in that order.

Our functional model is compatible with existing evidence drawn from a wide range of sources, including laboratory experiments, studies of everyday errors, and studies of patients with different types of cerebral injury. For many of the components, these different areas provide converging evidence for the organization we propose. For some components, evidence is currently available from only one source (e.g. the proposal that facial speech analysis is independent of expression analysis and person identification rests entirely on clinical evidence at present).

The fact that the model can encompass such diverse types of evidence is one example of its usefulness. Another example comes from the way such a model can be used to clarify the similarities and differences between processes responsible for object, word, and face recognition. However, the true measure of the value of an explicit model of this type lies in its capacity to stimulate the research that will lead to further improvements in our understanding. In this respect the model presented here makes several obvious predictions concerning the results of conventional laboratory experiments, and the types of disorder that should be found in brain-injured patients. In addition, we have devoted some space to spelling out areas which we see as important for future research.

As we said in our introduction, the account we have presented is a synthesis and extension of several current models of face recognition. Together with other authors we feel that this kind of approach will prove fruitful for understanding how we identify people from their faces, and why face recognition sometimes fails.

References

Assal, G., Aubert, C., and Buttet, J. (1981). Asymétrie cérébrale et reconnaissance de la voix. *Revue Neurologique*, **137**, 255–68.

Baddeley, A. D. and Hitch, G. J. (1974). Working memory. In *The psychology of learning and motivation*, vol. 8, (ed. G. Bower). Academic Press, New York.

Baron, R. J. (1979). A bibliography on face recognition. *The SISTM Quarterly Incorporating The Brain Theory Newsletter*, **II**, 27–36.

Baron, R. J. (1981). Mechanisms of human facial recognition. *International Journal of Man-Machine Studies*, **15**, 137–78.

Beales, S. A. and Parkin, A. J. (1984). Context and facial memory: the influence of different processing strategies. *Human Learning*, **3**, 257–64.

Benton, A. L. (1980). The neuropsychology of facial recognition. *American Psychologist*, **35**, 176–86.

Blanc-Garin, J. (1984). Perception des visages et reconnaissance de la physionomie dans l'agnosie des visages. *L'Année Psychologique*, **84**, 573–98.

Bodamer, J. (1947). Die Prosop-Agnosie. *Archiv für Psychiatrie und Nervenkrankheiten*, **179**, 6–53.

Bornstein, B. (1963). Prosopagnosia. In *Problems of dynamic neurology*, (ed. L. Halpern), pp. 283–318. Hadassah Medical School, Jerusalem.

Bower, G. H. and Karlin, M. B. (1974). Depth of processing pictures of faces and recognition memory. *Journal of Experimental Psychology*, **103**, 751–7.

Bowers, D., Bauer, R. M., Coslett, H. B., and Heilman, K. M. (1985). Processing of faces by patients with unilateral hemisphere lesions: 1. Dissociation between judgements of facial affect and facial identity. *Brain and Cognition*, **4**, 258–72.

Bruce, V. (1977). Processing and remembering pictorial information. PhD thesis, Cambridge University.

Bruce, V. (1979). Searching for politicians: an information-processing approach to face recognition. *Quarterly Journal of Experimental Psychology*, **31**, 373–95.

Bruce, V. (1981). Visual and semantic effects in a serial word classification task. *Current Psychological Research*, **1**, 153–62.

Bruce, V. (1982). Changing faces: visual and non-visual coding processes in face recognition. *British Journal of Psychology*, **73**, 105–16.

Bruce, V. (1983). Recognizing faces. *Philosophical Transactions of The Royal Society of London*, **B302**, 423–36.

Bruce, V. and Valentine, T. (1985). Identity priming in the recognition of familiar faces. *British Journal of Psychology*, **76**, 373–83.

Bruce, V. and Valentine, T. (1986). Semantic priming of familiar faces. *Quarterly Journal of Experimental Psychology*, **38A**, 125–50.

Bruyer, R., Laterre, C., Seron, X., Feyereisen, P., Strypstein, E., Pierrard, E., and Rectem, D. (1983). A case of prosopagnosia with some preserved covert remembrance of familiar faces. *Brain and Cognition*, **2**, 257–84.

Campbell, R. and Dodd, B. (1980). Hearing by eye. *Quarterly Journal of Experimental Psychology*, **32**, 85–99.

Campbell, R., Landis, T., and Regard, M. (1986). Face recognition and lipreading: a neurological dissociation. *Brain*, **109**, 509–21.

Caramazza, A. and Berndt, R. S. (1978). Semantic and syntactic processes in aphasia: a review of the literature. *Psychological Bulletin*, **85**, 898–918.

Cicone, M., Wapner, W., and Gardner, H. (1980). Sensitivity to emotional expressions and situations in organic patients. *Cortex*, **16**, 145–58.

Damasio, A. R., Damasio, H., and Van Hoesen, G. W. (1982). Prosopagnosia: anatomic basis and behavioral mechanisms. *Neurology*, **32**, 331–41.

Davies, G., Ellis, H., and Shepherd, J. (1981). *Perceiving and remembering faces*. Academic Press, London.

Deffenbacher, K. A., Carr, T. H., and Leu, J. R. (1981). Memory for words, pictures and faces: retroactive interference, forgetting and reminiscence. *Journal of Experimental Psychology: Human Learning & Memory*, **7**, 299–304.

Dodd, B. (1979). Lipreading in infants: attention to speech presented in- and out-of-synchrony. *Cognitive Psychology*, **11**, 478–84.

Ekman, P. and Oster, H. (1979). Facial expressions of emotion. *Annual Review of Psychology*, **30**, 527–54.

Ellis, A. W. (1984). *Reading, writing and dyslexia: a cognitive analysis*. Erlbaum, London.

Ellis, A. W., Young, A. W., and Hay, D. C. (1987). Modelling the recognition of faces and words. In *Modelling cognition*, (ed. P. E. Morris), pp. 269–97. Wiley, London.

Ellis, H. D. (1975). Recognizing faces. *British Journal of Psychology*, **66**, 409–26.

Ellis, H. D. (1981). Theoretical aspects of face recognition. In *Perceiving and remembering faces*, (ed. G. Davies *et al.*). Academic Press, London.

Ellis, H. D. (1983). The role of the right hemisphere in face perception. In *Functions of the right cerebral hemisphere*, (ed. A. W. Young), pp. 33–64. Academic Press, London.

Ellis, H. D. (1986a). Processes underlying face recognition. In *The neuropsychology of face perception and facial expression*, (ed. R. Bruyer), pp. 1–27. Erlbaum, Hillsdale, NJ.

Ellis, H. D. (1986b). Disorders of face recognition. In *Neurology: Proceedings of the 13th World Congress of Neurology*, (ed. K. Poeck, H. J. Freund, and H. Gänshirt), pp. 179–87. Springer, Berlin.

Ellis, H. D., Shepherd, J. W., and Davies, G. M. (1979). Identification of familiar and unfamiliar faces from internal and external features: Some implications for theories of face recognition. *Perception*, **8**, 431–9.

Endo, M., Takahashi, K., and Maruyama, K. (1984). Effects of observer's attitude on the familiarity of faces: using the difference in cue value between central and peripheral facial elements as an index of familiarity. *Tohoku Psychologica Folia*, **43**, 23–34.

Etcoff, N. L. (1984). Selective attention to facial identity and facial emotion. *Neuropsychologia*, **22**, 281–95.

Etcoff, N. L. (1986). The neuropsychology of emotional expression. In *Advances in clinical neuropsychology*, Vol. 3, (ed. G. Goldstein and R. E. Tarter), pp. 127–79. Plenum, New York.

Glaser, W. R. and Düngelhoff, F. J. (1984). The time course of picture-word interference. *Journal of Experimental Psychology: Human Perception & Performance*, **10**, 640–54.

Goodglass, H. (1980). Disorders of naming following brain injury. *American Scientist*, **68**, 647–55.

Hansch, E. C. and Pirozzolo, F. J. (1980). Task relevant effects on the assessment of cerebral specialisation for facial emotion. *Brain and Language*, **10**, 51–9.

Harmon, L. D. (1973). The recognition of faces. *Scientific American*, **229**, 70–82.

Hay, D. C. and Young, A. W. (1982). The human face. In *Normality and pathology in cognitive functions*, (ed. A. W. Ellis), pp. 173–202. Academic Press, London.

Hécaen, H. (1981). The neuropsychology of face recognition. In *Perceiving and remembering faces*, (ed. G. Davies, H. Ellis and J. Shepherd), pp. 39–54. Academic Press, London.

Hécaen, H. and Angelergues, R. (1962). Agnosia for faces (prosopagnosia). *Archives of Neurology*, **7**, 92–100.

Jeeves, M. A. (1984). The historical roots and recurring issues of neurobiological studies of face perception. *Human Neurobiology*, **3**, 191–6.

Klatzky, R. L., Martin, G. L., and Kane, R. A. (1982*a*). Influences of social-category activation on processing of visual information. *Social Cognition*, **1**, 95–109.

Klatzky, R. L., Martin, G. L., and Kane, R. A. (1982*b*). Semantic interpretation effects on memory for faces. *Memory and Cognition*, **10**, 195–206.

Kuhl, P. K. and Meltzoff, A. N. (1982). The bimodal perception of speech in infancy. *Science*, **218**, 1138–41.

Kurucz, J. and Feldmar, G. (1979). Prosopo-affective agnosia as a symptom of cerebral organic disease. *Journal of the American Geriatrics Society*, **27**, 225–30.

Kurucz, J., Feldmar, G., and Werner, W. (1979). Prosopo-affective agnosia associated with chronic organic brain syndrome. *Journal of the American Geriatrics Society*, **27**, 91–5.

Laughery, K. R., Fessler, P. K., Lenorovitz, D. R., and Yoblick, D. A. (1974). Time delay and similarity effects in facial recognition. *Journal of Applied Psychology*, **59**, 490–6.

Ley, R. G. and Bryden, M. P. (1979). Hemispheric differences in processing emotions and faces. *Brain and Language*, **7**, 127–38.

Lindsay, P. H. and Norman, D. A. (1977). *Human information processing*. Academic Press, New York.

McClelland, J. L. and Rumelhart, D. E. (1985). Distributed memory and the representation of general and specific information. *Journal of Experimental Psychology: General*, **114**, 159–88.

McGurk, H. and MacDonald, J. (1976). Hearing lips and seeing voices. *Nature*, **264**, 746–8.

Mackain, K. S., Studdert-Kennedy, M., Spieker, S., and Stern, D. (1983). Infant intermodal speech perception is a left hemisphere function. *Science*, **219**, 1347–9.

McKenna, P. and Warrington, E. K. (1980). Testing for nominal dysphasia. *Journal of Neurology, Neurosurgery, and Psychiatry*, **43**, 781–8.

McWeeny, K. H. (1985). Face processing: an investigation of everyday problems in learning and recognising faces and names. MPhil thesis, Lancaster University.

Malone, D. R., Morris, H. H., Kay, M. C., and Levin, H. S. (1982). Prosopagnosia: a double dissociation between the recognition of familiar and unfamiliar faces. *Journal of Neurology, Neurosurgery, and Psychiatry*, **45**, 820–2.

Marr, D. (1982). *Vision*. Freeman, San Francisco.

Marr, D. and Nishihara, K. (1978). Representation and recognition of the spatial organisation of three-dimensional shapes. *Proceedings of the Royal Society of London*, **B200**, 269–94.

Matthews, M. L. (1978). Discrimination of identikit constructions of faces: evidence for a dual processing strategy. *Perception and Psychophysics*, **23**, 153–61.

Memon, A. and Bruce, V. (1983). The effects of encoding strategy and context change on face recognition. *Human Learning*, **2**, 313–26.

Memon, A. and Bruce, V. (1985). Context effects in episodic studies of verbal and facial memory. *Current Psychological Research and Reviews*, **4**, 349–69.

Meyer, D. E. and Schvaneveldt, R. W. (1971). Facilitation in recognising pairs of words: evidence of a dependence between retrieval operations. *Journal of Experimental Psychology*, **90**, 227–34.

Morton, J. (1969). Interaction of information in word recognition. *Psychological Review*, **76**, 165–78.

Morton, J. (1979). Facilitation in word recognition: experiments causing change in the logogen model. In *Processing of visible language*, (ed. P. A. Kolers, M. Wrolstad, and H. Bouma), pp. 259–68. Plenum, New York.

Morton, J. (1984). Naming. In *Dysphasia*, (ed. S. Newman and R. Epstein), pp. 217–30. Churchill Livingstone, Edinburgh.

Morton, J., Hammersley, R. H., and Bekerian, D. A. (1985). Headed records: a model for memory and its failures. *Cognition*, **20**, 1–25.

Nelson, D. L. and Reed, V. S. (1976). On the nature of pictorial encoding: a levels of processing analysis. *Journal of Experimental Psychology: Human Learning & Memory*, **2**, 49–57.

Nelson, D. L., Reed, V. S., and McEvoy, C. L. (1977). Learning to order pictures and words: a model of sensory and semantic encoding. *Journal of Experimental Psychology: Human Learning & Memory*, 3, 485–97.

Palmer, S. E. (1975). The effects of contextual scenes on the identification of objects. *Memory and Cognition*, 3, 519–26.

Patterson, K. E. and Baddeley, A. D. (1977). When face recognition fails. *Journal of Experimental Psychology: Human Learning & Memory*, 3, 406–17.

Perrett, D. I., Rolls, E. T., and Caan, W. (1982). Visual neurones responsive to faces in the monkey temporal cortex. *Experimental Brain Research*, 47, 329–42.

Perrett, D. I., Smith, P. A. J., Potter, D. D., Mistlin, A. J., Head, A. S., Milner, A. D., and Jeeves, M. A. (1984). Neurones responsive to faces in the temporal cortex: studies of functional organisation, sensitivity to identity and relation to perception. *Human Neurobiology*, 3, 197–208.

Perrett, D. I., Smith, P. A. J., Potter, D. D., Mistlin, A. J., Head, A. S., Milner, A. D., and Jeeves, M. A. (1985). Visual cells in the temporal cortex sensitive to face view and gaze direction. *Proceedings of the Royal Society of London*, B223, 293–317.

Pizzamiglio, L., Zoccolotti, P., Mammucari, A., and Cesaroni, R. (1983). The independence of facial identity and facial expression recognition mechanisms: relationship to sex and cognitive style. *Brain and Cognition*, 2, 176–88.

Potter, M. C. and Faulconer, B. A. (1975). Time to understand pictures and words. *Nature*, 253, 437–8.

Ratcliff, G. and Newcombe, F. (1982). Object recognition: some deductions from the clinical evidence. In *Normality and pathology in cognitive functions*, (ed. A. W. Ellis), pp. 147–71. Academic Press, London.

Read, D. J. and Bruce, D. (1982). Longitudinal tracking of difficult memory retrievals. *Cognitive Psychology*, 14, 280–300.

Reason, J. T. and Lucas, D. (1984). Using cognitive diaries to investigate naturally occurring memory blocks. In *Everyday memory, actions and absentmindedness*, (ed. J. Harris and P. E. Morris), pp. 53–70. Academic Press, London.

Reason, J. T. and Mycielska, K. (1982). *Absent-minded? The psychology of mental lapses and everyday errors*. Prentice-Hall, Englewood Cliffs, NJ.

Rhodes, G. (1985). Lateralized processes in face recognition. *British Journal of Psychology*, 76, 249–71.

Rosch, E. (1978). Principles of categorization. In *Cognition and categorization*, (ed. E. Rosch and B. Lloyd), pp. 27–48. Erlbaum, Hillsdale, NJ.

Rosch, E., Mervis, C. B., Gray, W. D., Johnson, D. M., and Boyes-Braem, P. 19976). Basic objects in natural categories. *Cognitive Psychology*, 8, 382–439.

Rosinski, R. R., Golinkoff, R. M., and Kukish, K. S. (1975). Automatic semantic processing in a picture-word interference task. *Child Development*, 46, 247–53.

Schwartz, M. F., Marin, O. S. M. and Saffran, E. M. (1979). Dissociations of language function in dementia: a case study. *Brain and Language*, 7, 277–306.

Schwartz, M. F., Saffran, E. M., and Marin, O. S. M. (1980). Fractionating the reading process in dementia: Evidence for word-specific print-to-sound associations. In *Deep dyslexia*, (ed. M. Coltheart, K. Patterson, and J. C. Marshall). Routledge & Kegan Paul, London.

Sergent, J. (1984). An investigation into component and configural processes underlying face perception. *British Journal of Psychology*, **75**, 221–42.

Seymour, P. H. K. (1979). *Human visual cognition*. Collier Macmillan, London.

Shuttleworth, E. C. Jr, Syring, V., and Allen, N. (1982). Further observations on the nature of prosopagnosia. *Brain and Cognition*, **1**, 307–22.

Smith, M. C. and Magee, L. E. (1980). Tracing the time course of picture-word processing. *Journal of Experimental Psychology: General*, **109**, 373–92.

Sperber, R. D., McCauley, C., Ragain, R., and Weil, C. (1979). Semantic priming effects on picture and word processing. *Memory and Cognition*, **7**, 339–45.

Strauss, E. and Moscovitch, M. (1981). Perception of facial expressions. *Brain and Language*, **13**, 308–32.

Suberi, M. and McKeever, W. F. (1977). Differential right hemispheric memory storage of emotional and non-emotional faces. *Neuropsychologia*, **15**, 757–68.

Tulving, E. and Thomson, D. M. (1973). Encoding specificity and retrieval processes in episodic memory. *Psychological Review*, **80**, 352–73.

Valentine, T. and Bruce, V. (1986). The effect of race, inversion and encoding activity upon face recognition. *Acta Psychologica*, **61**, 259–73.

Van Lancker, D. R. and Canter, G. J. (1982). Impairment of voice and face recognition in patients with hemispheric damage. *Brain and Cognition*, **1**, 185–95.

Wagstaff, G. F. (1982). Context effects in eyewitness reports. Paper presented at the Law and Psychology Conference, Swansea, Wales.

Warren, C. and Morton, J. (1982). The effects of priming on picture recognition. *British Journal of Psychology*, **73**, 117–29.

Warrington, E. K. and James, M. (1976). An experimental investigation of facial recognition in patients with unilateral cerebral lesions. *Cortex*, **3**, 317–26.

Whiteley, A. M. and Warrington, E. K. (1977). Prosopagnosia: a clinical psychological and anatomical study of three patients. *Journal of Neurology, Neurosurgery, and Psychiatry*, **40**, 395–403.

Williams, M. D. and Hollan, J. D. (1981). The process of retrieval from very long-term memory. *Cognitive Science*, **5**, 87–119.

Williams, M. and Smith, H. V. (1954). Mental disturbances in tuberculous meningitis. *Journal of Neurology, Neurosurgery, and Psychiatry*, **17**, 173–82.

Winograd, E. and Rivers-Bulkeley, N. J. (1977). Effects of changing context on remembering faces. *Journal of Experimental Psychology: Human Learning & Memory*, **3**, 397–405.

Yarmey, A. D. (1973). I recognise your face but I can't remember your name: further evidence on the tip-of-the-tongue phenomenon. *Memory and Cognition*, **1**, 287–90.

Yin, R. K. (1969). Looking at upside-down faces. *Journal of Experimental Psychology*, **81**, 141–5.

Young, A. W. (1984). Right cerebral hemisphere superiority for recognizing the internal and external features of famous faces. *British Journal of Psychology*, **75**, 161–9.

Young, A. W. (1986). Subject characteristics in lateral differences for face processing by normals: age. In *The neuropsychology of face perception and facial expression*, (ed. R. Bruyer), pp. 167–200. Erlbaum, Hillsdale, NJ.

Young, A. W., Hay, D. C., McWeeny, K. H., Flude, B. M., and Ellis, A. W. (1985a). Matching familiar and unfamiliar faces on internal and external features. *Perception*, **14**, 737–46.

Young, A. W., Hay, D. C., and Ellis, A. W. (1985b). The faces that launched a thousand slips: everyday difficulties and errors in recognizing people. *British Journal of Psychology*, **76**, 495–523.

Young, A. W., Hay, D. C., and McWeeny, K. H. (1985c). Right cerebral hemisphere superiority for constructing facial representations. *Neuropsychologia*, **23**, 195–202.

Young, A. W., McWeeny, K. H., Hay, D. C., and Ellis, A. W. (1986a). Access to identity-specific semantic codes from familiar faces. *Quarterly Journal of Experimental Psychology*, **38A**, 271–95.

Young, A. W., McWeeny, K. H., Ellis, A. W., and Hay, D. C. (1986b). Naming and categorizing faces and written names. *Quarterly Journal of Experimental Psychology*, **38A**, 297–318.

Young, A. W., Hay, D. C., and Ellis, A. W. (1986c). Getting semantic information from familiar faces. In *Aspects of face processing*, (ed. H. D. Ellis, M. A. Jeeves, F. Newcombe, and A. W. Young). Martinus Nijhoff, Dordrecht.

4

Applicability of the theoretical model

Reprinted in slightly modified form from Young, A. W. (1994), Face recognition, in *International Perspectives on psychological science, Vol. 2: The state of the art* (ed. G. d'Ydewalle, P. Eelen and P. Bertelson), pp. 1–27, Lawrence Erlbaum, Hove, East Sussex. With kind permission of Psychology Press (Erlbaum UK, Taylor & Francis).

Summary

The ease with which we usually recognize familiar faces can hide an interesting perceptual feat. Faces form a class of stimuli with high inter-item similarity (two eyes, nose, mouth, in similar positions) and often with an arbitrary mapping to semantic information (the face gives little away as to whether its bearer is an actor or a stockbroker), yet because of their overwhelming social importance we are highly expert at identifying them.

Here, I examine what recent studies have taught us about the organization of face processing abilities. As well as considering everyday and laboratory recognition of familiar faces, I pay attention to the implications of face recognition impairments caused by brain injury, and the importance of the interaction between data from investigations of normal and disordered recognition in advancing our understanding.

Face processing as an important achievement

Any member of a species with a complex social organization needs to be able to recognize other individuals, in order to be able to interact with them in different ways. For humans, the face is especially important to recognition. In addition, a wealth of social information other than identity can be derived from the face. We use this to infer moods and feelings, to regulate social interaction through eye contact and facial gestures, to support speech comprehension by lip-reading (even people with normal hearing do this without realizing it), to determine age and sex, and to attribute characteristics on the basis of social stereotypes.

These uses of facial information have a long evolutionary history (Grüsser and Landis 1991). They are well developed even in infancy, and are probably built up from a basis of innately specified components. Newborn babies are attentive to faces (Johnson *et al.* 1991), they can perceive different emotional expressions (Field *et al.* 1982), and they will imitate both emotional and relatively conventional facial gestures (Field *et al.* 1982; Meltzoff and Moore 1983; Vinter 1985).

We also know a little about the neural substrate for face processing from neurophysiological studies (Desimone 1991; Gross and Sergent 1992; Heywood and Cowey 1992; Perrett *et al.* 1992; Sergent *et al.* 1992). The cerebral cortex contains many neurones that are maximally responsive to faces, especially in the temporal lobes, though there is as yet no evidence of any sizeable region in which there are exclusively 'face' cells.

Even without this evolutionary and biological background, there are reasons to suggest that faces form a special class of visual stimuli (Ellis and Young 1989). In particular, there are different environmental demands between the tasks of recognizing people's faces and many other visual objects. Everyday objects often need to be assigned to relatively broad categories that maximize the visual and functional similarity between exemplars; if you are knocking a nail into a wall, it is important to know that a particular object is *a* hammer, knowing *which* hammer it might be is not always necessary. Face recognition presents a quite different type of problem. Galton (1883) pointed out that faces form a visual stimulus category that contains many similar items; each with two eyes, nose, mouth, and so on in roughly the same general arrangement. But recognizing a face as a face does not get us very far. Instead, we need to know which individual's face we are looking at, and the smallest of differences may be crucial in determining this.

The relation between form and function is also different. The shapes of manufactured objects are generally closely related to the functions they must perform, so that one could expect to tell fairly easily whether a novel object was likely to be a tool or a piece of furniture. This is much less true for faces. Although there are some pointers (pop stars are usually young people with exuberant hairstyles, etc.), there is a fundamentally arbitrary mapping to semantic information; you can't really know whether the face of an unfamiliar young person with an exuberant hairstyle is that of a would-be pop star, actor, student, or hairdresser.

For all of these reasons, investigations of face processing present an important opportunity to study some of our most highly developed visual abilities with stimuli that are rich in social meaning. Here, I will examine what recent studies have taught us about the organization of face processing abilities, and the recognition of familiar faces in particular. As well as considering everyday and laboratory recognition of familiar faces, I will examine some of the implications of face recognition impairments caused by brain injury, and the importance of the interaction between data from investigations of normal and disordered recognition in advancing our understanding.

Functional models of face processing

One of the dominant themes of 1980s work on face recognition was the attempt to map out the functional organization of the face processing system in a simple schematic form. The aim of this was not to pretend that we had solved the problem, but to provide a convenient way of synthesizing what was known and guiding further investigation (Bruyer 1987).

The model proposed by Bruce and Young (1986) is shown in Fig. 4.1. They maintained that recognition of identity, expression, lip-reading, and directed visual processing can all be achieved independently. Hence Bruce and Young claimed that one does not need to interpret a person's facial expression in order to lip-read, or to determine their sex in order to recognize their identity, and so on.

Instead, Bruce and Young (1986) proposed that recognition involves sequential stages of perceptual classification (by domain-specific face recognition units), semantic classification (involving domain-independent person identity nodes which can access previously learnt semantic information from the person's face, voice, or name), and name retrieval. This was meant as an idealized sequence, and would be compatible with a 'cascade' mode of operation. Bruce and Young based these claims on a range of mutually corroborative sources of information, including the results of work on the different patterns of impairment that can follow brain injury, experiments with normal subjects, and studies of everyday errors. Reviews of this evidence can be found elsewhere (Ellis 1992*a*; Young 1992; Young and Bruce 1991), and I will only reiterate some of the main points here.

Recognition and other face processing abilities

One of the most important claims made by the Bruce and Young (1986) model is that different types of information are extracted in parallel from the faces we see. I will examine briefly four of these putative

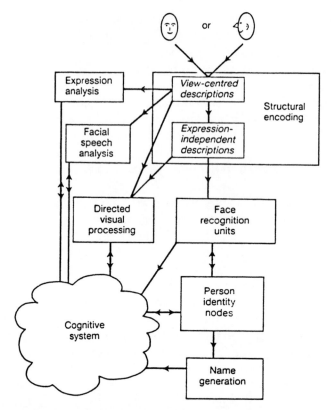

Fig. 4.1 Bruce and Young's (1986) model of face recognition.

dissociations. These involve identity and expression, sex and identity, familiar face recognition and unfamiliar face matching, and lip-reading. A more detailed discussion is given by Young and Bruce (1991).

Identity and expression

Studies of normal subjects have found that people can classify or match the expressions of unfamiliar faces just as quickly as familiar faces (Bruce 1986a; Young et al. 1986a). This lack of any influence of face familiarity on expression processing is consistent with the view that independent systems are involved in determining identity and expression.

The same conclusion follows from neuropsychological studies. There are some brain-injured patients who remain able to understand emotional facial expressions, despite being unable to recognize familiar faces (Bruyer et al. 1983; Tranel et al. 1988). The opposite dissociation has also been reported, with impaired comprehension of facial expressions even though the identities of the people can be recognized (Kurucz and Feldmar 1979; Parry *et al.* 1991).

Sex and identity

Some prosopagnosic patients are correctly able to determine the sex of seen faces, even though they can no longer recognize their identities (Bruyer *et al.* 1983; Tranel *et al.* 1988), but the opposite dissociation (recognition of familiar faces by someone who cannot determine the sex of unfamiliar faces) has not yet been reported in neuropsychological cases. These neuropsychological findings thus leave open the possibility of a perceptual hierarchy in which the face's sex is determined before its identity.

However, findings with normal subjects favour the view that sex and identity are determined independently. Bruce *et al.* (1987) asked people to classify faces as familiar or unfamiliar, or as male or female. They found that faces whose sex was difficult to determine were recognized as familiar just as quickly as faces whose sex was easy to determine, which is inconsistent with any hierarchy in which sex must be determined before identity. Similarly, Roberts and Bruce (1988) noted that masking various facial features had different effects on determining a face's sex or familiarity; concealing the eyes had the greatest detrimental effect on determining familiarity, whereas it was concealing the nose area which had the greatest effect on determining sex.

Roberts and Bruce's (1988) findings show neatly that judgements about sex and identity may dissociate because these draw on cues which primarily involve different regions of the face. They are consistent with other evidence indicating that the face's three-dimensional structure is particularly important as a source of information for the person's sex (Bruce 1990; Enlow 1982). For example, Enlow (1982) has pointed out that the relatively larger lung capacity of males creates the need for larger nasal passages and thus a more convex facial profile. We will return to this point later, when we consider the roles of pattern and surface-based information.

Familiar face recognition and unfamiliar face matching

From his review of neuropsychological studies, Benton (1980) argued that identification of familiar faces and discrimination of unfamiliar faces involve different cerebral mechanisms. Warrington and James (1967) had demonstrated that impairments affecting the processing of familiar or unfamiliar faces were associated with different lesion sites, and there were several reports that prosopagnosic patients (whose recognition of familiar faces is severely impaired) were successfully able to perform face matching tasks. Benton's position has been supported by more recent studies, which have reported contrasting patterns of impairment of ability to recognize familiar faces or match views of unfamiliar faces (Malone *et al.* 1982; Parry *et al.* 1991).

However, Newcombe (1979) has pointed out that we need to know not only that prosopagnosic patients can match unfamiliar faces successfully, but also that they achieve this in the normal way. There are grounds at present for suspecting that at least some use idiosyncratic strategies to compensate for their problems with unfamiliar face matching tasks.

Despite this caveat concerning the neuropsychological evidence, the independence of certain aspects of familiar and unfamiliar face processing is supported by studies of normal subjects (Bruce 1988; Young and Bruce 1991). A clue to at least one of the reasons for differences between familiar and unfamiliar face processing lies in the finding that somewhat different facial features are involved (Ellis *et al* 1979; Young *et al.* 1985*a*). The internal features (eyes, nose, mouth) are particularly important in the processing of familiar faces, whereas with unfamiliar faces we make relatively more use of external features (hair, face shape). The differential salience may accrue to the internal features of familiar faces because these remain unaffected by changes in hairstyle or from the attention paid to them because of their expressive characteristics.

Lip-reading

McGurk and MacDonald (1976) described a remarkable illusion in which a mismatch between heard and seen phonemes results in the perceiver blending the two. For example, when watching a video of a person mouthing the phoneme 'ga', which is synchronized to the soundtrack 'ba', most people hear the fusion as 'da'. Yet neither the visual nor the auditory recording track carries the signal 'da'; it is a genuine fusion. The reason why we possess this lip-reading skill is not yet known with certainty. An appealing possibility is that it relates to the demands of learning to decode speech in infancy, when a lot of time is spent watching people talking (Studdert-Kennedy 1983). Lip-reading would then be particularly useful, because some of the sounds which are difficult to distinguish auditorily are among those which are relatively easy to lip-read. However, recent findings of cross-modal influences on speech perception for stimuli which could not have pre-existing association in memory show that this is not in itself a full explanation of the phenomenon (Fowler and Dekle 1991).

A dissociation between lip-reading and the processing of facial expression and identity has been demonstrated in a neuropsychological study by Campbell *et al.* (1986). One patient (with a posterior lesion of the right cerebral hemisphere) was unable to recognize familiar faces and could not categorize facial expressions correctly. Yet she could judge correctly what phonemes were being mouthed in photographs of faces, and she was susceptible to the McGurk illusion. The second patient (with a posterior lesion of the left hemisphere) was impaired at making phoneme judgements to face stimuli and was not susceptible to the McGurk illusion, yet had no difficulties in recognizing faces or facial expressions.

The dissociation of lip-reading and expression processing is particularly important, since both types of information are derived from a similar area of the face; the main difference is that for expression, eyes and eyebrows are involved as well as mouth and lips. Hence, in this case it seems to be the use to which the information is put, rather than the region of the face being analysed, which is crucial in determining whether or not a separable functional subsystem is dedicated to the task.

The nature of the representations used to effect recognition

A feature that makes some people uneasy about functional models of the type shown in Fig. 4.1 is that they (deliberately) sidestep difficult questions concerning the nature of the representations used to effect recognition of familiar faces. We are still a long way from a satisfactory answer to such questions, but some useful pointers have emerged.

Representation of wholes and parts

Carey and Diamond (1977) suggested that the differences between faces can be considered in terms of differences in the individual features (different eyes, noses, mouths, etc.) or differences in the way these features are arranged with respect to each other – the *configuration*. In some publications, the same idea is described in terms of first-order features (eyes, nose mouth, etc.) and second-order features characterizing the spatial relations between first-order features (the configuration).

The importance of individual features seems obvious, but recent studies have also shown that the configuration can have a powerful effect. Hosie *et al.* (1988) took photographs of well known faces and used image manipulation techniques to move features upwards or downwards and

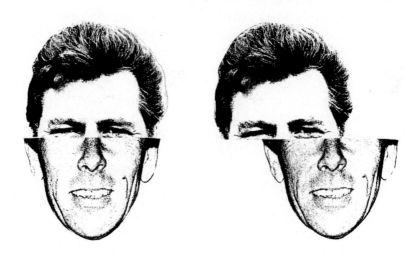

Fig. 4.2 Examples of composite and non-composite stimuli, as used by Young *et al.* (1987).

inwards or outwards; the effect on appearance was very marked. This technique caused some alteration to the features themselves, but it primarily affected the configuration, thus providing powerful evidence of the importance of the configuration as well as the individual features.

Further evidence of the importance of configurations comes from a simple technique in which the top and bottom halves of two familiar faces are assembled into a crude montage; people tend to see the resulting composite as a novel, unfamiliar face (Carey 1992; Young *et al.* 1987). Figure 4.2 shows an example, and a corresponding non-composite in which the same components are misaligned. Experiments in which people are asked to identify the components of such stimuli (e.g. if they are asked to name the top half or to name the bottom half) have shown that it is much easier to do this for non-composites than for composites (see Table 4.1); the novel facial configuration of the composites makes identification of the constituent parts more difficult.

Patterns or surfaces?

Many approaches to face recognition assume, implicitly or explicitly, that the question can be reduced to one of recognizing a two-

Table 4.1 Reaction times (ms) for correct identification of the top and bottom halves of composite and non-composite stimuli (Young *et al.* 1987)

	Composite	Non-composite
Top half	1297	1041
Bottom half	1282	1123

dimensional pattern, and assign no special role to the face's three-dimensional structure. This is a convenient assumption in work which often relies on photographic stimuli, but it was questioned by Bruce (1988), who pointed out that the visual system may be able to make use of the face's three-dimensional structure.

To examine this possibility, Bruce and her colleagues have described a series of studies involving laser scanning of many locations on the head and face, which are then rendered into a three-dimensional model using computer graphics programs (Bruce 1990; Bruce *et al.* 1989, 1991, 1992*a*). This gives an accurate rendition of the face as a three-dimensional *surface*, devoid of pigmentation. The results have been intriguing. Bruce *et al.* (1989) showed that the cardioidal strain transformation, which is known to affect the perception of age (Mark and Todd 1983; Pittenger and Shaw 1975), would also work for these three-dimensional models, and Bruce (1990) has reported that altering the shape of the nose affects the perception of the face's sex, which bears out Roberts and Bruce's (1988) finding that masking the nose area seriously affects the determination of sex from photographs.

However, although recognition of the identity of these three-dimensional head models is above-chance, it is noticeably poor (Bruce *et al.* 1991). This suggests that surface pigmentation is quite important in conveying identity. Although three-dimensional cues are heavily utilized in conveying socially important information about age and sex, they may be less central to recognition of the face's identity.

Instance-based or abstractive?

Theoretical models produced in the 1980s took their inspiration from Morton's (1979) logogen model of word recognition, and proposed that the representations which underlie recognition are able to *abstract* the essential qualities of a particular face's appearance, so that it can be recognized across a wide range of transformations of pose, viewing angles, and so on. Such models propose a single recognition unit for each known face, with each of these recognition units holding a description of the appropriate face (Bruce and Young 1986; Hay and Young 1982).

A challenge to this type of conception comes from models which are more *instance-based*, and only store the details of every particular encounter with a face. The most well known of these are connectionist models based on distributed representations (McClelland and Rumelhart 1985). Although some of these theoretical differences may reflect stylistic changes in emphasis (Broadbent 1985), the results of experiments have tended to demonstrate the usefulness of the instance-based conception. Repetition priming studies show this most clearly.

Repetition priming tasks investigate the facilitatory effect of having previously encountered a particular stimulus on subsequent recognition. Consider, for example, an experiment reported by Bruce and Valentine (1985). Their subjects saw faces or names of familiar people in a pre-training part of the experiment, and were then asked to make familiarity decisions (familiar *v.* unfamiliar person) to faces in a second part of the experiment. The mean reaction times for correct familiarity decisions are shown in Table 4.2.

Note that there was a facilitation of reaction time to the face if it had been seen previously (same view and different view *v.* unprimed), but there was no significant effect of previously seeing a name or recognizing the person's face (name seen *v.* unprimed). Repetition effects are domain-specific. There was, though, additional benefit from seeing the same view rather than a different view of the face in Bruce and Valentine's (1985) experiment, which they attributed to an effect of visual memory of the specific photograph used.

One reason why repetition priming effects are domain-specific is that they are based on the degree of physical similarity between prime and test items. Ellis *et al.* (1987) showed that repetition priming transfers from one photograph of a face to another in proportion to the degree of similarity between the two views (see Table 4.3). A simple way of accounting for such graded-similarity effects is to conclude that the recognition system operates in a way that allows it to store records of previously encountered instances (McClelland and Rumelhart 1985), rather than the relatively abstractive conception we had initially put forward (Bruce and Young 1986; Hay and Young 1982).

A striking feature of models based on distributed representations is that presentation of part of a familiar pattern will activate the representation of the whole pattern; that is, they can show pattern completion (McClelland and Rumelhart 1985). This property is found in repetition priming. Table 4.4 shows reaction times for familiarity

Table 4.2 Mean reaction times (ms) for correct familiarity decisions to familiar faces (Bruce and Valentine 1985)

Same view as pre-training	Different view from pre-training	Name seen in pre-training	Unprimed
893	952	1000	1032

Table 4.3 Gradient of similarity in the priming of reaction times (ms) for familiarity decisions to familiar faces (Ellis *et al.* 1987)

Primed by the same photograph	Primed by a similar photograph	Primed by a dissimilar photograph	Unprimed
664	697	756	860

Table 4.4 Mean correct reaction times (ms) for familiarity decisions to familiar faces that had previously been recognised from internal features, external features, or the whole face (Brunas *et al.* 1990)

Primed by internal features	Primed by external features	Primed by whole face	Unprimed
713	703	708	860

decisions to familiar faces that had previously been recognized from internal features, external features, or the whole face (Brunas *et al.* 1990); it is clear that viewing part of a familiar face on a previous occasion was as effective at priming recognition as seeing the whole face.

Taken together, these studies of the nature of the representations used to effect recognition show the importance of instance-based representations of the configuration of facial features in recognition, but they also imply that there is probably no simple, unidimensional solution. In general, information about individual features and about configurations, about patterns and about surfaces, will be readily available and can be flexibly used and given differential weight according to the task in hand.

Face-specific processes, and the importance of expertise

There has been considerable interest in the issue of how face recognition might differ from other types of visual recognition, and whether a specialized, face-specific system is involved (Ellis and Young 1989). The issue is not yet fully resolved, but important pointers have come from work on prosopagnosia and on acquired expertise in normal people.

Specificity of the recognition impairment in prosopagnosia

In cases of prosopagnosia caused by brain injury, there is a very severe impairment of face recognition, in which even the most familiar faces (famous faces, friends, family, and the patient's own face when seen in a mirror) are not recognized overtly. Despite this, a number of prosopagnosic patients can read, and can recognize many everyday objects, so the deficit does not compromise all aspects of visual recognition. But is it only face recognition which is impaired?

In most cases, the answer is clearly 'no'. For instance, Bornstein (1963) described a prosopagnosic patient who had also lost the ability to identify species of birds which had formerly been well known to her. She commented that 'all the birds look the same'. Similarly, Bornstein et al. (1969) reported the case of a prosopagnosic farmer who could no longer identify his own livestock. Previously, he had been able to recognize his cows as individuals, but he could no longer do this.

There are at least two different ways of interpreting such reports; both may draw attention to important factors, but neither seems in itself to give a full account of the patterns observed. First, the patients had some special expertise with another visual category. When they became prosopagnosic, they lost their expertise as well as their expertise with faces. Second, what they seem to have lost is the ability to recognize the individual members of categories that contain several items of similar appearance. Ability to identify the general category to which the items belong (faces, birds, cows, etc.) is preserved, but ability to achieve within-category recognition is lost.

Damasio et al. (1982) emphasized the second interpretation, and maintained that prosopagnosia is a deficit of within-category recognition. For several patients, this description does seem to fit, but there are also reports of dissociable impairments affecting different types of within-category recognition (Assal et al. 1984; Bruyer et al. 1983). A very compelling example is given by McNeil and Warrington (1993), whose prosopagnosic patient later became a farmer and was able to recognize his sheep.

De Renzi and his colleagues have described two cases for whom the deficit did seem to be remarkably specific to face recognition, with many other types of within-category recognition being well preserved (De Renzi 1986; De Renzi et al. 1991). Despite being severely impaired at face recognition, these patients could pick out their own belongings when they were mixed in with several distractor objects chosen to resemble them, recognize cars in a car park, and sort domestic coins from foreign coins.

These studies show that the within-category recognition deficit hypothesis cannot provide a complete explanation of prosopagnosia. However, there is some evidence that the degree of expertise we all have with faces may be an important contributory factor. This comes from investigations of the effects of inversion.

Expertise and inversion

A curious property of faces is that they are difficult to recognize when seen upside-down (Valentine 1988). The explanation for the effect of inversion on faces does not simply lie in the fact that we are used to seeing them the right way up, since Yin (1969) and others have shown that the effect of inversion is larger for faces than for other stimuli we are used to encountering in a fixed orientation.

Yin (1970) thought that the explanation must be that the brain has specialized perceptual mechanisms for faces, and it is these that are particularly sensitive to inversion. His findings suggested that posterior areas of the right cerebral hemisphere are critically involved in these specialized abilities, and he tended to think of these as if they were assigned to faces for purely biological reasons. More recent studies, though, have tended to emphasize that the crucial variable may be degree of expertise (Diamond and Carey 1986; Rhodes *et al.* 1989). Because of their social importance, we are highly expert at face perception.

This point is neatly demonstrated in Diamond and Carey's (1986) study. They used recognition memory tasks with upright and inverted pictures of faces and dogs. In the 'dogs' part of the task, subjects had to recognize the particular dog seen on the previous trial from two members of the same breed. Some of Diamond and Carey's (1986) subjects knew little about dogs (novices), but the others were breeders who were breeding the exact type of dog used in the memory test (experts). Both dog experts and dog novices showed a marked effect of inversion on face recognition. This is to be expected as both groups can be considered expert with faces. The dog novices, however, showed little effect of inversion on dog recognition, whereas the dog experts showed a marked effect of inversion on their recognition memory for the dog pictures; this effect was as large as the inversion effect they had shown to faces.

These findings show that expertise plays an important role in inversion effects, suggesting that disruption of this expertise, which we all have for faces, might also underlie prosopagnosia. Note, though, that McNeil and Warrington's (1993) patient was later able to acquire expertise in recognizing sheep, yet he could not re-acquire his ability to recognize faces. This again implies that expertise is not the only factor involved.

Recent studies, then, have shown that in rare cases recognition impairments can be remarkably specific to faces. We do not yet know precisely why this can happen, but such findings are consistent with the hypothesis of an evolved neural substrate for face recognition. Expertise seems to be also an important factor, but is not in itself sufficient to account for all of the findings. Of course, the expertise hypothesis is not necessarily antagonistic to the idea of an evolved neural substrate for face recognition; such a neural substrate would facilitate the acquisition of this expertise for faces, and it might even be the case that acquisition of other types of visual expertise is to some extent achieved by 'parasitizing' on parts of this system.

Distinctiveness and caricature

A well known finding from work on eyewitnessing and recognition memory has been that some faces are easier to remember than others because they are more *distinctive*. In contrast, faces which look much like the average face (*typical* faces) are less well remembered.

Valentine and Bruce (1986) showed that distinctiveness also affects the recognition of faces which are highly familiar. They asked people to decide as quickly as possible whether or not faces were familiar, and recorded their reaction times. Reaction times to familiar faces were faster for distinctive than for typical faces (see Table 4.5). Valentine and Bruce argued that we may encode faces by reference to the average of the faces we have seen, so that what is used for recognition are

Table 4.5 Reaction times (ms) to distinctive and typical familiar faces in familiarity decision and face *v.* non-face classification tasks (Valentine and Bruce 1986)

	Distinctive faces	Typical faces
Familiarity decision	661	707
Face v. non-face decision	608	561

differences from the average, making typical faces (which are less different from the average) harder to recognize. If this theory is correct, one would expect typical faces to show an advantage over distinctive faces if we changed the task to one of deciding whether or not a stimulus is a face (i.e. whether it is close to the average). As Table 4.5 shows, this result was found by Valentine and Bruce with a face versus non-face (scrambled face) classification task.

Further evidence consistent with Valentine and Bruce's (1986) position can be found in work on caricature. Rhodes *et al.* (1987) reported experiments using caricatures generated by a computer, and showed that these were identified more quickly and rated as better likenesses than were exact line drawings or anti-caricatures. The program used by Rhodes *et al.* takes as its input a number of points specifying the locations of various parts of the face. These points are then compared to the average location of the same points in a set of faces, and any differences from the average are increased to create a caricature, or decreased to create an anti-caricature (Brennan 1982). Subsequent work by Benson and Perrett (1991*a*, *b*) has shown that the same principles can be extended to create caricatures of photographs.

These findings therefore show that exaggerating differences from the average (in effect, increasing the face's distinctiveness) produces a representation which is a 'better likeness' than the original. Valentine has developed these observations by proposing a theoretical framework in which faces are represented as points in a multidimensional space (Valentine 1991); typical faces would then lie in a very densely populated part of this space, making them hard to recognize because the presence of close neighbours means that they are not easily assigned to a unique region.

Two main ways of implementing a multidimentional space theory can be distinguished (Valentine 1991): in one ('norm-based coding'), each face's deviation from the average is represented explicitly; in the other ('exemplar-based') , a norm is not abstracted as such, but arises as a by-product of storing specific faces. Valentine and Endo (1992) argued that comparison to an explicitly stored norm is not necessary, and Valentine and Ferrara (1991) showed that at least one variant of an exemplar-based approach can readily be simulated with a parallel distributed processing model.

Impressively, the multidimensional space theory can also encompass the known effects of race and inversion on recognition (Valentine 1991; Valentine and Endo 1992). This ability to provide a unified account of effects which might otherwise seem entirely diverse (distinctiveness, race, inversion) makes it very powerful.

Recognition as a hierarchic process

Although functional models of face recognition claim that recognition proceeds in parallel with other types of face processing, recognition itself is generally seen as a multi-stage hierarchic process (Bruce and Young 1986; Ellis 1986; Hay and Young, 1982). Bruce and Young (1986) based this claim in part on the fact that studies of everyday difficulties and errors show that many of them reflect breakdown at different levels of recognition (Young *et al* 1985*b*). For example:

1. We may completely fail to recognise a familiar face, and mistakenly think that the person is unfamiliar.
2. We may recognize the face as familiar, but be unable to bring to mind any other details about the person, such as her or his occupation or name.
3. We may recognize the face as familiar and remember appropriate semantic information about the person, while failing to remember her or his name.

The orderliness of these types of everyday error suggests that the face recognition system itself uses some form of sequential access to different types of information, in the order familiarity then semantics then name retrieval. Experiments with normal subjects have given strong support to this suggestion (Bruce 1988; Bruce and Young 1986; Young and Ellis 1989). Additional confirmation has come from studies of errors made under laboratory conditions, and the types of cue needed to resolve them (Hanley and Cowell, 1988; Hay *et al* 1991). These studies can eliminate reporting biases, yet still find only the types of error predicted by the sequential access view.

Each of these types of error can also arise after neuropsychological impairment. In such cases, a brain-injured patient will make her or his characteristic error to many or almost all seen faces. In prosopagnosia, for example, known faces seem unfamiliar (Meadows 1974), which corresponds to error type 1. We have reported a case in which known faces only were familiar (de Haan 1991*a*), corresponding to error type 2. In anomia, name retrieval to known faces may become problematic even though semantic information can be properly accessed (Flude *et al.* 1989), as in error type 3.

We thus have converging evidence from studies of everyday errors, laboratory errors, experiments, and neuropsychological case studies, indicating that the functional organization of the face recognition system involves sequential access to different types of information.

Recent work has therefore concentrated on providing a simulation of how this might be achieved (Bruce *et al*. 1992*b*; Burton *et al*. 1990).

Modelling the functional organization of the recognition system

Priming effects have provided useful ways of examining the organization of mechanisms involved in the recognition of familiar people. In particular, comparisons of repetition and semantic priming have been instructive.

Repetition and semantic priming

As we have noted, repetition priming involves the facilitation of recognition of a previously seen stimulus. For example, recognition of Prince Charles's face is faster if his face has appeared previously in the experiment than if it has not come up before (Bruce and Valentine 1985; Ellis *et al*. 1987; Young *et al*. 1986*b*). Repetition priming effects are long lasting (being found across intervals of several minutes in existing published studies, and as long as three months in as yet unpublished work of our own) and domain specific (recognition of Prince Charles's face is not facilitated by previously having recognized the name 'Prince Charles').

The effects of repetition seem to be located in the face recognition system itself, since decisions about the face's expression or sex, which can be made without needing to recognize the person, do not show repetition priming. Table 4.6 shows data from an experiment reported by Ellis *et al*. (1990), in which subjects saw photographs of faces during the pre-training phase and then were later asked to make decisions about the familiarity, expression, or sex of these faces in a second phase of the experiment. Although exactly the same photographs were used in

Table 4.6 Reaction times (ms) for familiarity, expression or sex decisions to familiar faces which were seen (primed) or not seen (unprimed) in a pre-training phase of the experiment (Ellis *et al*. 1990)

	Primed faces	Unprimed faces
Familiarity decision	709	862
Expression decision	552	566
Sex decision	636	638

Table 4.7 reaction times (ms) for familiarity decisions to face targets preceded by related, neutral or unrelated face primes presented 250, 500, or 1000 ms before each target (Bruce and Valentine 1986)

Stimulus onset asynchrony	Related prime	Neutral prime	Unrelated prime
250 ms	782	848	855
500 ms	705	804	816
1000 ms	662	828	805

the pre-training and test phases, only reaction times for familiarity decisions showed any benefit.

Semantic priming tasks investigate the effect of having previously recognized a closely associated stimulus; for example, the effect of having recently recognized Princess Diana's face on recognition of Prince Charles's face (Bruce 1983, 1986b; Bruce and Valentine 1986; Young et al. 1988). Table 4.7 shows data from a study in which Bruce and Valentine (1986) examined reaction times in a face familiarity decision task (this involves deciding whether or not faces are those of familiar people). Each of the familiar target faces could be preceded by a *related* face prime (e.g. Ronnie Barker's face preceding the target face of Ronnie Corbett; both are British comedians who often appeared together), a *neutral* prime (an unfamiliar face), or an *unrelated* face prime (e.g. Sebastian Coe's face preceding the target face of Ronnie Corbett; Coe was an athlete). These primes were presented with stimulus onset asynchronies (SOAs) of 250, 500, or 1000 ms before each target. As can be seen, recognition was facilitated by related primes at all SOAs.

In contrast to repetition priming effects, the facilitation produced by semantic priming is very short lived (generally dissipating within seconds), yet can cross stimulus domains (for example, from recognition of Princess Diana's face to recognition of Prince Charles's name).

These differences between repetition priming and semantic priming effects are widely taken to indicate that the sources of facilitation arise at different loci in the recognition system in each case (Bruce 1986b; Young and Ellis 1989), but more precise specification of the underlying reasons for the differences has proved difficult. However, Burton et al. (1990) have developed an interactive activation model which is able to simulate the effects of repetition and semantic priming and the differences between them.

Modelling repetition and semantic priming

Burton and co-workers' (1990) model is particularly important, since it can account for a number of effects reported in the literature with very few assumptions. For example, it gives a very neat account of priming effects.

The basic structure of the Burton *et al.* (1990) model is shown in schematic form in Fig. 4.3. The model is couched in interactive activation terms. It consists of active units connected to each other by modifiable links, which can be excitatory (increasing the unit's activation) or inhibitory (decreasing the unit's activation); in the absence of such input, each unit's level of activation is set to decay slowly at a standard rate. As in other interactive activation models, 'pools' of functional units are interconnected by bidirectional excitatory links, and within each pool the rival units compete by inhibiting each other. This inhibition becomes greater as units in a pool gain in activation. There are pools of units corresponding to individual faces (face recognition units, or FRUs), seen names (name input units, or NIUs) and items of semantic information (SIUs; politician, teacher, etc.). These are connected to each other via person identity nodes (PINs), with one identity node for each person being linked to the appropriate FRU and NIU, and to whichever SIUs

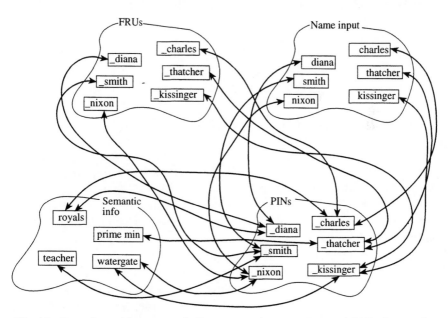

Fig. 4.3 Central architecture of Burton and co-workers' (1990) interactive activation model.

are appropriate. The idea is that there is one PIN for each known person, and that this is connected to the FRU for that person's face, the NIU for the person's name, and to whichever SIUs are appropriate.

The Burton *et al.* (1990) model can be considered to be an implementation of part of Bruce and Young's (1986) model, though it also involves certain differences. The most important of these concern the PINs. Burton *et al.* (1990) see these as providing an interface to semantic information (the SIUs), rather than holding semantic information themselves. In addition, the PINs are held to form the level at which an input can be classified as familiar, rather than the FRUs or NIUs, as Bruce and Young (1986) had envisaged. This simple model provides a neat simulation of the properties of semantic priming and repetition priming, if we assume that familiarity is recognized when activation at the PIN crosses an arbitrary threshold.

We will look first at semantic priming. Consider what happens at the PINs for Prince Charles and Princess Diana when activation is increased at the 'Charles' FRU (the equivalent of seeing Prince Charles's face). Obviously, the 'Charles' PIN crosses the threshold of recognition quite quickly, but Burton *et al.* (1990) showed that activation at the 'Diana' PIN also increases (but remains below threshold). This happens because activation is passed back to the PINs from the SIUs shared by Charles and Diana. However, this activation does not bring the 'Diana' PIN to threshold, because it is simultaneously being inhibited by the more active 'Charles' PIN. After the input ceases, activation at both the 'Charles' and 'Diana' PINs decays a little, but does not return to resting level. This means that a subsequent presentation of Charles or Diana will be recognized more quickly than if the activation in these PINs was at resting level.

In the Burton *et al.* (1990) simulation, then, the mechanism for semantic priming lies in the interaction of the PINs and SIUs. This explains why semantic priming will cross input domains, because the PINs can receive input from FRUs or NIUs. The short duration of semantic priming is accounted for by the fact that subsequent presentation of any face (or name) other than Charles or Diana will drive the 'Charles' and 'Diana' PINs back to resting level, because of the within-pool inhibitory links.

The mechanism for repetition priming in the Burton *et al.* (1990) model is that the connection strengths between units which activate each other are increased every time they do this. So although the 'Charles' PIN may have returned to resting level, the strength of the excitatory connection between the 'Charles' FRU and the 'Charles' PIN will be increased if Charles's face was previously recognized. Repetition of the face then leads to faster recognition. This explains why repetition priming effects are domain specific, because it is the links between input units (FRUs or NIUs) and PINs which are strengthened, and why they are long lasting (within-pool inhibition does not affect these).

Burton *et al.* (1990) also suggest a simple account of distinctiveness, based on whether or not faces share features, which we will not look at in detail here.

Although Burton *et al.* (1990) were thus able to show that this implementation can simulate several reported results on face recognition, at first sight there is no mechanism to account for problems in accessing name output codes (since a separate store for these is not built into the model). However, Burton and Bruce (1992) noticed that the model shown in Fig. 4.3 can already account for problems in name retrieval, if it is assumed that names are stored along with other types of semantic information. A name like 'Richard Nixon' would then be linked to a single PIN (for Richard Nixon), whereas most items of semantic information would be linked to several PINs (e.g. 'politician' to PINs for Richard Nixon, John Major, Neil Kinnock, etc.). It is a property of this type of architecture that the less interconnectivity as item has, the less easy it is to boost its activation. Hence, Burton and Bruce (1992) point out that problems of name retrieval may simply reflect the status of names as relatively unique items of semantic information.

Covert recognition in prosopagnosia

A further strength of the Burton *et al.* (1990) model is that it can provide an account of the otherwise puzzling phenomenon of covert recognition found in some cases of prosopagnosia. Prosopagnosic patients usually fail all tests of overt recognition of familiar faces (Hécaen and Angelergues 1962; Meadows 1974). They cannot name the face, give the person's occupation, or other biographical details, or even state whether or not a face is that of a familiar person (all faces seem unfamiliar). Surprisingly, though, there is substantial evidence of covert recognition from physiological and behavioural measures (Bruyer 1991; Young and de Haan 1992).

In a very elegant study, Bauer (1984) measured skin conductance while a prosopagnosic patient, L.F., viewed a familiar face and listened to a list of five names. When the name belonged to the face L.F. was looking at, there was a greater skin conductance change than when someone else's name was read out. Yet if L.F. was asked to choose which name in the list was correct for the face, his performance was at chance level. The same effect was found to personally known faces (L.F.'s family) and famous faces he would only have encountered in the mass media.

A number of other indices of covert recognition in prosopagnosia have also been developed. For example, priming has been found from 'unrecognized' faces on to the recognition of name targets (de Haan *et al.* 1992; Young *et al.* 1988).

Findings of covert recognition in prosopagnosia show responses based on the unique identities of familiar faces, even though overt recognition of these faces is not achieved. A simulation of this pattern can be made by halving the connection strengths between FRUs and PINs in the Burton *et al.* (1990) model (Burton *et al.* 1991). The network is then no longer able to classify face inputs as familiar, yet it continues to display semantic priming from 'unrecognized' faces because the PIN–SIU links can still pass excitation to each other even at these sub-threshold levels. The problem of understanding how covert responses can be preserved when there is no overt discrimination may thus be less intractable than it at first appeared.

An interesting feature of this simulation is that it implies that the failure of recognition seen in cases of prosopagnosia need not be absolute, and this has been borne out by recent work. Sergent and Poncet (1990) observed that their patient, P.V., could achieve overt recognition of some faces if several members of the same semantic category were presented together. This only happened when P.V. could determine the category herself. For the categories P.V. could not deter-mine, she continued to fail to recognize the faces overtly even when the occupational category was pointed out to her. This phenomenon of overt recognition provoked by multiple exemplars of a semantic category has been replicated for another patient, P.H. (de Haan *et al.* 1991*b*). Both P.V. and P.H. were very surprised at being able to recognize faces overtly.

Sergent and Poncet (1990) suggested that their demonstration shows that 'neither the facial representations nor the semantic information were critically disturbed in PV, and her prosopagnosia may thus reflect faulty connections between faces and their memories'. They thought that the simultaneous presentation of several members of the same category may have temporarily raised the activation level above the appropriate threshold.

Such findings show that the boundary between overt recognition and lack of any awareness of recognition is not as completely impassable as it seems to the patients' everyday experience. The face that certain types of stimulation can trigger the experience of overt recognition that they no longer enjoy routinely, fits readily with a model in which activation must cross some form of threshold before it can result in awareness (Burton *et al.* 1991; Sergent and Poncet 1990). However, the circumstances under which this has been found to happen are at present very limited.

Conclusions

The functional modelling approach was introduced to provide a simple way of integrating the findings of studies of face recognition and guiding further investigations (Bruce and Young 1986; Bruyer 1987; Hay and Young 1982). In this, it has succeeded well beyond our expectations. We know a lot more about the recognition of familiar faces than we did 10 years ago, and much of the work has shown that the models of Hay and Young (1982) and of Bruce and Young were reasonable first approximations. The development of an implemented version by Burton *et al.* (1990) has brought enhanced explanatory power and an account of otherwise very puzzling phenomena such as covert recognition in prosopagnosia (Burton *et al.* 1991). Work with image manipulation techniques has significantly increased our understanding of the representations which might underlie recognition (Bruce 1990) and the effects of distinctiveness and caricature (Benson and Perrett 1991*a*; Rhodes *et al.* 1987). Valentine's development of the multidimensional space theory has allowed it to encompass phenomena that might otherwise be considered entirely diverse (Valentine 1991).

In addition to the use of a relatively widely shared theoretical perspective, one of the strengths of work on familiar face recognition has been a willingness to draw on an eclectic range of sources of evidence. As well as considering everyday and laboratory recognition of familiar faces, I have been able to consider here the implications of face recognition impairments caused by brain injury, and this interaction between data from investigations of normal and disordered recognition has been most useful. Moreover, the approach is being extended even further, into investigations of recognition memory (Bartlett and Fulton 1991; Bartlett *et al.* 1991), ageing (Bartlett and Fulton 1991; Bartlett *et al.* 1991; Maylor 1990), the development of face processing abilities (Ellis 1992*b*) and delusional misidentifications that have been considered the province of psychiatry (Ellis and Young 1990; Young *et al.* 1993). Hence there is good reason to hope that the interplay between these different sources of evidence and explicit functional models will continue to enhance our understanding.

References

Assal, G., Favre, C., and Anderes, J.P. (1984). Non-reconnaissance d'animaux familiers chez un paysan: zoo-agnosie ou prosopagnosie pour les animaux. *Revue Neurologique*, **140**, 580–4.

Bartlett, J. and Fulton, A. (1991). Familiarity and recognition of faces in old age. *Memory and Cognition*, **19**, 229–38.

Bartlett, J., Strater, L., and Fulton, A. (1991). False recency and false fame of faces in young adulthood and old age. *Memory and Cognition*, **19**, 177–88.

Bauer, R. M. (1984). Autonomic recognition of names and faces in proso-pagnosia: a neuropsychological application of the guilty knowledge test. *Neuropsychologia*, **22**, 457–69.

Benson, P. J. and Perrett, D. I. (1991*a*). Perception and recognition of photo-graphic quality facial caricatures: implications for the recognition of natural images. *European Journal of Cognitive Psychology*, **3**, 105–35.

Benson, P. J. and Perrett, D. I. (1991*b*). Synthesising continuous-tone caricatures. *Image and Vision Computing*, **9**, 123–9.

Benton, A. L. (1980). The neuropsychology of facial recognition. *American Psychologist*, **35**, 176–86.

Bornstein, B. (1963). Prosopagnosia. In *Problems of dynamic neurology*, (ed. L. Halpern), pp. 283–318. Hadassah Medical School, Jerusalem.

Bornstein, B., Sroka, H., and Munitz, H. (1969). Prosopagnosia with animal face agnosia. *Cortex*, **5**, 164–9.

Brennan, S. E. (1982). Caricature generator: dynamic exaggeration of faces by computer. *Leonardo*, **18**, 170–8.

Broadbent, D. E. (1985). A question of levels: comment on McClelland and Rumelhart. *Journal of Experimental Psychology: General*, **114**, 189–92.

Bruce, V. (1983). Recognizing faces. *Philosophical Transactions of the Royal Society, London*, **B302**, 423–36.

Bruce, V. (1986*a*). Influences of familiarity on the processing of faces. *Perception*, **15**, 387–97.

Bruce, V. (1986*b*). Recognizing familiar faces. In *Aspects of face processing*, (ed. H. D. Ellis, M. A. Jeeves, F. Newcombe, and A. Young), pp. 107–17. Martinus Nijhoff, Dordrecht.

Bruce, V. (1988). *Recognising faces*. Lawrence Erlbaum, London.

Bruce, V. (1990). Perceiving and recognising faces. *Mind and Language*, **5**, 342–64.

Bruce, V. and Valentine, T. (1985). Identity priming in the recognition of familiar faces. *British Journal of Psychology*, **76**, 363–83.

Bruce, V. and Valentine, T. (1986). Semantic priming of familiar faces. *Quarterly Journal of Experimental Psychology*, **38A**, 125–50.

Bruce, V. and Young, A. (1986). Understanding face recognition. *British Journal of Psychology*, **77**, 305–27.

Bruce, V., Ellis, H. D., Gibling, F., and Young, A. W. (1987). Parallel processing of the sex and familiarity of faces. *Canadian Journal of Psychology*, **41**, 510–20.

Bruce, V., Burton, M., Doyle, T., and Dench, N. (1989). Further experiments on the perception of growth in three dimensions. *Perception and Psychophysics*, **46**, 528–36.

Bruce, V., Healey, P., Burton, M., Doyle, T., Coombes, A., and Linney A. (1991). Recognising facial surfaces. *Perception*, **20**, 755–69.

Bruce, V., Burton, M., and Doyle, T. (1992a). Faces as surfaces. In *Processing images of faces*, (ed. V. Bruce and A. M. Burton), pp. 228–48. Ablex, Norwood, NJ.

Bruce, V., Burton, A. M., and Craw, I. (1992b). Modelling face recognition. *Philosophical Transactions of the Royal Society, London*, **B335**, 121–8.

Brunas, J., Young, A. W., and Ellis, A. W. (1990). Repetition priming from incomplete faces: Evidence for part to whole completion. *British Journal of Psychology*, **81**, 43–56.

Bruyer, R. (1987). *Les mecanismes de reconnaissance des visages*. Presses Universitaires de Grenoble.

Bruyer, R. (1991). Covert face recognition in prosopagnosia: a review. *Brain and Cognition*, **15**, 223–35.

Bruyer, R., Laterre, C., Seron, X., Feyereisen, P., Strypstein, E., Pierrard, E., and Rectem, D. (1983). A case of prosopagnosia with some preserved covert remembrance of familiar faces. *Brain and Cognition*, **2**, 257–84.

Burton, A. M. and Bruce, V. (1992). I recognise your face but I can't remember your name: a simple explanation? *British Journal of Psychology*, **83**, 45–60.

Burton, A. M., Bruce, V., and Johnston, R. A. (1990). Understanding face recognition with an interactive activation model. *British Journal of Psychology*, **81**, 361–80.

Burton, A. M., Young, A. W., Bruce, V., Johnston, R., and Ellis, A. W. (1991). Understanding covert recognition. *Cognition*, **39**, 129–66.

Campbell, R., Landis, T., and Regard, M. (1986). Face recognition and lipreading: a neurological dissociation. *Brain*, **109**, 509–21.

Carey, S. (1992). Becoming a face expert. *Philosophical Transactions of the Royal Society, London*, **B335**, 95–103.

Carey, S. and Diamond, R. (1977). From piecemeal to configurational representation of faces. *Science*, **195**, 312–14.

Damasio, A. R., Damasio, H., and Van Hoesen, G. W. (1982). Prosopagnosia: anatomic basis and behavioral mechanisms. *Neurology*, **32**, 331–41.

de Haan, E. H. F., Young, A. W., and Newcombe, F. (1991a). A dissociation between the sense of familiarity and access to semantic information concerning familiar people. *European Journal of Cognitive Psychology*, **3**, 51–67.

de Haan, E. H. F., Young, A. W., and Newcombe, F. (1991b). Covert and overt recognition in prosopagnosia. *Brain*, **114**, 2575–91.

de Haan, E. H. F., Bauer, R. M., and Greve, K. W. (1992). Behavioural and physiological evidence for covert face recognition in a prosopagnosic patient. *Cortex*, **28**, 77–95.

De Renzi, E. (1986). Current issues in prosopagnosia. In *Aspects of face processing*, (ed. H. D. Ellis, M. A. Jeeves, F. Newcombe, and A. Young), pp. 243–52. Martinus Nijhoff, Dordrecht.

De Renzi, E., Faglioni, P., Grossi, D., and Nichelli, P. (1991). Apperceptive and associative forms of prosopagnosia. *Cortex*, **27**, 213–21.

Desimone, R. (1991). Face-selective cells in the temporal cortex of monkeys. *Journal of Cognitive Neuroscience*, **3**, 1–8.

Diamond, R. and Carey, S. (1986). Why faces are and are not special: an effect of expertise. *Journal of Experimental Psychology: General*, **115**, 107–17.

Ellis, H. D. (1986). Processes underlying face recognition. In *The neuro-psychology of face perception and facial expression*, (ed. R. Bruyer), pp. 1–27. Lawrence Erlbaum, Hillsdale, NJ.

Ellis, A. W. (1992*a*). Cognitive mechanisms of face processing. *Philosophical Transactions of the Royal Society, London*, **B335**, 113–19.

Ellis, H. D. (1992*b*). The development of face processing skills. *Philosophical Transactions of the Royal Society, London*, **B335**, 105–11.

Ellis, H. D. and Young, A. W. (1989). Are faces special: In *Handbook of research on face processing*, (ed. A. W. Young and H. D. Ellis), pp. 1–26. North-Holland, Amsterdam.

Ellis, H. D. and Young, A. W. (1990). Accounting for delusional mis-identifications. *British Journal of Psychiatry*, **157**, 239–48.

Ellis, H. D., Shepherd, J. W., and Davies, G. M. (1979). Identification of familiar and unfamiliar faces from internal and external features: some implications for theories of face recognition. *Perception*, **8**, 431–9.

Ellis, A. W., Young, A. W., Flude, B. M., and Hay, D. C. (1987). Repetition priming of face recognition. *Quarterly Journal of Experimental Psychology*, **39A**, 193–210.

Ellis, A. W., Young, A. W., and Flude, B. M. (1990). Repetition priming and face processing: Priming occurs within the system that responds to the identity of a face. *Quarterly Journal of Experimental Psychology*, **42A**, 495–512.

Enlow, D. H. (1982). *Handbook of facial growth*. W. B. Saunders, Philadelphia, PA.

Field, T. M., Woodson, R., Greenberg, R., and Cohen, D. (1982). Discrimination and imitation of facial expressions by neonates. *Science*, **218**, 179–81.

Flude, B. M., Ellis, A. W., and Kay, J. (1989). Face processing and name retrieval in an anomic aphasic: names are stored separately from semantic information about familiar people. *Brain and Cognition*, **11**, 60–72.

Fowler, C. A. and Dekle, D. J. (1991). Listening with eye and hand: cross-modal contributions to speech perception. *Journal of Experimental Psychology: Human Perception and Performance*, **17**, 816–28.

Galton, F. (1883). *Inquiries into human faculty and its development*. Macmillan, London.

Gross, C. G. and Sergent, J. (1992). Face recognition. *Current Opinion in Neurobiology*, **2**, 156–61.

Grüsser, O.-J. and Landis, T. (1991). *Visual agnosias and other disturbances of visual perception and cognition*. Vol. 12 in *Vision and visual dysfunction*, (ed. J. R. Cronly-Dillon). Macmillan, Basingstoke.

Hanley, J. R. and Cowell, E. S. (1988). The effects of different types of retrieval cues on the recall of names of famous faces. *Memory and Cognition*, **16**, 545–55.

Hay, D. C. and Young, A. W. (1982). The human face. In *Normality and pathology in cognitive functions*, (ed. A. W. Ellis), pp. 173–202. Academic Press, London.

Hay, D. C., Young, A. W., and Ellis, A. W. (1991). Routes through the face recognition system. *Quarterly Journal of Experimental Psychology*, **43A**, 761–91.

Hécaen, H. and Angelergues, R. (1962). Agnosia for faces (prosopagnosia). *Archives of Neurology*, **7**, 92–100.

Heywood, C. A. and Cowey, A. (1992). The role of the 'face-cell' area in the discrimination and recognition of faces by monkeys. *Philosophical Transactions of the Royal Society, London*, **B335**, 31–8.

Hosie, J. A., Ellis, H. D., and Haig, N. D. (1988). The effect of feature displacement on the perception of well-known faces. *Perception*, **17**, 461–74.

Johnson, M. H., Dziurawiec, S., Ellis, H., and Morton, J. (1991). Newborns' preferential tracking of face-like stimuli and its subsequent decline. *Cognition*, **40**, 1–19.

Kurucz, J. and Feldmar, G. (1979). Prosopo-affective agnosia as a symptom of cerebral organic disease. *Journal of the American Geriatrics Society*, **27**, 225–30.

McClelland, J. L. and Rumelhart, D. E. (1985). Distributed memory and the representation of general and specific information. *Journal of Experimental Psychology: General*, **114**, 159–88.

McGurk, H. and MacDonald, J. (1976). Hearing lips and seeing voices. *Nature*, **264**, 746–8.

McNeil, J. E. and Warrington, E. K. (1993). Prosopagnosia: a face specific disorder. *Quarterly Journal of Experimental Psychology*, **46A**, 1–10.

Malone, D. R., Morris, H. H., Kay, M. C., and Levin, H. S. (1982). Prosopagnosia: a double dissociation between the recognition of familiar and unfamiliar faces. *Journal of Neurology, Neurosurgery, and Psychiatry*, **45**, 820–2.

Mark, L. S. and Todd, J. T. (1983). The perception of growth in three dimensions. *Perception and Psychophysics*, **33**, 193–6.

Maylor, E. A. (1990). Recognizing and naming faces: aging, memory retrieval, and the tip of the tongue state. *Journal of Gerontology: Psychological Sciences*, **45**, 215–26.

Meadows, J. C. (1974). The anatomical basis of prosopagnosia. *Journal of Neurology, Neurosurgery, and Psychiatry*, **37**, 489–501.

Meltzoff, A. N. and Moore, M. K. (1983). Newborn infants imitate adult facial gestures. *Child Development*, **545**, 702–9.

Morton, J. (1979). Facilitation in word recognition: experiments causing change in the logogen model. In *Processing of visible language*, Vol. 1, (ed. P. A. Kolers, M. Wrolstad, and H. Bouma), pp. 259–68. Plenum Press, New York.

Newcombe, F. (1979). The processing of visual information in prosopagnosia and acquired dyslexia: functional versus physiological interpretation. In

Research in psychology and medicine, Vol. 1, (ed. D. J. Oborne, M. M. Gruneberg, and J. R. Eiser), pp. 315–22. Academic Press, London.

Parry, F. M., Young, A. W., Saul, J. S. M., and Moss, A. (1991). Dissociable face processing impairments after brain injury. *Journal of Clinical and Experimental Neuropsychology*, **13**, 545–58.

Perrett, D. I., Hietanen, J. K., Oram, M. W., and Benson, P. J. (1992). Organization and functions of cells responsive to faces in the temporal cortex. *Philosophical Transactions of the Royal Society, London*, **B335**, 23–30.

Pittenger, J. B. and Shaw, R. E. (1975). Aging faces as viscal-elastic events: implications for a theory of nonrigid shape perception. *Journal of Experimental Psychology: Human Perception and Performance*, **1**, 374–82.

Rhodes, G., Brennan, S. E., and Carey, S. (1987). Identification and ratings of caricatures: implications for mental representations of faces. *Cognitive Psychology*, **19**, 473–97.

Rhodes, G., Brake, S., Taylor, K., and Tan, S. (1989). Expertise and configural coding in face recognition. *British Journal of Psychology*, **80**, 313–31.

Roberts, T. and Bruce, V. (1988). Feature saliency in judging the sex and familiarity of faces. *Perception*, **17**, 475–81.

Sergent, J. and Poncet, M. (1990). From covert to overt recognition of faces in a prosopagnosic patient. *Brain*, **113**, 989–1004.

Sergent, J., Ohta, S., and MacDonald, B. (1992). Functional neuroanatomy of face and object processing: a positron emission tomography study. *Brain*, **115**, 15–36.

Studdert-Kennedy, M. (1983). On learning to speak. *Human Neurobiology*, **2**, 191–5.

Tranel, D., Damasio, A. R., and Damasio, H. (1988). Intact recognition of facial expression, gender, and age in patients with impaired recognition of face identity. *Neurology*, **38**, 690–6.

Valentine, T. (1988). Upside-down faces: a review of the effect of inversion upon face recognition. *British Journal of Psychology*, **79**, 471–91.

Valentine, T. (1991). A unified account of the effects of distinctiveness, inversion, and race in face recognition. *Quarterly Journal of Experimental Psychology*, **43A**, 161–204.

Valentine, T. and Bruce, V. (1986). The effects of distinctiveness in recognising and classifying faces. *Perception*, **15**, 525–35.

Valentine, T. and Endo, M. (1992). Towards an exemplar model of face processing: the effects of race and distinctiveness. *Quarterly Journal of Experimental Psychology*, **44A**, 671–703.

Valentine, T. and Ferrara, A. (1991). Typicality in categorization, recognition and identification: evidence from face recognition. *British Journal of Psychology*, **82**, 87–102.

Vinter, A. (1985). La capacité d'imitation à la naissance: elle existe, mais que signifie-t-elle? *Canadian Journal of Psychology*, **39**, 16–33.

Warrington, E. K. and James, M. (1967). An experimental investigation of facial recognition in patients with unilateral cerebral lesions. *Cortex*, **3**, 317–26.

Yin, R. K. (1969). Looking at upside-down faces. *Journal of Experimental Psychology*, **81**, 141–5.

Yin, R. K. (1970). Face recognition by brain-injured patients: a dissociable ability? *Neuropsychologia*, **8**, 395–402.

Young, A. W. (1992). Face recognition impairments. *Philosophical Transactions of the Royal Society, London*, **B335**, 47–54.

Young, A. W. and Bruce, V. (1991). Perceptual categories and the computation of 'grandmother'. *European Journal of Cognitive Psychology*, **3**, 5–49.

Young, A. W. and de Haan, E. H. F. (1992). Face recognition and awareness after brain injury. In *The neuropsychology of consciousness*, (ed. A. D. Milner and M. D. Rugg), pp. 69–90. Academic Press, London.

Young, A. W. and Ellis, H. D. (1989). Semantic processing. In *Handbook of research on face processing*, (ed. A. W. Young and H. D. Ellis), pp. 235–62. North-Holland, Amsterdam.

Young, A. W., Hay, D. C., McWeeny, K. H., Flude, B. M., and Ellis, A. W. (1985*a*). Matching familiar and unfamiliar faces on internal and external features. *Perception*, **14**, 737–46.

Young, A. W., Hay, D. C., and Ellis, A. W. (1985*b*). The faces that launched a thousand slips: everyday difficulties and errors in recognizing people. *British Journal of Psychology*, **76**, 495–523.

Young, A. W., McWeeny, K. H., Hay, D. C., and Ellis, A. W. (1986*a*). Matching familiar and unfamiliar faces on identity and expression. *Psychological Research*, **48**, 63–8.

Young, A. W., McWeeny, K. H., Hay, D. C., and Ellis, A. W. (1986*b*). Access to identity-specific semantic codes from familiar faces. *Quarterly Journal of Experimental Psychology*, **38A**, 271–95.

Young, A. W., Hellawell, D., and Hay, D. C. (1987). Configurational information in face perception. *Perception*, **16**, 747–59.

Young, A. W., Hellawell, D., and de Haan, E. H. F. (1988). Cross-domain semantic priming in normal subjects and a prosopagnosic patient. *Quarterly Journal of Experimental Psychology*, **40A**, 561–80.

Young, A. W., Reid, I., Wright, S., and Hellawell, D. (1993). Face processing impairments and Capgras delusion. *British Journal of Psychiatry*, **162**, 695–8.

5

Everyday errors in face recognition

Reprinted in slightly modified form from Young, A. W. (1993),
Recognising friends and acquaintances, in *Memory in everyday life*, (ed.
G. M. Davies and R. H. Logie), pp. 325–50, North-Holland, Amsterdam.
With kind permission of Elsevier Science – NL, Sara Burgerhartstraat 25,
1055 KV Amsterdam, The Netherlands.

Species which depend heavily on social interaction need to be able to
recognize other individuals. Without this ability, we would not be able
to react differently to different people, modifying our behaviour
according to what we know about them.

For humans, face recognition is particularly important. It provides a
way of identifying people which is usually effective (there are not so
many identical twins in the world), which is not affected by changes in
clothing, and which can cope with a reasonable range of other transformations, such as altered hairstyles, beards, and so on (at least for
highly familiar people). Of course, what we are primarily concerned to
do is to identify *people*, so we also rely on voice, gait, clothing, context,
and any other appropriate source of information to some extent, and
occasionally (for example, on the telephone) one of these will play a
primary role.

The apparent ease with which we recognize faces can be deceptive.
Searle (1984, p. 52) used face recognition as an example of an ability
that happens quite effortlessly and which he considered may not require
complex computation. Instead, Searle argued that it could be 'as simple
and automatic as making footprints in the sand'. However, there are
quite serious problems with this view, not the least of which is that
there is no evidence that sand can *recognize* your footprints (Ellis *et al.*
1987). In fact, there are many occasions in everyday life when misidentifications and other forms of error can happen (Young *et al.* 1985).
Although these mistakes mostly occur outside our conscious control,
they reflect the organization of a system which is nothing like as simple
as Searle implied.

A variety of different sources of evidence can be used to gain insight into the organization of the recognition system. These include everyday errors, errors induced in the laboratory, errors due to brain pathology, and performance in 'real-life' or laboratory-based tasks. I will draw on all of these methods. None of them is free from problems of interpretation, but such interpretive problems are mostly quite different between one method and another. This allows us to be reasonably confident about conclusions which are supported by more than one source of evidence, and it is pleasing that these divergent types of study have pointed toward consistent conclusions.

Long-term memory for people

Important examples of the 'real-life' approach come from the work of Bahrick et al. (1975) and Bahrick (1984), who have reported studies of memory for people across long intervals, using faces or names of former students or classmates.

Bahrick et al. (1975) examined recognition of the names and faces of people taken from high school yearbooks. In this way, they were able to test the recognition abilities of groups of subjects across mean intervals ranging from 3 months to 48 years since graduation. Subjects were tested on several tasks, including their ability to recognize whether or not names were of former classmates, to recognize whether or not faces were of former classmates, and to name a given face.

Table 5.1 shows percentages of faces and names correctly recognized, and of faces which could be named by groups of subjects in Bahrick et al.'s (1975) study. These percentages have been statistically adjusted to take into account what would otherwise be uncontrolled variables, such as differences in the sizes of the classes in different years. It is clear that the ability to recognize faces and names of former classmates remains good for many years after graduation. For faces, there is virtually

Table 5.1 Percentages of faces and names correctly recognized, and of faces which could be named, by subjects in Bahrick et al.'s (1975) study

	Years since graduation								
	0.25	0.75	2	4	7	15	26	34	48
Name recognition	91	91	79	93	87	93	78	74	77
Face recognition	89	91	78	94	92	92	93	90	73
Face naming	68	59	36	64	57	41	53	47	18

Table 5.2 Percentages of faces and names of former students correctly recognized, and of faces which could be named, by college teachers in Bahrick's (1984) study

	Years since class was taught			
	0.03	1.13	4.15	8.08
Name recognition	88	76	59	52
Face recognition	69	48	31	26
Face naming	36	6	3	0

unimpaired performance across a 34 year interval, whereas performance for names begins to fall after 15 years. Face naming is never as good as face recognition, and shows a gradual decline as the years go by. Of course, face naming can be considered a recall task, and recall is often poorer than recognition, but as we will see later there are other reasons which also contribute to the difficulty of face naming.

Although one cannot but be impressed by the levels of performance achieved across such long retention intervals, there is no doubt that the faces and names used in Bahrick *et al.*'s (1975) study would mostly have been very thoroughly learnt at high school, and some subjects may have engaged in modest amounts of rehearsal during the retention interval (by reminiscing, or even consulting their yearbooks, though this was one of the variables Bahrick *et al.* took into account).

Subsequent work by Bahrick (1984) looked at what happens when the people have been much less well learnt, by using an introductory University class which had met 3–5 times per week across a 10 week period. Table 5.2 gives percentages of faces and names of former students which could be correctly recognized by people who had taught this class, and percentages of faces which could be named. As might be expected, there was much poorer retention for these less familiar people. The better recognition of names than faces probably reflects the fact that the teachers would come across the students' names more often than their faces (in class lists, and when marking essays, tests, and so on).

Recognition errors and their implications

Bahrick's work demonstrates that people who have initially been very thoroughly learnt can be recognized across remarkable periods of time. In everyday life, however, we are often dealing with people who are much less well known to us, or who can crop up in different or unusual

Table 5.3 Examples of main types of everyday error noted by Young *et al.* (1985)

	Number of records
Person misidentified:	314
'I was driving under a bridge in Lancaster: it was a bit dark. I saw a person with a dog and I thought it was a dog owner I sometimes see there. It was the wrong type of dog: I thought he must have got a new one!'	
Person unrecognized:	114
'I was going through the doors to B floor of the library when a friend said, 'Hello'. I at first ignored him, thinking that he must have been talking to the person behind me.'	
Person seemed familiar only:	233
'I was in the bank, waiting to be served. I saw a person and I knew there was something familiar immediately. After a few seconds I realized she was from a shop on campus or a secretary of one of the departments. I eventually remembered by a process of elimination.'	
Difficulty in retrieving full details of person:	190
'I saw a poster advertising a film. I knew what films the actress was in and knew she does a lot of Beckett, but it was another minute before I could remember her name.'	
Decision problems:	35
'I was going into my house, when I thought I saw Steve Duck outside. I wouldn't expect to see him there, and I decided it wasn't him. I became sure it wasn't him, but then he spoke to me.'	

contexts. Errors and mistakes in recognition therefore occur with appreciable frequency, though they are often quickly corrected.

Young *et al.* (1985) collected a corpus of everyday errors by carrying out a 'diary' study in which 22 people took notes on mistakes they made in recognizing people across an eight-week period. To standardized these records, they were made on forms which provided a checklist of things to note. After discounting the records made during the first week (this was considered to be the time needed to learn how to use the record sheets properly), there were 922 records of difficulties and errors. Most of these records could readily be grouped into different types, and Table 5.3 gives examples of the main types.

The most common form of error (314 records) involved mis-identifications of one person for another. In most of these cases (272 records), an unfamiliar person was misidentified as someone familiar, and often highly familiar (54 per cent). A substantial proportion of such misidentifications of an unfamiliar person as someone familiar (55 per cent) were associated with poor viewing or hearing conditions, and were quickly corrected (69 per cent within 10 seconds), usually when a better view was obtained (76 per cent).

Other common types of error noted by Young *et al.* (1985) can be considered to reflect breakdown at different levels of recognition:

1. Failure to recognize a familiar person, who is mistakenly thought to be unfamiliar (114 records). This type of error is readily understandable when the person was of low familiarity, seen under poor conditions, or when the error was quickly corrected, but there were also a proportion of records for which such factors did not seem to apply (42 per cent involved familiar people, for 82 per cent conditions were not described as poor, and 58 per cent lasted more than 10 seconds).

2. Recognizing a person as familiar, but being unable to bring to mind any other details, such as her or his occupation or name (233 records). This problem was often felt to be due to meeting someone who was not very well known in an unexpected context. In the cases where the person's identity was successfully discovered (135 records) only 13 per cent involved highly familiar people, and only 16 per cent happened in contexts where that person would be expected.

3. Recognizing the person as familiar and remembering appropriate semantic information about them, whilst failing to remember certain other details, such as her or his name (190 records). Of the cases where this problem was successfully resolved (135 records) the overwhelming majority (99 per cent) involved inability to remember the person's name. This could happen even to highly familiar people (33 per cent of these records), and usually lasted for some time (71 per cent over 10 seconds).

Young *et al.* (1985) pointed out that the orderliness of these types of everyday error is consistent with the idea that the recognition system uses some form of sequential access to different types of information, in the order familiarity, then semantics, then name retrieval. This had first been suggested by Hay and Young (1982), and it has since been more fully developed by Bruce and Young (1986) and partially implemented in slightly modified form as an interactive activation model by Burton *et al.* (1990) and Burton and Bruce (1992). We will return to consider this interactive activation simulation later.

The model suggested by Young *et al.* (1985) is shown in Fig. 5.1. They

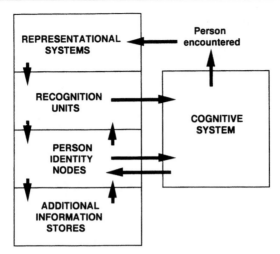

Fig. 5.1 Outline of the model of person recognition proposed by Young *et al.* (1985).

proposed that representional systems create descriptions of the person encountered (face, build, clothing, voice, etc.). These are used to activate recognition units that signal the degree of resemblance to known people, and can access information about the person's identity, and then additional information such as the person's name. Recognition of a person thus involves sequential stages of perceptual classification as a familiar visual or auditory pattern (by domain-specific recognition units for faces, voices, seen or heard names, etc.), semantic classification (involving domain-independent person identity nodes which can access previously learnt semantic information from the person's face, voice, or name), and access to additional but less essential information, which would include name retrieval. This is only meant as an idealized sequence, and would be compatible with a 'cascade' mode of operation. Note that in this model, recognition from facial and non-facial sources of information (such as hearing the person's voice, or hearing or reading their name) is achieved by domain-specific input systems (for faces, voices, names, etc.) which can feed into the common set of domain-independent person identity nodes.

Young *et al.* (1985) also suggested that the cognitive system is involved in evaluating information given by the recognition system. A number of the records arising from their 'diary' study involved decision problems. For example, diarists were sometimes uncertain about whether or not they had correctly identified a particular person (35 records), often because the context made that person unlikely (see Table 5.3). Hence, we can see that we are constantly monitoring the results of more automatic aspects of recognition, to correct errors we sometimes make, and also because different types of information must sometimes be intentionally combined and evaluated. Inappropriate context is a particularly clear example of this, but so is the encountered person's behaviour. Thomson (1986) mentions a field study, in which the daughter of an Australian couple was asked to stand outside a London hotel when her parents thought she was in Australia. They recognized their daughter, but when she (deliberately) did not respond, her father apologized; 'I am terribly sorry, I thought you were someone else'.

A further reason for emphasizing the importance of decision processes involves the phenomenon of resemblance. Young *et al.* (1985) found that most of their diarists noted experiences which were not really errors as such, but based on 'resemblance only'. Table 5.4 gives examples, which parallel some of the types of everyday error noted in Table 5.3.

Most diarists commented that they could not keep systematic records of these 'resemblance' experiences, because the criterion for what was or was not a noteworthy resemblance tended to shift around. But the fact that they happen at all is of interest. In general, they seem to be based on correct rejections of resemblances signalled by outputs from recognition units or person identity nodes. The basis of such rejections could involve an insufficient degree of resemblance ('it didn't look quite like her'), conflict between resemblances ('her hair was like her but the face wasn't'), or inappropriate context ('I knew she was abroad'). The descriptions of these experiences often pointed out that under different

Table 5.4 Examples of experiences involving 'resemblance' which paralleled some of the types of everyday error noted by Young *et al.* (1985)

Person misidentified:
  I saw someone I didn't know in the town centre in Preston. I thought he looked very like Mike Read (a disc jockey and television personality). I might have thought it was Mike Read in different circumstances where I might have expected to see him.'

Person seemed familiar only:
  'I thought he looked like someone I knew, but I couldn't think who. It took me a couple of minutes to work out who he looked like.'

Difficulty in retrieving full details of person:
  'I was watching a film on television. An actor reminded me of someone; I knew it was an American actor he reminded me of, but I couldn't get the name. I thought of Cary Grant and Gregory Peck. I finally had to ask the name of the actor I was thinking of (Rock Hudson).'

circumstances a genuine error might have been made, which is consistent with our suggestion that they reflect decision processes.

Errors in the laboratory

We have seen that everyday errors can be readily assimilated to the model shown in Fig. 5.1. However, diary studies suffer a number of limitations which might affect this conclusion (Reason and Lucas 1984). The most important of these are that diarists' reports might show biases, perhaps because they only report the errors they find particularly striking or easy to interpret themselves, or because they deliberately or unintentionally distort the errors in ways that make them seem more clear-cut than was actually the case.

Additional confirmation of the findings of diary studies of everyday errors has therefore been obtained from studies of errors made under laboratory conditions (Hanley and Cowell 1988; Hay *et al*. 1991). These studies can eliminate reporting biases, because errors can be examined systematically as they are made, yet still find the types of error predicted by the sequential access view.

Hay *et al*. (1991) showed 190 slides of famous and unfamiliar faces to 12 subjects who were asked whether or not each face was a familiar person, what the person's occupation was, and what the person's name was. All of the errors made fell into patterns which would be expected from a 'sequential access' model (such as Fig. 5.1), and examples were found for all of the types of error predicted by such a model. More importantly, there were no examples of any of the types of error which would be incompatible with a sequential access model. For example, the sequential access model does not permit errors in which a subject can name a particular face without being able to give the person's occupation. Reassuringly, this never happened (such errors were not found in Young *et al*.'s diary study, either).

In a further study, Hay *et al*. (1991) examined more carefully just what information was available when subjects made different types of error, and explored the types of cue needed to correct difficulties arising at each stage. Results were again compatible with a sequential access model.

A similar cueing technique has been used very effectively by Hanley and Cowell (1988), and Table 5.5 shows some of the data from their study. Subjects who found a face they should have recognized to be unfamiliar, familiar only, or who knew who the person was but couldn't remember the name, were cued by giving them semantic information about the person (e.g. 'Brilliant cavalier Spanish golfer whose raw

Table 5.5 Percentages of names successfully retrieved after cueing by semantic information or initials in Hanley and Cowell's (1988) study

	Initial knowledge state		
	Face unfamiliar	Face familiar only	Face familiar, and occupation known
Semantic cue	41	52	35
Initials cue	12	22	47

ability and adventurous play have carried him to the top of the sport') or a card containing the initials of four famous people (one being the person in question), with blank spaces for the remaining letters (S– – – B– – – – – – – – – –, etc.). As is clear from Table 5.5, the semantic cue was most effective at promoting correct naming when subjects found the face familiar only, whereas cueing with the initials was more effective when the occupation was already known. This is exactly as would be expected from a sequential access model, since people who find the face familiar only would be 'blocked' at the stage where semantic information would normally be retrieved (and hence assisted by a semantic cue more than an initials cue), whereas people who can already access the occupation but are still searching for the name should derive more benefit from an initials cue than a semantic cue (they have the semantic information already).

An interesting extension of the cueing technique was made by Brennen *et al.* (1990), who induced tip-of-the-tongue states by asking subjects to name famous people from snippets of semantic information (e.g. 'The nervous man with the knife, in the shower scene in Hitchcock's *Psycho*'). When subjects felt sure that they knew the name, but could not recall it (the tip-of-the-tongue state, or TOT; see Brown 1991) they were cued either by giving the target person's initials, by showing the person's face, or by repeating the question (to control for the possibility that more time, or a second attempt, is all that is required). Results are shown in Table 5.6. The important point is that

Table 5.6 Percentages of tip-of-the-tongue states resolved by different types of cue in Brennen *et al.'s* (1990) study

Initials cue	Face cue	Repeat question
47	15	11

cueing from seeing the person's face had no effect, since no more TOTs were resolved by this than by simply repeating the question. This is as a sequential access model would predict (the face can only access the same pool of semantic information as the original question, but the 'block' occurs later).

Experiments with normal subjects

Studies of everyday and laboratory errors have produced a number of findings which fit a sequential access model of recognition. Experiments with normal subjects have also given strong support to this suggestion (for reviews see Bruce and Young 1986; Bruce 1988; Young and Ellis 1989). For example, speeded reaction time tasks have shown that faces can be classified as familiar more quickly than they can be classified by occupation, and that categorizations based on occupations or other semantic properties can be achieved more quickly than categorizations which require access to the person's name. Such findings hold even when task demands and response requirements are carefully equated (Young *et al.* 1986*a*, *b*, 1988; Johnston and Bruce 1990).

Another way to explore the sequential access model is through its implications for ability to remember faces. Bruce (1982, 1983) suggested that episodic memory for faces would depend on the number of different memory codes available at test. One could consider activation of a face recognition unit as requiring a structural code, accessing occupation and other biographical information as involving semantic codes, and name retrieval as requiring access to a name output code. If access to each of these codes from the face occurs in a fixed sequence, we would expect better retention when people are asked to name faces than when they are asked to decide their occupations, and that this would in turn lead to better retention than merely assessing the face's familiarity, since fewer distinct codes need to be generated in each case. Exactly this result was found by Hanley *et al.* (1990), both in recall and recognition tests.

As Hanley *et al.* (1990) note, this result is less easy to reconcile with some other views about memory. For example, there is no particular reason (other than the sequential access model) for proposing that naming a face would lead to more 'deep' processing than accessing the bearer's occupation, so that a 'levels of processing' framework (Craik and Lockhart 1972) can only apply if the properties of the sequential access model are assumed. Similarly, transfer appropriate processing (Morris *et al.* 1977) does not provide an adequate account, because the same advantage for named faces was found when subjects had to recall their occupations at test (i.e. memory for faces that have been named on initial presentation is better regardless of whether one is tested on recalling names or occupations).

Although there is evidence of sequential access within the face recognition system, other types of facial information may be determined independently from identity (Bruce and Young 1986; Parry *et al.* 1991). It is not necessary to analyse the facial expression before a person's identity can be known, or vice versa; there are parallel systems for extracting these different types of information from seen faces. Studies of normal subjects and people with brain injuries support this conclusion (for reviews, see Bruce and Young 1986; Young and Bruce 1991). For example, Young *et al.* (1986c) and Bruce (1986) found that analysis of expressions was no faster for familiar faces than for unfamiliar faces, whereas familiarity did influence decisions when the person's identity was involved (faster matching of the identities of photographs of familiar than unfamiliar faces, etc.).

As has been pointed out, Fig. 5.1 emphasizes not only sequential access to different types of information from seen faces, but also the importance of decision processes. Further support for this view has come from the work of Bartlett and Fulton (1991) and Bartlett *et al.* (1991), who have shown how it can help to account for age differences in recognition memory for faces.

The particular difficulty of name retrieval

Everybody recognizes the irritating top-of-the-tongue (TOT) state, when we seem to know everything relevant except the word we are looking for, and it does seem that inability to bring to mind people's names is a common cause of TOTs (Brown 1991).

Diary and laboratory studies have been able to reveal a number of interesting features of TOTs involving problems in name retrieval (Yarmey 1973; Williams and Hollan 1981; Read and Bruce 1982; Reason and Mycielska 1982; Reason and Lucas 1984; Young *et al.* 1985; Cohen and Faulkner 1986; Hanley and Cowell 1988; Brennen *et al.* 1990; Maylor 1990). Like other TOTs, they often involve partial information states in which quite a lot is known about the intended target name. Cohen and Faulkner (1986) described a person searching for the name 'Kepler' who managed to generate the candidates Keller, Klemperer, Kellet, and Kendler. Although all of these were rejected, this person knew that the target was foreign-sounding, and that Keller was the closest to it.

Another feature of many TOTs is that recall of the correct name is blocked by an incorrect name that is persistently brought to mind. Reason and Lucas (1984) have shown that these blocking items usually share structural, contextual, or semantic features with the target, but tend to be items that have been more recently and more frequently encountered than the target itself. They suggested that blocked TOT states thus show the susceptibility to strong habit intrusions previously noted in several other types of everyday error by Reason and Mycielska (1982).

Why should it be so hard to remember names? The question is deceptively simple, and we still don't have a definitive answer. Although I have emphasized here the importance of the sequential access account, which holds that information is accessed from seen faces in the order familiarity, then semantics, then name, this does not in itself account for why name retrieval should come last in this sequence.

Bahrick's work (Bahrick *et al.* 1975; Bahrick 1984) showed that there is no evidence of anything like comparable difficulty for name *recognition*; when we read or hear the name 'Buddy Holly', we don't usually have any trouble remembering who he was. Bruce and Young (1986) therefore drew a careful distinction between *name input* codes which allow us to recognize a seen or heard name, and the *name output* codes involved in saying (or writing) that name. Problems arise when we have to generate a name output code in response to a face, voice, or some other cue which contains no information about what the name might be.

Of course, we noted earlier that face naming can be considered a recall task, and recall is often poorer than recognition. However, remembering an arbitrary fact, such as that Buddy Holly was American rather than British, is just as much a recall task, yet it does not usually cause the same type of problem (Johnston and Bruce 1990). A satisfactory explanation must be sought elsewhere.

One promising approach has been to study how names and occupations are learnt in the laboratory. Cohen and Faulkner (1986) constructed brief biographical descriptions of fictitious people. Each biography contained a person's name, the name of a place associated with that person, the person's occupation, and the person's hobby; for example, 'a well-known amateur photographer, Ann Collins, lives near Bristol where she works as a health visitor'. As Table 5.7 shows, recall of the people's names from these biographies was poorer than recall of the other types of information. Notice, too, that the place names were recalled relatively well; it is not simply the fact that names are proper nouns which somehow accounts for our problems in remembering them.

Table 5.7 Percentages of each type of target correctly recalled by 26 year-olds in Cohen and Faulkner's (1986) study

First names	Surnames	Places	Occupations	Hobbies
31	30	62	69	68

A similar study was carried out by McWeeny *et al.* (1987), who taught subjects a fictitious surname and occupation to each of 16 unfamiliar faces. The surnames were found to be much harder to learn than the occupations, and this was true even for items which can be used as names or occupations (Baker, Cook, etc.). It is more difficult to recall that a person's surname is Farmer than to recall that she or he is a farmer. Hence the explanation of differences between the ease of recall of names and occupations does not lie in properties of the items themselves, such as imageability, frequency, and so on.

Cohen and Faulkner (1986) suggested that occupations, hobbies, and place names like Glasgow or Bristol may be semantically richer than people's names, which remain essentially arbitrary labels. There are some points in favour of this view. Cohen (1990) found that subjects could remember people's possessions (e.g. that Mr Hobbs has a dog) as well as they could remember their occupations (Mr Hobbs is a pilot), but that recall of nonsense possessions (Mr Hobbs has a blick) was as poor as recall of names. Furthermore, when Cohen (1990) paired potentially meaningful names (e.g. Mr Baker) with meaningless occupations (Mr Baker is a ryman), it was the occupations which were worse recalled. Hence, subjects can make use of the imageability and meaningfulness of names, but only if this does not conflict with other semantic information about the person.

A related view was suggested by Young *et al.* (1988), who proposed that names are stored separately from other semantic information because they are nowadays arbitrary labels which are only occasionally required; when we see a face, we want to know who that person is, but it would be unnecessary and inconvenient if the name were constantly brought to mind.

An alternative possibility has been suggested by Burton and Bruce (1992), based on the interactive activation simulation of the Bruce and Young (1986) model developed by Burton *et al.* (1990). The basic architecture of this simulation is shown in Fig. 5.2. For present purposes, its key features are that it allows input systems for recognizing seen faces (FRUs) or names (Name input) to converge on a common set of person identity nodes (PINs) which are in turn linked to items of

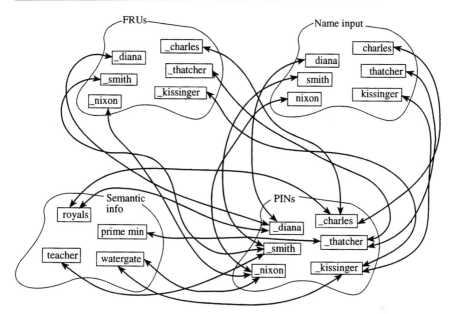

Fig. 5.2 Central architecture of Burton and co-workers' (1990) interactive activation model.

semantic information. Unlike the type of model shown in Fig. 5.1, this implementation proposes a clear separation of PINs and semantic information; decisions about a face or name's familiarity are then taken at the PINs.

Burton *et al.* (1990) were able to show that this implementation can simulate several reported results on face recognition. However, at first sight there is no mechanism to account for problems in accessing name output codes, since a separate store for these is not built in to the model.

In fact, Burton and Bruce (1992) noticed that the model shown in Fig. 5.1 can already account for problems in name retrieval, if it is assumed that names are stored along with other types of semantic information. A name like 'Richard Nixon' would then be linked to a single PIN (for Richard Nixon), whereas most items of semantic information would be linked to several PINs (e.g. 'politician' to PINs for Richard Nixon, John Major, Neil Kinnock, etc.). It is a property of this type of architecture that the less interconnectivity an item has, the less easy it is to boost its activation. Hence, Burton and Bruce (1992) point out that problems of name retrieval may simply reflect the status of names as relatively unique items of semantic information.

This proposal is appealingly simple. More importantly, it makes clear predictions which can be confirmed or falsified. For example, it suggests that people will be as poor at recalling other facts which are unique to individuals as they are at remembering names, and this could be tested in TOT states or brain-injured patients. The results of such studies are awaited with interest.

Normal and pathological errors

The point that errors can correspond to breakdowns arising at different stages or levels of recognition can also be demonstrated in cases of neuropsychological impairment (Young 1992). In such cases, a brain-injured patient will make characteristic errors to many seen faces. To investigate this, my colleagues and I have developed 'line-up' tasks in which faces or names are presented one at a time, and subjects are asked to rate familiarity, provide information about the person's identity (such as occupation), and (for faces only) give the person's name. The tasks we have used most often include faces and names of 20 highly familiar famous people, 20 less familiar people, and 20 unknown people. Table 5.8 presents data from the highly familiar faces and names in these line-up tasks for three cases with contrasting patterns of impairment.

PH (who had occipito-temporal lesions caused by a closed head injury; de Haan *et al.* 1987) shows the 'prosopagnosic' pattern of impaired recognition of faces with relatively well preserved recognition of familiar people from their names. For ME (vasculitic disorder; de Haan *et al.* (1991a) the sense of familiarity of faces or names was well preserved, but access to semantic information and name retrieval (from the face) were severely compromised. For EST (surgery to remove a left temporal lobe tumour; Flude *et al.* 1989) only name retrieval seemed to be affected.

The published reports on these cases present other data to substantiate the patterns seen in Table 5.8. The findings are consistent with a hierarchy of impairments corresponding to the idea that access to familiarity, occupation, and name retrieval involve sequential stages. There are breakdowns at each level, but those at the earlier levels affect later stages: without a sense of the face's familiarity, occupation and name cannot be retrieved (PH); if the face is familiar but the occupation cannot be retrieved, then it can't be named either (ME); and name retrieval impairments can exist even when familiarity and occupation are available (EST). These neuropsychological impairments thus parallel some of the patterns of error which arise as transitory phenomena for normal people in everyday life (Young *et al.* 1985).

Turning to the names line-up, ME shows the same pattern of im-

Table 5.8 Recognition of highly familiar people in line-up tasks by PH (de Haan *et al.* 1987), ME (de Haan *et al.* 1991*a*), and EST (Flude *et al.* 1989) (Asterisked scores are more than 3.10 standard deviations below the control mean, $p < 0.001$.)

	Faces line-up			Names line-up	
	Familiarity (1–7 rating scale)	Occupation (max. = 20)	Name (max. = 20)	Familiarity (1–7 rating scale)	Occupation (max. = 20)
PH	1.2***	0***	0***	6.0	19
ME	5.7	7***	7***	6.2	8***
EST	5.2	17	3***	6.9	19
Control subjects ($N = 28$)					
Mean	5.98	18.86	16.25	6.27	19.66
SD	0.51	1.15	2.81	0.63	0.84

pairment as for faces, whereas PH does not. Hence there is a difference between impairments which primarily affect the recognition of faces, and those which seem to involve person recognition regardless of the input domain. In line with Bruce and Young's (1986) suggestion that it is the earlier stages of recognition that are domain specific, when there is a problem with recognition from faces and not names (as for PH), all stages of face recognition (familiarity, occupation, and name retrieval) are affected.

Also important are patterns of impairment which do not occur. As for everyday and laboratory errors, we have never found a brain-injured person for whom name retrieval was normal from seen faces but access to occupations was impaired. Such a case would clearly violate the proposed hierarchy, and therefore be of considerable theoretical importance.

There may also be neuropsychological cases which involve impaired decision mechanisms. Young *et al.* (1990) reported the case of SP, who showed severe impairments on face recognition tasks yet did not think that she had any problems in face recognition. SP continued to show lack of insight into this impairment even when directly confronted with its consequences on formal testing. Her errors mostly involved either failures to find a face familiar at all, or misidentification as another familiar person.

In contrast to her unawareness of her face recognition problems, SP showed adequate insight into other physical and cognitive impairments produced by her illness. Young *et al.* (1990) proposed that her lack of insight into her face recognition problems was due to impairment of

domain-specific monitoring abilities needed to monitor our own performance in everyday life. As we have seen from everyday errors,
monitoring is necessary to correct the mistakes we sometimes make,
and also because different types of information must sometimes
intentionally be combined and evaluated.

As Bisiach *et al.* (1986) point out, the existence of such a deficit-
specific loss of insight suggests that this monitoring does not involve a
common central monitoring mechanism, but is to some degree
decentralized.

Overview

We have seen that there is a rich interplay between naturalistic and
laboratory studies of person recognition, and that it is possible to arrive
at closely comparable conclusions from studies of everyday errors,
errors in the laboratory, effects of brain injury, and laboratory experiments involving learning or speeded decisions. This interplay is highly
desirable, and greatly enhances the confidence we can place in the
conclusions reached. Computational studies and simulations (Burton *et
al.* 1990; Burton and Bruce 1992) are now adding enhanced precision
and predictive power.

I have discussed in detail the sequential access model of recognition
derived initially from Hay and Young's (1982) proposals (see Fig. 5.1).
This model may not necessarily be correct, but it has proved valuable in
stimulating studies whose results will have to be encompassed by any
more adequate theory, and the sequential access view remains readily
consistent with most of the available findings.

Many of the properties of person recognition revealed by these
investigations show obvious parallels to other forms of recognition and
memory. For example, although TOT errors seem to be very common in
person recognition, there are no obvious differences between TOTs
involving people's names and TOTs caused in any other way. Similarly,
the sequential access model shown in Fig. 5.1 has parallels with more
general models of object recognition (see Bruce and Young 1986).

So is there anything special about recognition of people? To some
extent, it depends on what one means by special (Hay and Young
1982; Ellis and Young 1989). However, there are some clear pointers
from the neuropsychological literature, where quite specific deficits are
occasionally reported.

In most cases of brain injury involving impaired recognition of people,
there are also other problems. Considering the cases shown in Table 5.8,

PH was poor at recognizing stimuli from other visual categories with many similar exemplars (e.g. cars and flowers; de Haan *et al.* 1987, 1991*b*), ME showed long-term memory deficits on several tasks, though her other cognitive abilities were well preserved (de Haan *et al.* 1991*a*), and EST had severe word-finding difficulties (Flude *et al.* 1989). However, it is always risky to infer that one deficit causes the other in cases with co-occurring neurological impairments, and more powerful evidence comes in the form of fractionation of deficits which often co-occur, showing that their association is not inevitable (Ellis and Young 1988; Shallice 1988).

Such fractionations have been reported for face and person recognition impairments. De Renzi (1986) and De Renzi *et al.* (1991) described prosopagnosic patients whose problems did seem to affect faces only, and Ellis *et al* (1989) investigated a patient who showed impaired recognition of familiar people despite good performance of many memory tests. Semenza and Zettin (1988, 1989) described cases of impaired name retrieval for proper names only, and McKenna and Warrington (1980) reported a case of impaired ability to retrieve people's names with relatively well preserved retrieval of other proper names.

Thus there is some evidence that recognition impairments can take face- or person-specific forms. As we began by noting, the brain may develop specialized recognition and memory systems to underpin the need to be able to interact differently with different individuals.

References

Bahrick, H. P. (1984). Memory for people. In *Everyday memory, actions and absent-mindedness*, (ed. J. E. Harris and P. E. Morris), pp. 19–34. Academic Press, London.

Bahrick, H. P., Bahrick, P. O., and Wittlinger, R. P. (1975). Fifty years of memory for names and faces: a cross-sectional approach. *Journal of Experimental Psychology: General*, **104**, 54–75.

Bartlett, J. and Fulton, A. (1991). Familiarity and recognition of faces in old age. *Memory and Cognition*, **19**, 229–38.

Bartlett, J., Strater, L., and Fulton, A. (1991). False recency and false fame of faces in young adulthood and old age. *Memory and Cognition*, **19**, 177–88.

Bisiach, E., Valler, G., Perani, D., Papagno, C., and Berti, A. (1986). Unawareness of disease following lesions of the right hemisphere: anosognosia for hemiplegia and anosognosia for hemianopia. *Neuropsychologia*, **24**, 471–82.

Brennen, T., Baguley, T., Bright, J., and Bruce, V. (1990). Resolving semantically induced top-of-the-tongue states for proper nouns. *Memory and Cognition*, **18**, 339–47.

Brown, A. S. (1991). A review of the tip-of-the-tongue experience. *Psychological Bulletin*, **109**, 204–23.

Bruce, V. (1982). Changing faces: visual and non-visual coding processes in face recognition. *British Journal of Psychology*, **73**, 105–16.

Bruce, V. (1983). Recognizing faces. *Philosophical Transactions of the Royal Society of London*, **B302**, 423–36.

Bruce, V. (1986). Influences of familiarity on the processing of faces. *Perception*, **15**, 387–97.

Bruce, V. (1988). *Recognising faces*. Erlbaum, London.

Bruce, V. and Young, A. (1986). Understanding face recognition. *British Journal of Psychology*, **77**, 305–27.

Burton, A. M. and Bruce, V. (1992). I recognise your face but I can't remember your name: a simple explanation? *British Journal of Psychology*, **83**, 45–60.

Burton, A. M., Bruce, V., and Johnston, R. A. (1990). Understanding face recognition with an interactive activation model. *British Journal of Psychology*, **81**, 361–80.

Cohen, G. (1990). Why is it difficult to put names to faces? *British Journal of Psychology*, **81**, 287–97.

Cohen, G. and Faulkner, D. (1986). Memory for proper names: age differences in retrieval. *British Journal of Developmental Psychology*, **4**, 187–97.

Craik, F. I. M. and Lockhart, R. S. (1972). Levels of processing: a framework for memory research. *Journal of Verbal Learning and Verbal Behavior*, **11**, 671–84.

De Haan, E. H. F., Young, A., and Newcombe, F. (1987). Face recognition without awareness. *Cognitive Neuropsychology*, **4**. 385–415.

De Haan, E. H. F., Young, A. W., and Newcombe, F. (1991a). A dissociation between the sense of familiarity and access to semantic information concerning familiar people. *European Journal of Cognitive Psychology*, **3**, 51–67.

De Haan, E. H. F., Young, A. W., and Newcombe, F. (1991b). Covert and overt recognition in prosopagnosia. *Brain*, **114**, 2575–91.

De Renzi, E. (1986). Current issues in prosopagnosia. In *Aspects of face processing*, (ed. H. D. Ellis, M. A. Jeeves, F. Newcombe, and A. Young), pp. 243–53. Nijhoff, Dordrecht.

De Renzi, E., Faglioni, P., Grossi, D., and Nichelli, P. (1991). Apperceptive and associative forms of prosopagnosia. *Cortex*, **27**, 213–21.

Ellis, A. W. and Young, A. W. (1988). *Human cognitive neuropsychology*. Erlbaum, London.

Ellis, H. D. and Young, A. W. (1989). Are faces special? In *Handbook of research on face processing*, (ed. A. W. Young and H. D. Ellis), pp. 1–26. North-Holland, Amsterdam.

Ellis, A. W., Young, A. W., and Hay, D. C. (1987). Modelling the recognition of faces and words. In *Modelling cognition*, (ed. P. E. Morris), pp. 269–97. Wiley, Chichester.

Ellis, A. W. and Young, A. W., and Critchley, E. M. R. (1989). Loss of memory for people following temporal lobe damage. *Brain*, **112**, 1469–83.

Flude, B. M., Ellis, A. W., and Kay, J. (1989). Face processing and name retrieval in an anomic aphasic: names are stored separately from semantic information about familiar people. *Brain and Cognition*, **11**, 60–72.

Hanley, J. R. and Cowell, E. S. (1988). The effects of different types of retrieval cues on the recall of names of famous faces. *Memory and Cognition*, **16**, 545–55.

Hanley, J. R., Pearson, N. A., and Howard, L. A. (1990). The effects of different types of encoding task on memory for famous faces and names. *Quarterly Journal of Experimental Psychology*, **42A**, 741–62.

Hay, D. C. and Young, A. W. (1982). The human face. In *Normality and pathology in cognitive functions*, (ed. A. W. Ellis), pp. 173–202. Academic Press, London.

Hay, D. C., Young, A. W., and Ellis, A. W. (1991). Routes through the face recognition system. *Quarterly Journal of Experimental Psychology*, **43A**, 761–91.

Johnston, R. A. and Bruce, V. (1990). Lost properties? Retrieval differences between name codes and semantic codes for familiar people. *Psychological Research*, **52**. 62–7.

McKenna, P. and Warrington, E. K. (1980). Testing for nominal dysphasia. *Journal of Neurology, Neurosurgery, and Psychiatry*, **43**, 781–8.

McWeeny, K. H., Young, A. W., Hay, D. C., and Ellis, A. W. (1987). Putting names to faces. *British Journal of Psychology*, **78**, 143–9.

Maylor, E. A. (1990). Recognizing and naming faces: aging, memory retrieval, and the tip of the tongue state. *Journal of Gerontology: Psychological Sciences*, **45**, 215–26.

Morris, C. D., Bransford, J. D., and Franks, J. J. (1977). Levels of processing versus transfer appropriate processing. *Journal of Verbal Learning and Verbal Behavior*, **16**, 519–33.

Parry, F. M., Young, A. W., Saul, J. S. M., and Moss, A. (1991). Dissociable face processing impairments after brain injury. *Journal of Clinical and Experimental Neuropsychology*, **13**, 545–58.

Read, J. D. and Bruce, D. (1982). Longitudinal tracking of difficult memory retrievals. *Cognitive Psychology*, **14**, 280–300.

Reason, J. and Lucas, D. (1984). Using cognitive diaries to investigate naturally occurring memory blocks. In *Everyday memory, actions and absentmindedness*, (ed. J. E. Harris and P. E. Morris), pp. 53–70. Academic Press, London.

Reason, J. and Mycielska, K. (1982). *Absent-minded? The psychology of mental lapses and everyday errors*. Prentice-Hall, New Jersey.

Searle, J. (1984). *Minds, brains and science: The 1984 Reith lectures*. British Broadcasting Corporation, London.

Semenza, C. and Zettin, M. (1988). Generating proper names: a case of selective inability. *Cognitive Neuropsychology*, **5**, 711–21.

Semenza, C. and Zettin, M. (1989). Evidence from aphasia for the role of proper names as pure referring expressions. *Nature*, **342**, 678–9.

Shallice, T. (1988). *From neuropsychology to mental structure*. Cambridge University Press.

Thomson, D. M. (1986). Face recognition: more than a feeling of familiarity? In *Aspects of face processing*, (ed. H. D. Ellis, M. A. Jeeves, F. Newcombe, and A. Young), pp. 118–22. Nijhoff, Dordrecht.

Williams, M. D. and Hollan, J. D. (1981). The process of retrieval from very long-term memory. *Cognitive Science*, **5**, 87–119.

Yarmey, A. D. (1973). I recognize your face but I can't remember your name: further evidence on the tip-of-the-tongue phenomenon. *Memory and Cognition*, **1**, 287–90.

Young, A. W. (1992). Face recognition impairments. *Philosophical Transactions of the Royal Society of London*, **B335**, 47–54.

Young, A. W. and Bruce, V. (1991). Perceptual categories and the computation of 'grandmother'. *European Journal of Cognitive Psychology*, **3**, 5–49.

Young, A. W. and Ellis, H. D. (1989). Semantic processing. In *Handbook of research on face processing*, (ed. A. W. Young and H. D. Ellis), pp. 235–62. North-Holland, Amsterdam.

Young, A. W., Hay, D. C., and Ellis, A. W. (1985). The faces that launched a thousand slips: everyday difficulties and errors in recognizing people. *British Journal of Psychology*, **76**, 495–523.

Young, A. W., McWeeny, K. H., Ellis, A. W., and Hay, D. C. (1985*a*). Naming and categorizing faces and written names. *Quarterly Journal of Experimental Psychology*, **38A**, 297–318.

Young, A. W., McWeeny, K. H., Hay, D. C., and Ellis, A. W. (1986*b*). Access to identity-specific semantic codes from familiar faces. *Quarterly Journal of Experimental Psychology*, **38A**, 271–95.

Young, A. W., McWeeny, K. H., Hay, D. C., and Ellis, A. W. (1986*c*). Matching familiar and unfamiliar faces on identity and expression. *Psychological Research*, **48**, 63–8.

Young, A. W., Ellis, A. W., and Flude, B. M. (1988). Accessing stored information about familiar people. *Psychological Research*, **50**, 111–15.

Young, A. W., de Haan, E. H. F., and Newcombe, F. (1990). Unawareness of impaired face recognition. *Brain and Cognition*, **14**, 1–18.

6

Dissociable deficits after brain injury

Reprinted in slightly modified form from Young, A. W., Newcombe, F., de Haan, E. H. F., Small, M., and Hay, D. C. (1993). Face perception after brain injury: selective impairments affecting identity and expression. *Brain*, **116**, 941–59. With kind permission of co-authors and Oxford University Press.

Summary

Current theoretical models of face perception postulate separate routes for processing information needed in the recognition of a familiar face, for matching photographs of unfamiliar faces, and for the analysis of facial expressions. The present study investigated this claim in a group of ex-servicemen who had sustained unilateral brain injuries affecting posterior areas of the left or right cerebral hemisphere. Care was taken to confirm the nature of impairment by using two different tasks to assess each of the three theoretically defined abilities (leading to a total of six tasks). We adopted a stringent application of the double dissociation methodology to investigate the pattern of performance across tasks of individual ex-servicemen. A selective impairment was defined as a significantly impoverished performance on both tests of a specific ability, while all other tasks were performed within normal limits. In addition, we used both accuracy and response latency measures to substantiate evidence for spared or defective abilities. The results showed selective impairments of all three abilities on accuracy scores. Response latency data confirmed the finding of a selective deficit in the processing of facial expressions, but produced evidence suggesting that impairments affecting familiar face recognition and unfamiliar face matching were not completely independent from each other in this group of ex-servicemen.

Introduction

Faces form the source for a multitude of inferences. From a perceived face we are able to determine gender, age, and whether we would buy a used car from the person in question. We can assess the emotional state of the person, and by observing the movements of the lips and tongue we gain additional information regarding any verbal message which the speaker is trying to convey. Finally, the face constitutes the principal cue for visual identification of people we know.

Functional models based on evidence from experimental psychology and neuropsychology have proposed that the processes involved in these different abilities are to some extent independent from each other. As an example we take the model of Bruce and Young (1986), but there are a number of similar suggestions (e.g. Hay and Young 1982; Ellis 1983, 1986; Rhodes 1985). Figure 6.1 shows schematically the arrangement of functional components involved in processing the different types of

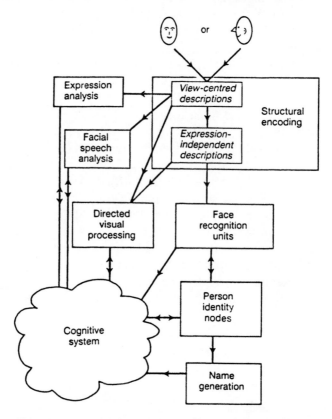

Fig. 6.1 Bruce and Young's (1986) model of face recognition.

information which can be derived from a seen face, according to Bruce and Young (1986). They propose that the processing of facial expressions, the recognition of familiar faces, and the matching of unfamiliar faces (to decide whether two photographs are of the same or different people) involve different cognitive processes, and that each utilizes a distinct functional pathway. Facial expression analysis is held to be dependent upon view-centred descriptions created at the structural encoding stage, whereas familiar face recognition requires access to face recognition units via expression-independent descriptions. Unfamiliar face matching is dependent upon both view-centred and expression-independent descriptions, which are utilized by the directed visual processing module. Thus, according to Bruce and Young (1986), the pathway needed for unfamiliar face matching is different from that used in facial expression recognition, which in turn is distinct from the pathway used in familiar face recognition.

Although there are data from studies of normal subjects to support this putative organization (see Bruce and Young 1986; Bruce 1988; Young and Bruce 1991), one of the principal sources of supporting evidence comes from neuropsychological studies, where there is evidence of dissociable impairments affecting different types of face processing ability. The strongest clinical evidence of independent functional components comes in the form of double dissociations (Teuber 1955; Weiskrantz 1968; Shallice 1988); if Patient X has problems with ability A but is normal on ability B and patient Y shows the reverse pattern it is inferred that A and B rely at least in part on different processes. In terms of the Bruce and Young (1986) model it is thought that cerebral injury can cause specific face processing impairments, including dissociable impairments for expression analysis, familiar face recognition, and unfamiliar face matching. Of particular importance in the present context is the claim that familiar face recognition, directed visual processing (needed for matching views of unfamiliar faces), and facial expression analysis are independent of each other. This heterarchic organization is counterintuitive for many people, but it is suggested by a number of clinical reports.

Of course, a term like 'facial expression analysis' may well cover a collection of separate abilities which are themselves susceptible to further fractionation. For example, it is noticeable that in the Bruce and Young (1986) model, where the recognition of familiar faces was of primary interest, a number of functional components was held to underlie familiar face recognition, whereas expression analysis was much less precisely specified. But this broad brush treatment forms a useful level of description for an initial characterization of face processing impairments, and there are reports in the literature consistent with a division of impairments into those affecting familiar face recognition, unfamiliar face matching, and expression analysis.

Evidence for a dissociation between the recognition of familiar faces and the processing of facial expressions was reported by Bornstein (1963), and has been confirmed by Tranel *et al.* (1988), who found that some patients with severe impairments of facial identity recognition showed relatively intact ability to recognize facial expressions. Conversely, Kurucz *et al.* (1979) and Kurucz and Feldmar (1979) reported findings indicating that disoriented patients were impaired at recognizing facial expressions and at recognizing American presidents, but the identity and expression impairments did not correlate with each other.

There is also evidence for distinct processing pathways involved in the recognition of facial expressions and the matching of unfamiliar faces. For example, Bowers *et al.* (1985) tested patients with left hemisphere lesions, right hemisphere lesions, and people with no neurological disease. They were given a series of perceptual and associative facial affect and identity judgement tasks, and tasks requiring naming of emotions and pointing to named emotions. The patients with right hemisphere lesions were significantly impaired on all the affect and identity tasks. However, their impairment on facial affect tasks remained even when their perceptual identity performance was statistically partialled out. Bowers *et al.* (1985) thus showed that this impairment in interpreting facial expressions could not be entirely due to a visuoperceptual deficit, but was instead, to some extent, dependent upon different cognitive processes to those necessary for matching views of faces. Other reports of dissociable impairments of facial expression recognition and unfamiliar face matching after brain injury have been made by Cicone *et al.* (1980), Pizzamiglio *et al.* (1983), and Etcoff (1984).

The literature also supports the idea of differences between pathways for the recognition of familiar faces and processing of unfamiliar faces. This was suggested by Warrington and James (1967) from a study of the effects of unilateral cerebral lesions. Later, Benton and Van Allen (1972) reported a case of prosopagnosia in which performance on an unfamiliar face matching task was well within the normal range. Similar findings in prosopagnosic cases were made by Rondot *et al.* (1967), Assal (1969), and several subsequent authors. Conversely, patients with unfamiliar face matching impairments often are not clinically prosopagnosic (Tzavaras *et al.* 1970). Benton (1980) thus emphasized the independence of impairments affecting familiar face recognition and unfamiliar face matching, and this has been confirmed in subsequent reports by Malone *et al.* (1982) and McNeil and Warrington (1991).

The studies we have considered so far provide evidence of dissociable face processing abilities when examining various permutations of two of the three face processing abilities of interest here (facial expression, familiar face recognition, and unfamiliar face matching). However, some limited evidence has also been reported when measuring all three abilities in one test session. Parry *et al.* (1991) tested a group of head-injured patients, using a common forced-choice procedure to examine facial expression recognition, familiar face recognition, and unfamiliar face matching. The use of a common general procedure ensured that each task was equivalent in its demands and response requirements. Cases of dissociable impairment affecting only one of the face processing tasks were reported by Parry *et al.* (1991), though none of these dissociable impairments was particularly severe in the group of patients investigated.

Taking all of this evidence together, it can be concluded that, although there is substantial support for the existence of dissociable impairments of face processing, there are limitations which make some of the findings difficult to interpret unequivocally. We will draw attention here to five such problems, which the present study seeks to eliminate.

Limitations of comparisons across different reports

The comparisons needed to establish a double dissociation are often made across single dissociations noted in two separate reports. Thus, one study might describe a patient with normal perception of expression but with problems in identifying familiar faces. A separate report published some years later may then describe the opposite pattern. The problem is that different tests will usually have been used to assess the abilities in question, which makes it difficult to compare the patients directly. This problem is exacerbated when the comparisons concerned do not involve what Shallice (1988) calls 'classical' dissociations. In a classical dissociation, the preserved abilities are within the normal range of performance. Many of the reports in the literature do not meet this ideal, since they describe patients for whom one ability is more obviously impaired than another, but neither ability is demonstrably normal.

Double dissociations are only double

The Bruce and Young (1986) model claims at least three independent functional routes. However, the dissociations on which this proposal is built have often been noted from comparisons of only two abilities. Farah (1991) has drawn attention to the fact that such pairwise comparisons can conceal potentially important associations between what might otherwise be considered separate impairments. Therefore, if one wants to test the theoretical hypothesis of three independent pathways for different types of facial information, the appropriate technique must be to examine dissociations between all three types of ability in the same study.

The chance that it happened by chance

Single case studies have assumed a privileged role in cognitive neuro-psychology (Marshall and Newcombe 1984; Ellis and Young 1988; Shallice 1988; McCarthy and Warrington 1990) because of the emphasis now placed on dissociable impairments. However, it is clear that group studies will continue to be appropriate for answering certain types of question (Newcombe and Marshall 1988), but few studies have addressed issues like the size of the group of patients from which a particular case was drawn in relation to the significance levels of the impairment. This problem is not particularly evident in investigations of single cases with severe, stable, and long-standing impairment (Shallice 1979), but it does arise when striking, single-case examples are drawn from a group study, as is sometimes done.

The dangers of equating tests and abilities

In a number of studies a functional deficit has been inferred from the performance on a single test. It is clear, however, that there are a number of reasons, apart from a defect in the hypothesized function, why a patient may fail a certain test (Shallice 1988). One way to avoid spurious dissociations created by this problem is to ensure that the different tests used are closely comparable in terms of demands and response requirements (Parry *et al.* 1991). Alternatively, one could deliberately choose two very different tests of the same ability, and consider that a brain-injured person is impaired on that ability only if he/she performs poorly on both tests. This is the procedure used here, since we are concerned to establish dissociations between quite broadly specified abilities (such as familiar face recognition, unfamiliar face matching, and analysis of expressions). It also has the advantage of addressing 'The chance that it happened by chance' (*above*), since impairment on two different tests of the same ability and on no other tests is a most unlikely chance pattern.

Strategies and trade-offs

This point is well illustrated by the research on preserved unfamiliar face matching skills in patients with face recognition problems. As Newcombe (1979) indicated, patients often apply idiosyncratic strategies to compensate for their matching problem (such as careful use of feature-based comparisons, which has been noted in several of the published reports). They can then reach normal levels of performance on accuracy scores by what may well be abnormal means. Since these alternative strategies tend to be time-consuming, it is possible to control for this problem by measuring response latency as well as accuracy scores. The use of response latencies also allows evaluation of whether brain-injured patients will trade speed for accuracy in tasks which are sensitive to their impaired abilities. The use of idiosyncratic strategies forms an example of the more general possibility of speed–accuracy trade-offs.

The present study was designed to investigate the hypothesis of independent routes for familiar face identification, unfamiliar face matching, and expression analysis. In order to avoid the problems raised above, we employed the following procedures. The study was carried out with an unselected group of brain-injured people known to have unilateral missile wound lesions affecting posterior areas of the left or right cerebral hemisphere. Two separate tests using different techniques were used to assess each of the three abilities (i.e. there were two different tests of face identification, two different tests of unfamiliar face matching, and two different tests of expression analysis). Where possible, both accuracy and response latency measures were taken, so that the possibilities of trade-offs of speed against accuracy and use of unusual but time-consuming strategies could be evaluated. Finally, we made use of an important modification to the concept of double dissociation; that of *selective impairment*, which was defined as a significantly reduced performance on tests of that ability, but with a normal performance on all tests of the other abilities.

Methods

Subjects

Ex-servicemen who had sustained a penetrating missile injury to the brain during World War II (32 cases) or subsequent military service (a further two cases) participated in this study. This experimental group is particularly valuable for scientific research because of the well defined, traumatic lesions incurred at a similar age in what were previously young, healthy brains (Newcombe 1969). All of the ex-servicemen were right-handed, and all had suffered injuries leading to unilateral lesions involving the posterior half of the brain, as confirmed by operation reports and/or CT scan. Lesion locations were assessed in terms of side affected (i.e. affecting the left or the right cerebral hemisphere) and site within the hemisphere, on the basis of all available neurological information, which could include autopsy, CT, and surgical records for different cases. All men who had suffered further head injury or neurological incident since the initial missile wound were excluded from the investigation.

The main tests reported here were carried out during the years 1983–1989, as part of a larger investigation of the ex-servicemen's visual and spatial abilities. During this period, ex-servicemen attended the Neuropsychology Unit at the Radcliffe Infirmary to participate in a series of tests spread across sessions lasting two or more days. Some of the ex-servicemen attended for more than one such test series. A set of face processing tasks formed part of this investigation, and the initial set of tasks was added to at later stages, as new tasks were developed for different purposes. The tasks of interest to the present report will be described later, but it is probably useful to note at this point that the face identification ('faces line-up') task, Benton test and sequential matching task formed part of the original set of tasks with which we began the study in 1983, the two expression tasks were added somewhat later, and the familiarity decision task later still. All of the tasks included an accuracy measure, and we also collected response latency measurements where possible.

The data presented here are for all of the ex-servicemen with unilateral lesions involving posterior brain areas who had performed all of the six tasks of principal interest at some point during this time period. It is important to note that these data thus relate to ex-servicemen chosen only on the basis that they had unilateral injuries affecting posterior regions of one hemisphere, and that they had completed all of the tasks. There has been no attempt to create matched groups with equivalent left- and right-sided lesions for this report; instead, our aim is to present all the data relevant to considering putative selective impairments in individual ex-servicemen.

Full data were available across the six tasks for 34 ex-servicemen with unilateral posterior lesions. Fifteen ex-servicemen had suffered a right hemisphere lesion, and the remaining 19 had left-sided damage. Thirty-two healthy subjects who were comparable to the experimental group with respect to age, educational background and general intellectual abilities served as controls. Given the age of the participants (most of the ex-servicemen are now in their 60s and 70s) it was thought prudent to screen all subjects with tests of verbal and non-verbal intelligence, using the Mill Hill synonyms test and the standard progressive matrices tests, respectively. Scores fell within normal ranges for the age groups concerned; there was no evidence of generalized intellectual deterioration.

The work received approval from the Central Oxford Research Ethics Committee and all participants gave informed consent.

Tasks

Our intention was to examine impairments affecting the recognition of familiar faces, unfamiliar face matching, and the analysis of facial expressions. For each of these abilities, we chose two separate tests which involved different procedures.

Familiar face recognition

We assessed ability to identify highly familiar faces by providing the name or appropriate semantic information, and ability to classify faces as familiar or unfamiliar.

Face identification: This task involved 20 black-and-white slides of highly familiar famous faces, presented one at a time with unlimited exposure duration. These 20 faces were selected from an original item pool of 190 face photographs on the basis of good recognition performance for 12 normal subjects. Correct identification of each face was inferred when the subject was able to give the name or the exact occupation of the bearer of the face, or any other information that would uniquely identify the person.

This task forms part of the faces line-up we have used in single case studies (e.g. Young *et al.* 1990; de Haan *et al.* 1991). The score used here was the number of faces (out of the possible maximum of 20) successfully identified. Because a certain amount of negotiation and questioning could be needed to establish that a face really had been identified as belonging to a specific person (vague comments like 'something to do with politics' were not accepted), the task could not be timed.

Familiarity decision: The stimuli consisted of 32 black-and-white photographs of faces, 16 familiar and 16 unfamiliar, presented one at a time in a pseudo-random order on back-projected slides. Each face subtended a visual angle of approximately 10°, and appeared on the screen for 4 s. Subjects were instructed to decide as quickly and as accurately as possible whether the face was familiar or not. They made their responses by moving a lever situated at the vertical midline of their body. The lever could be moved away from ('familiar face') or towards the body ('unfamiliar face') in order to signal the two possible responses. Large paper signs marked 'FAMILIAR' and 'UNFAMILIAR' were positioned at each end of the lever's travel to indicate the appropriate direction. At stimulus onset an Electronic Developments timer was started, and this was stopped by the subject moving the response lever in either direction.

The task began with eight practice trials, after which reaction times and errors to each of the 32 test faces were noted, allowing the calculation of an overall accuracy score (for the 32 trials) and mean reaction time for correct responses for each subject. For a more detailed description of this task, see Newcombe *et al.* (1989).

Unfamiliar face matching

Two separate tests were used to assess efficiency in matching photographs of unfamiliar faces on identity. These were the Benton test of facial recognition, which uses simultaneous presentation of a target and multiple choices, and a sequential matching task in which the target was removed before a single comparison face was presented.

Benton test: This is a well standardized simultaneous matching task, using unfamiliar faces and a multiple-choice format (Benton *et al.* 1983). In the first six trials the identical view to the target face has to be found among five foils. The remaining 16 items require the subject to select three out of six photographs shown simultaneously, as being the same person as shown in the target photograph. These photographs differ from the target in either orientation or in lighting conditions.

The Benton test is scored in terms of the total number of items correctly matched. However, because of our concern about the possible use of idiosyncratic strategies or speed–accuracy trade-offs, the time spent on each target item was also recorded by hand with a stopwatch.

Sequential matching task: The second unfamiliar face matching task involved a series of 32 trials in which two slides were presented one after the other for 4 s each, with an inter-stimulus interval of 1 s. The visual angle of the stimuli was approximately 10° for each face. In half of the trials, the two slides were of different people, while in the other half two different views of the same face were shown. The slides were black-and-white photographs of male students' faces, so that age and sex were homogeneous, and members of 'different' pairs were matched to have similar hairstyles. The first slide was always a full-face view, whereas the second slide was a three-quarter view (turned to the left in half the trials, and to the right in the other half). Because the two views shown to subjects differed in orientation, a purely pictorial match would be insufficient for accurate performance (cf. Hay and Young 1982); the task demanded the construction of a more abstract representation of the face, and directed visual processing.

Subjects were instructed to make a 'same person' versus 'different person' decision, and the task began with eight practice trials. They were asked to be as accurate as possible, and the task was not timed. Accuracy scores (out of a possible maximum of 32 correct) were recorded.

Facial expression analysis

Tests which required matching and recognition of emotional facial expressions were used.

Expression matching: A photograph of a target face displaying one of six possible emotions (anger, sadness, happiness, disgust, surprise, fear) had to be matched against four simultaneously presented alternatives (another view of the target emotion, and three distractors selected from the remaining possibilities). All five photographs (target + alternatives) were of faces of five different people of the same sex, taken from the Ekman and Friesen (1976) series. They were mounted in a vertical arrangement on a sheet of paper, with the target face slightly separated from the others at the top of the page, and the four alternative choices in line below it, as described by Gainotti (1989).

Subjects were asked to point to the face which showed the same expression as the target face, and the task began with four practice trials, followed by 18 experimental trials (three using each of the six emotions as target). A score out of a possible maximum of 18 correct choices was recorded, and response latencies to each target were taken by hand with a stopwatch.

This task was kindly made available to us by Professor Gainotti, Professor Pizzamiglio, and Dr Zoccolotti of Rome University, with the consent of their collaborator Professor Paul Ekman of the University of California.

Expression recognition: In the second expression task, subjects were shown a photograph of a face from the Ekman and Friesen (1976) series, displaying one of the six possible emotional expressions (anger, sadness, happiness, disgust, surprise, fear). The names of the six emotions were printed below the photograph in a vertical alignment, with the order of these emotion names randomized across trials. The subject was asked to decide which of the emotion names best described the facial expression shown.

There were six practice trials and 24 experimental trials (four for each of the six emotions), leading to an accuracy score out of a possible maximum of 24 correct choices. Again, response latencies to each target were taken by hand with a stopwatch.

The photographs of facial expressions used as targets in this task were chosen because they were all accurately recognized in the norms published by Ekman and Friesen (1976). Mean accuracies for our chosen targets are: anger = 98 per cent; sadness = 96 per cent; happiness = 100 per cent; disgust = 96 per cent; surprise = 96 per cent; fear = 93 per cent. None of the target photographs had been used as targets in the expression matching task.

Results

Our aim was to identify selective impairments affecting familiar face recognition, unfamiliar face matching, and facial expression analysis. There were two separate tests to assess each ability, with accuracy scores for all tests and response latency data available from four of the six tests.

To evaluate the individual performances of the ex-servicemen, means and standard deviations of the control group were calculated for all six tests. These were used to derive cut-offs for scores which differed from the control mean at 0.05 ($z > 1.65$), 0.01 ($z > 2.33$), and 0.001 ($z > 3.10$) levels of statistical significance. A full listing of each ex-serviceman's scores on each of the measures used is given in Appendix 1.

As Appendix 1 shows, there were quite a number of impaired scores for particular tasks in the group of ex-servicemen. However, there are also a large number of observations tabulated in Appendix 1, so that some of these impairments might arise 'by chance', and we have also already noted that there will be many potential reasons as to why any one person might fail any particular test, since no attempt was made to match the demands and response requirements across the different tasks. Here, though, we are concerned with *selective impairments* affecting familiar face recognition, unfamiliar face matching, or facial expression analysis. We therefore adopted a stringent criterion, in which a selective impairment was inferred only when an ex-serviceman performed with an accuracy significantly below the control mean (at least at a 0.05 level) on both tasks directed at measuring a specific ability, while his performance was within the normal range on all (four) other tests. Here we report data for all of the ex-servicemen who met this criterion, considering the accuracy data first, and then response latencies. We then consider a few other cases with interesting patterns of performance.

Background information for all of the individual cases we discuss is given in Appendix 2, which includes details concerning visual field defects, epilepsy, motor and somatosensory defects, ages, Mill Hill vocabulary scale IQs, and raw scores on the standard progressive matrices (raw scores are given for this test, rather than IQ equivalents, because of concern that the original published norms may now overestimate performance).

Accuracy data

There were seven ex-servicemen whose pattern of performance met our criteria for selective impairment when their response accuracies were examined. Their performances are summarized in Table 6.1, with additional background information in Appendix 2. P.G. was severely impaired at recognizing familiar faces, but his accuracies for matching unfamiliar faces and inferring emotional state from a person's face were normal. Conversely, S.J. was selectively impaired in accuracy of matching unfamiliar faces, while G.M., V.M., W.M., T.R., and A.S. only had problems in processing facial expressions. Hence, using accuracy scores, we found in our group of ex-servicemen at least one example of each of the three possible types of selective impairment, with one man showing impaired recognition of familiar faces, one showing impaired matching of unfamiliar faces, and no less than five men showing impaired analysis of facial expressions.

Table 6.1 Accuracy scores for the control group and seven ex-servicemen who showed selective impairments of performance on familiar face recognition, unfamiliar face matching, and expression analysis tasks

	Familiar face recognition		Unfamiliar face matching		Expression analysis	
	Familiarity decision	Identification	Benton test	Sequential matching	Matching	Recognition
Right hemisphere lesions						
P.G.: familiar face recognition impaired	23***	10***	40	26	16	20
S.J.: unfailiar face matching impaired	31	18	38*	22***	17	23
Left hemisphere lesions						
V.M.: expression analysis impaired	32	18	42	27	13*	16**
A.S.: expression analysis impaired	30	20	48	28	12*	18*
T.R.: expression analysis impaired	30	17	45	26	11**	18*
W.M.: expression analysis impaired	32	19	42	30	13*	18*
G.M.: expression analysis impaired	31	16	42	28	9***	15***
Control subjects ($n = 32$)						
Mean	31.30	18.34	44.22	28.42	16.23	20.93
Standard deviation	1.38	1.56	3.07	2.01	1.91	1.70
Maximum possible score for each test	32	20	54	32	18	24

Asterisked scores are significantly below the control mean: *$p < 0.05$; **$p < 0.01$; ***$p < 0.001$.

From Table 6.1 it is also apparent that the man with the selective impairment of face recognition accuracy (P.G.) and the man with the unfamiliar face matching deficit (S.J.) both had right hemisphere lesions. All five patients with a selective expression impairment had left hemisphere damage.

Response latencies

In order to probe more deeply into the nature of the selective deficits found in the accuracy data, we proceeded to examine the response latencies of these seven men. These are summarized in Table 6.2. Unfortunately, two of the six tasks we used were untimed (sequential unfamiliar face matching and familiar face identification), but the four tasks that were timed included at least one task to represent each of the three types of face processing ability found to be susceptible to selective impairment of accuracy scores.

With regard to the selective deficit in expression analysis, the response times corroborated the accuracy data, with the exception of A.S., who was somewhat slow in his responses to the Benton (unfamiliar face matching) test. However, A.S.'s accuracy on the Benton was significantly *above* the control mean ($z = 1.88, p < 0.05$), suggesting that his increased time was due to his taking extra care with this task, rather than impaired performance *per se*.

For the other four men with selective impairments of expression analysis on accuracy scores, the response times simply confirmed the picture. This was especially clear for G.M. and W.M., whose response times were also impaired on both expression tasks, but normal for familiar face recognition (familiarity decision task) and unfamiliar face matching (Benton test). This corresponds exactly to the pattern found in the accuracy data. V.M. was only somewhat slower on the expression matching task, and for T.R. there was no significant increase in response times on any of the tasks. Even so, there was no evidence of any speed–accuracy trade-off affecting T.R.'s performance of expression tasks, since he was neither particularly slow nor particular fast when performing these. For these four men (G.M., V.M., W.M., and T.R.), then, there is strong evidence of selective impairment in facial expression analysis when the accuracy scores and response latencies are considered together.

This finding of a selective impairment of expression analysis in ex-servicemen with unilateral left hemisphere lesions is initially surprising, since a link between facial expression processing and the right hemisphere has often been noted in other clinical reports. We therefore

Table 6.2 Mean response latencies in seconds for the control group and the seven ex-servicemen who had shown selective deficits of performance accuracy on familiar face recognition, unfamiliar face matching, and expression analysis tasks

	Familiar face recognition (familiarity decision)	Unfamiliar face matching (Benton test)	Expression analysis	
			Matching	Recognition
Right hemisphere lesions				
P.G.: familiar face recognition accuracy impaired	2.3***	65.3***	11.6**	5.9*
S.J.: unfamiliar face matching accuracy impaired	2.3***	50.4***	6.5	3.7
Left hemisphere lesions				
V.M.: expression analysis accuracy impaired	1.5	24.1	8.8*	5.5
A.S.: expression analysis accuracy impaired	1.2	40.0*	6.8	4.1
T.R.: expression analysis accuracy impaired	1.0	32.8	3.1	3.1
W.M.: expression analysis accuracy impaired	1.1	25.3	9.5*	9.1***
G.M.: expression analysis accuracy impaired	1.3	33.1	12.0***	12.7***
Control subjects (n = 32)				
Mean	1.2	23.4	5.4	3.7
Standard deviation	0.3	8.3	2.0	1.3

Asterisked latencies are significantly below the control mean: *$p < 0.05$; **$p < 0.01$; ***$p < 0.001$.

considered whether it might reflect some form of naming problem. However, one of the expression tasks (facial expression matching) did not require name retrieval at all, and in the other expression task (facial expression recognition) the printed names of the six expressions were always in view, which would minimize the effects of any problem in name retrieval. Moreover, two cases with a specific defect in naming facial expressions have been described elsewhere (Bowers and Heilman 1984; Rapcsak *et al.* 1989), and both of these patients had a right hemisphere lesion. These cases are, however, different from the impairments of expression analysis described here, because they were both reported as being able to match facial expressions but unable to name them. Our ex-servicemen showed a selective impairment of expression analysis which encompassed *both* matching and choice of the correct label.

Table 6.3 shows data for the naming abilities of V.M., A.S., T.R., W.M., and G.M. from our series. It includes notes on the clinical presence of aphasia at the time of injury (1940s) and in the 1980s, details of performance on a standard picture naming task (Newcombe

Table 6.3 Naming abilities for the ex-servicemen with selective deficits of performance on expression analysis tasks

Clinical impression	Picture naming	Fluency		
		Objects	Animals	F, A, S
V.M.: some aphasia noted on discharge in 1940s; mild residual naming difficulty in 1980s	19/26[†]	11*	9*	26
A.S.: some aphasia noted on discharge in 1945; none apparent in 1980s	23/26	33	16	46
T.R.: some aphasia noted in 1940s; none apparent in 1980s	24/26	18	10	17
W.M.: some aphasia noted in 1940s; none apparent in 1980s	22/26	24	21	23
G.M.: some aphasia noted in 1940s; some expressive aphasia but good comprehension in 1980s	20/26	16	9*	NT
Control subjects				
Mean		30.20	16.95	46.19
Standard deviation		10.45	4.42	20.65

Asterisked scores are significantly below the control mean: *$p < 0.05$; **$p < 0.01$; ***$p < 0.001$.
[†]A score below the range for non-dysphasic patients from Newcombe *et al.* 1971.
NT indicates no data available.

et al. 1971), and verbal fluencies for generating object names (1 min), animal names (1 min), and words beginning with F, A, and S (1 min each). Norms for the object names and animal names come from 20 controls from the Radcliffe Infirmary series, those for F, A, and S letter fluency come from normal controls reported by Hanley *et al.* (1990).

Although all of these individuals were noted as having some degree of aphasia when they were injured in the 1940s, one needs to bear in mind that this would apply to most men with left hemisphere lesions; Russell and Espir (1961) noted that only 113 of 348 right-handers with left-sided brain lesions were recorded as not being clinically aphasic. The more important point is that in three of these cases there was no longer any clinical or test evidence of significant naming problems. We can therefore conclude that there are no compelling grounds for linking the selective deficits of expression analysis we observed to aphasic difficulties.

Although we were able to identify these clear cases of selective impairments of expression analysis, the position concerning the men with a selective deficit in accuracy of familiar face recognition and unfamiliar face matching became less clear-cut when their response times were considered. Both men showed significantly long response latencies on the tests which had also demonstrated the impairment on accuracy scores. In addition, however, they showed increased response times elsewhere. Specifically, P.G. (who had shown a selective impairment of familiar face recognition on accuracy scores) was impaired on all tasks where response times were taken, and S.J. (who had shown a selective impairment of accuracy of unfamiliar face matching) was also slow at recognizing familiar faces (face familiarity decision task). In these cases, then, we cannot rule out the possibility that some (S.J.) or even all (P.G.) of the tasks carried out with normal accuracy might have been achieved by diligent application of unusual strategies, or by using defective abilities with extra care (and hence a cost in speed).

Other cases with interesting patterns of performance

There are a few other men listed in Appendix 1 whose pattern of performance seems to us worth considering in more detail. These are R.G., L.H., R.T., and E.W. Further background information on these men is given in Appendix 2.

We have noted that, although P.G. showed a selective impairment of familiar face recognition on accuracy measures (Table 6.1), his response times indicated quite widespread problems which also affected unfamiliar face matching and expression analysis (Table 6.2). In fact, there are two further men in the right hemisphere group who would fit this characterization (and none in the left hemisphere group); R.G. and L.H. Both R.G. and L.H. proved to be *imparied for nearly every task in terms of either accuracy or response latency*. This pattern is consistent with a single locus of impairment affecting a relatively early stage of face processing.

We also noted that despite initial indications pointing to a selective impairment of unfamiliar face matching, S.J. was impaired in terms of accuracy or latency for both familiar face recognition and unfamiliar face matching, but remained unimpaired on the expression analysis tasks (*see* Tables 6.1, 6.2). R.T. is interesting because he also shows the same overall patterns of impairment on accuracy or time for all the familiar face recognition and unfamiliar face matching tasks, with preserved processing of facial expressions. This might thus best be considered an impairment affecting the processing of identity of familiar or unfamiliar people from the face.

For the sake of completeness, we also mention E.W., who showed impairment of familiar face recognition and expression analysis on accuracy measures, with preserved unfamiliar face matching and no problems for any of the latency measures.

Discussion

We set out to test the claim, made by most cognitive neuropsychological models of face perception, that the abilities to recognize familiar faces, to match unfamiliar faces, and to process facial expressions can be selectively impaired after brain injury. For this purpose, we assessed each of these three abilities in a group of ex-servicemen with unilateral posterior brain lesions, and defined a selective impairment as a significantly reduced performance on more than one test of that ability, but with a normal performance on all other tests.

For the accuracy scores, there was evidence of selective impairments of each of the three abilities. There was one ex-serviceman with a right hemisphere lesion who demonstrated severe problems in identifying familiar faces only. A second man, also with a right hemisphere lesion, was selectively impaired in accuracy of matching unfamiliar faces. Finally, a number of men with left hemisphere lesions were selectively impaired on the expression tasks.

Subsequent analysis of the response latencies available to four of the six tasks confirmed the suggestion of a selective disorder in the processing of information about facial expressions. Hence we have strong evidence of a selective impairment affecting some aspect of the processing of facial expressions. It is curious, though, that this finding was made for men with left hemisphere lesions, since a link between facial expression processing and the right hemisphere has often been noted in other clinical reports.

The resolution of this discrepancy may lie in the nature of the issues investigated. The evidence for right hemisphere involvement in expression processing is usually in the form of findings of greater impairments on specific expression tests after right than left hemisphere injury. But this is not the issue addressed by our data, which are directed toward questions of selective impairment of broadly specified abilities. There were indeed ex-servicemen in our group who had difficulties in the analysis of expressions after a right hemisphere lesion, but these impairments were either found for one of the expression tasks and not the other (and especially for the expression matching task; *see* Appendix 1), or the men had additional face processing impairments on tasks that did not involve expression analysis. Therefore, we are not seeking to question the link between the right hemisphere and the processing of facial expression information, which has been established in numerous studies [*see* Etcoff (1986), for a review]. It does appear, however, that with our very strict criteria a *selective* impairment affecting both of the tasks which we used to measure this ability is only found in our group after a left-sided lesion. This does not necessarily mean that the left hemisphere outperforms the right hemisphere in everything that is involved in facial expression analysis, but it does mean that it makes a distinct contribution to the process.

In fact, Etcoff (1984) noted that two of her 12 patients with right hemisphere lesions were impaired at matching facial expressions but were able to match unfamiliar faces. Some of our ex-servicemen in the right hemisphere group also showed this pattern (e.g. J.M.), but they did not have corresponding impairments affecting our expression recognition task. It may therefore be the case that it will be possible in future to achieve further fractionation of impairments affecting the analysis of facial expressions into different basic forms, and relate these to a more detailed model of expression processing.

Although there is strong evidence from our findings pointing toward a selective deficit of facial expression processing, the position is less clear for impairments of familiar face recognition and unfamiliar face matching. Selective impairments of these abilities were noted in the accuracy data, but these were not borne out by examination of response latencies for our cases. The ex-serviceman with a selective familiar face recognition problem in terms of his accuracy data (P.G.) showed prolonged response latencies on all of the face processing tasks which were timed, and the man who, on the accuracy scores, had only been impaired on unfamiliar face matching (S.J.) was slow on both unfamiliar face matching and deciding whether a face looks familiar or not. In both these cases one of the functions in question was disproportionately affected for accuracy, but there were difficulties in other areas that were apparent on response latencies only.

The two cases may be quite different in terms of the underlying impairments. For P.G., it seems that there could be an impairment to a relatively early face processing stage, such as Bruce and Young's (1986) 'structural encoding', and the degraded information then has a knock-on effect on more than one function. In fact, we have some evidence that this is so. P.G. was also one of the ex-servicemen reported in detail by Newcombe *et al.* (1989), who noted that he was impaired (in terms of reaction time) at a 'face decision' task which required him to decide whether or not a stimulus was a properly organized face, with eyes, nose, and mouth in the correct relative positions. This task was intended as a relatively pure measure of face perception, uncontaminated by memory or matching demands. The fact that P.G. performed poorly on this task (*see* Newcombe *et al.* 1989, Table 1; his mean response time was 2220 ms; control mean 1098 ms, SD 210 ms) is consistent with an impairment at a relatively early stage of face processing [cf. Bruce and Young's (1986) 'structural encoding']. Interestingly, though, this was not due to impaired basic visual abilities; P.G.'s spatial contrast sensitivity function was normal (*see* Newcombe *et al.* 1989, Table 1).

P.G.'s problems may thus reflect impairment to structural encoding, which then impairs all subsequent face processing operations to some extent. There are also two other men (both with right hemisphere lesions) who we have noted as showing quite general impairments that would fit this characterization; R.G. and L.H. (see Appendix 1).

S.J. did not show this impairment of an early stage of face processing. His spatial contrast sensitivity function was normal, but so was his ability to perform the face decision task (mean reaction time 1366 ms; control mean 1098 ms, SD 210 ms). Similarly, in the tasks reported here, it does not seem that there was any general loss of speed in face processing for S.J.; his reaction times for expression analysis were normal. Instead, S.J. was impaired on both speed and accuracy of unfamiliar face matching, but seemed to be able to trade speed for accuracy in familiar face recognition. To some extent, he may also have been trading speed for accuracy in unfamiliar face matching, since his time on the Benton test was noticeably more impaired than his accuracy score.

One way to think about S.J., then, is that he showed intact processing of facial expression, but impaired processing of facial identity, whether this was for unfamiliar faces or familiar faces. We have drawn attention to the point that R.T. (who also has a right hemisphere lesion) shows a comparable overall pattern of impairment on familiar face recognition and unfamiliar face matching, with intact performance for facial expression analysis (see Appendix 1).

We began this study with the assumption that analysis of the face's identity would fractionate into dissociable impairments affecting familiar face recognition and unfamiliar face matching. What we have found for our cases, though, are dissociable impairments for accuracy scores which were not fully borne out when response latencies were also considered. In interpreting this, however, two caveats must be noted. First, whilst a combination of normal accuracy and normal speed can provide strong evidence that a function is well preserved after brain injury, and unusual strategies will often lead to long response times, it is not necessarily the case that long response latencies must indicate defective performance of the ability in question. For example, they might sometimes simply indicate cautiousness created indirectly by other problems arising from the brain injury. We therefore conclude that whilst the combination of normal accuracy and normal speed should be regarded as the desirable ideal, there are many reasons why it might not always be achieved in practice.

A second caveat is that we have only tested a relatively small group of subjects in this study, so our findings do not disprove the possible existence of selective impairments in these two abilities, and we have noted that this finding has often been made in other studies. Hence, we accept that it is possible that these men had suffered impairments that simultaneously compromised two otherwise independent abilities; the strongest neuropsychological evidence always comes from dissociation rather than association of deficits.

In line with this possibility, some other studies have also measured both response time and accuracy and found dissociable deficits; one example is Sergent and Poncet's (1990) demonstration of preserved unfamiliar face matching in a case of prosopagnosia. However, Sergent and Poncet's (1990) patient represents only one-half of the putative double dissociation. It is important that there are such cases, but one might also turn the point round, and argue that it would also be desirable to show that the patients who are poor at unfamiliar face matching and yet can recognize familiar faces also show normal reaction times for familiar face recognition. In our own study, S.J. did not meet this stringent test, but we hope that later reports will be able to demonstrate cases that do meet it.

References

Assal, G. (1969). Régression des troubles de la reconnaissance des physionomies et de la mémoire topographique chez un malade opéré d'un hématome intracérébral pariéto-temporal droit. *Revue Neurologique*, **121**, 184–5.

Benton, A. L. (1980). The neuropsychology of facial recognition. *American Psychologist*, **35**, 176–86.

Benton, A. L. and Van Allen, M. W. (1972). Prosopagnosia and facial discrimination. *Journal of the Neurological Sciences*, **15**, 167–72.

Benton, A. L. Hamsher, K. de S., Varney, N., and Spreen, O. (1983). *Contributions to neuropsychological assessment: a clinical manual.* Oxford University Press.

Bornstein, B. (1963). Prosopagnosia. In *Problems of dynamic neurology*, (ed. L. Halpern), pp. 283–318. Hadassah Medical School, Jerusalem.

Bowers, D. and Heilman., K. M. (1984). Dissociation between the processing of affective and nonaffective faces: a case study. *Journal of Clinical Neuropsychology*, **6**, 367–79.

Bowers, D., Bauer, R. M., Coslett, H. B., and Heilman K. M. (1985). Processing of faces by patients with unilateral hemisphere lesions. 1. Dissociation between judgments of facial affect and facial identity. *Brain and Cognition*, **4**, 258–72.

Bruce, V. (1988). *Recognising faces.* Lawrence Erlbaum, Hove.

Bruce, V. and Young, A. (1986). Understanding face recognition. *British Journal of Psychology*, **77**, 305–27.

Cicone, M., Wapner, W., and Gardner, H. (1980). Sensitivity to emotional expressions and situations in organic patients. *Cortex*, **16**, 145–58.

de Haan. E. H. F., Young, A. W., and Newcombe, F. (1991). A dissociation between the sense of familiarity and access to semantic information concerning familiar people. *European Journal of Cognitive Psychology*, **3**, 51–67.

Ekman, P. and Friesen, W. V. (1976). *Pictures of facial affect.* Consulting Psychologists Press, Palo Alto, CA.

Ellis, A. W. and Young, A. W. (1988). *Human cognitive neuropsychology.* Lawrence Erlbaum, Hove.

Ellis, H. D. (1983). The role of the right hemisphere in face perception. In *Functions of the right cerebral hemisphere*, (ed. A. W. Young), pp. 33–64. Academic Press, London.

Ellis, H. D. (1986). Processes underlying face recognition. In *The neuropsychology of face perception and facial expression*, (ed. R. Bruyer), pp. 1–27. Lawrence Erlbaum, Hillsdale, NJ.

Etcoff, N. L. (1984). Selective attention to facial identity and facial emotion. *Neuropsychologia*, **22**, 281–95.

Etcoff, N. L. (1986). The neuropsychology of emotional expression. In *Advances in clinical neuropsychology*, Vol. 3, (ed. G. Goldstein and R. E. Tarter), pp. 127–79. Plenum Press, New York.

Farah, M. J. (1991). Patterns of co-occurrence among the associative agnosias:

implications for visual object representation. *Cognitive Neuropsychology*, **8**, 1–19.

Gainotti, G. (1989). The meaning of emotional disturbances resulting from unilateral brain injury. In *Emotions and the dual brain*, (ed. G. Gainotti and C. Caltagirone), pp. 147–67. Springer, Berlin.

Hanley, J. R., Dewick, H. C., Davies, A. D. M., Playfer, J. and Turnbull, C. (1990). Verbal fluency in Parkinson's disease. *Neuropsychologia*, **28**, 737–41.

Hay, D. C. and Young, A. W. (1982). The human face. In *Normality and pathology in cognitive functions*, (ed. A. W. Ellis), pp. 173–202. Academic Press, London.

Kurucz, J and Feldmar, G. (1979). Prosopo-affective agnosia as a symptom of cerebral organic disease. *Journal of the American Geriatrics Society*, **27**, 225–30.

Kurucz, J., Feldmar, G. and Werner, W. (1979). Prosopo-affective agnosia associated with chronic organic brain syndrome. *Journal of the American Geriatrics Society*, **27**, 1–5.

McCarthy, R. A. and Warrington, E. K. (1990). *Cognitive neuropsychology: a clinical introduction*. Academic Press, San Diego.

McNeil, J. E. and Warrington E. K. (1991). Prosopagnosia: a reclassification. *Quarterly Journal of Experimental Psychology*, **43A**, 267–87.

Malone, D. R., Morris, H. H., Kay, M. C. and Levin H. S. (1982). Prosopagnosia: a double dissociation between the recognition of familiar and unfamiliar faces. *Journal of Neurology, Neurosurgery, and Psychiatry*, **45**, 820–2.

Marshall, J. C. and Newcombe, F. (1984). Putative problems and pure progress in neuropsychological single-case studies. *Journal of Clinical Neuropsychology*, **6**, 65–70.

Newcombe, F. (1969). *Missile wounds of the brain: a study of psychological deficits*. Oxford University Press.

Newcombe, F. (1979). The processing of visual information in prosopagnosia and acquired dyslexia: functional versus physiological interpretation. In *Research in psychology and medicine*, Vol. 1, (ed. D. J. Oborne, M. M. Gruneberg, and J. R. Eiser), pp. 315–22. Academic Press, London.

Newcombe, F. and Marshall, J. C. (1988). Idealisation meets psychometrics: the case for the right groups and the right individuals. *Cognitive Neuropsychology*, **5**, 549–64.

Newcombe, F., Oldfield, R. C., Ratcliff, G. G. and Wingfield, A. (1971). Recognition and naming of object-drawings by men with focal brain wounds. *Journal of Neurology, Neurosurgery, and Psychiatry*, **34**, 329–40.

Newcombe, F., de Haan, E. H. F., Ross, J. and Young, A. W. (1989). Face processing, laterality and contrast sensitivity. *Neuropsychologia*, **27**, 523–38.

Parry, F. M., Young, A. W., Saul, J. S. M. and Moss, A. (1991). Dissociable face processing impairments after brain injury. *Journal of Clinical and Experimental Neuropsychology*, **13**, 545–58.

Pizzamiglio, L., Zoccolotti, P., Mammucari, A. and Cesaroni, R. (1983). The independence of face identity and facial expression recognition mechanisms: relationship to sex and cognitive style. *Brain and Cognition*, **2**, 176–88.

Rapcsak, S. Z., Kaszniak, A. W. and Rubens, A. B. (1989). Anomia for facial expressions: evidence for a category specific visual–verbal disconnection syndrome. *Neuropsychologia*, **27**, 1031–41.

Rhodes, G. (1985). Lateralized processes in face recognition. *British Journal of Psychology*, **76**, 249–71.

Rondot, P., Tzavaras, A. and Garcin, R. (1967). Sur un cas de prosopagnosie persistant depuis quinze ans. *Revenue Neurologique*, **117**, 424–8.

Russell, W. R and Espir, M. L. E. (1961). *Traumatic aphasia: a study of aphasia in war wounds of the brain.* Oxford University Press.

Sergent, J. and Poncet, M. (1990). From covert to overt recognition of faces in a prosopagnosic patient. *Brain*, **113**, 989–1004.

Shallice, T. (1979). Case study approach in neuropsychological research. *Journal of Clinical Neuropsychology*, **1**, 183–211.

Shallice, T. (1988). *From neuropsychology to mental structure.* Cambridge University Press.

Teuber, H-L. (1955). Physiological psychology. *Annual Review of Psychology*, **6**, 267–96.

Tranel, D., Damasio, A. R. and Damasio, H. (1988). Intact recognition of facial expression, gender, and age in patients with impaired recognition of face identity. *Neurology,* **38**, 690–6.

Tzavaras, A., Hécaen, H. and Le Bras, H. (1970). Le problème de la spécificité du déficit de la reconnaissance du visage humain lors des lésions hémisphériques unilatérales. *Neuropsychologia*, **8**, 403–16.

Warrington, E. K. and James, M. (1967). An experimental investigation of facial recognition in patients with unilateral cerebral lesions. *Cortex*, **3**, 317–26.

Weiskrantz, L. (1968). Some traps and pontifications. In *Analysis of behavioral change*, (ed. L. Weiskrantz), pp. 415–29. Harper and Row, New York.

Young, A. W. and Bruce, V. (1991). Perceptual categories and the computation of 'grandmother'. *European Journal of Cognitive Psychology*, **3**, 5–49.

Young, A. W., de Haan, E. H. F. and Newcombe, F. (1990). Unawareness of impaired face recognition. *Brain and Cognition*, **14**, 1–18.

Appendix 1

Accuracies and response latencies (in seconds) for all six tasks for the ex-servicemen

	Location of lesion	Familiar face recognition			Unfamiliar face matching			Expression analysis			
		FA	FT	IA	BA	BT	SA	MA	MT	RA	RT
Right hemisphere lesions											
E.B.	T,P	30	1.5	19	41	29.0	26	12*	3.3	19	2.8
L.C.	T,P	32	1.1	19	42	20.6	29	13*	4.0	20	2.4
P.G.	T,P	23***	2.3***	10***	40	65.3***	26	16	11.6**	20	5.9*
R.G.	T,P	29*	1.3	15*	40	39.0*	20***	11**	3.7	20	7.4**
J.O.	T,P	31	1.1	17	30***	15.9	28	12*	5.5	22	2.0
A.R.	T,P	27***	1.8*	18	42	67.6***	28	18	6.6	22	9.4***
G.S.	T,P	24***	2.2***	14**	38*	14.9	27	16	6.0	20	3.9
R.T.	T,P	32	2.1**	12***	31***	39.7*	23*	14	6.3	22	5.0
R.C.	O,P	32	1.3	19	48	42.3*	29	18	8.1	24	5.1
J.H.	O,P	29*	1.5	19	44	16.8	29	16	8.3	19	3.0
L.H.	O,P	28**	1.8*	17	35***	39.8*	24*	17	8.9*	13***	4.8
E.K.	O,P	32	1.9**	20	44	30.2	30	13*	9.8*	23	5.7
J.M.	O,P	32	1.2	20	42	32.4	29	11**	8.0	21	3.1
A.N.	O,P	30	1.4	20	46	27.3	29	13*	4.6	19	4.7
S.J.	F,P,O	31	2.3***	18	38*	50.4***	22***	17	6.5	23	3.7
Left hemisphere lesions											
V.M.	F,T,P	32	1.5	18	42	24.1	27	13*	8.8*	16**	5.5
A.J.	T,P	31	1.0	18	45	14.5	28	17	3.7	21	2.7
J.K.	T,P	30	1.2	14**	45	17.9	29	12*	4.9	16**	3.4
W.M.	T,P	32	1.1	19	42	25.3	30	13*	9.5*	18*	9.1***

T.R.	T, P	30	1.0	17	45	32.8	26	11**	3.1	18*	3.1
H.S.	T, P	32	1.2	19	44	25.9	29	11**	4.4	21	2.6
E.W.	T, P	29*	1.3	9***	40	18.2	29	12*	6.9	17*	4.8
J.A.	O, P	32	0.9	19	43	29.5	30	18	2.9	20	4.1
H.B.	O, P	32	1.2	20	46	22.2	29	17	3.4	18*	3.5
P.C.	O, P	29*	1.4	20	41	22.8	28	15	7.1	21	3.5
H.D.	O, P	30	1.3	15*	45	17.7	27	15	2.7	22	2.1
J.D.	O, P	30	1.4	13***	35***	21.3	29	15	9.9*	22	3.6
P.M.	O, P	32	1.0	20	39*	20.6	29	15	2.7	23	2.9
A.S.	O, P	30	1.2	20	48	40.0*	28	12*	6.8	18*	4.1
C.S.	O, P	32	1.2	17	41	37.6*	29	16	10.3**	23	6.1*
B.T.	O, P	31	1.5	19	37**	15.6	30	16	4.4	20	3.7
J.C.	F, P, O	31	1.1	20	51	46.5**	29	14	6.3	23	4.0
G.M.	F, P, O	31	1.3	16	42	33.1	28	9***	12.0***	15***	12.7***
P.O.	F, P, O	32	1.0	18	50	23.1	30	15	15.7***	22	13.9***

Asterisked scores are significantly below the control mean: $*p < 0.05$; $**p < 0.01$; $***p < 0.001$. O, P, T, F, refer to lesions involving occipital, parietal, temporal, and frontal lobes, respectively; FA = familiarity decision accuracy; FT = mean familiarity decision time; IA = familiar face identification accuracy; BA = Benton test accuracy; BT = mean time per item on Benton test; SA = sequential matching accuracy; MA = expression matching accuracy; MT = mean time per item on expression matching; RA = expression recognition accuracy; RT = mean time per item on expression recognition.

Appendix 2

Background information concerning individual cases discussed in the text; including visual field defects, age, verbal and non-verbal intelligence, and neurological symptoms as formerly assessed by Professor Ritchie Russell at initial follow-up within the first 2 years after injury (epilepsy, motor and somatosensory defects)

	Location of lesion	FD	E	M	S	A	MH	PM
Right hemisphere lesions								
P.G.	T, P	N	S	0	0	61	126	55
R.G.	T, P	LUQ	S	0	0	65	97	48
R.T.	T, P	LH	N	0	0	66	86	21
L.H.	O, P	LH	S	0	0	72	96	44
S.J.	F, P, O	N	N	2	2	71	126	38
Means for all right hemisphere cases						66.9	106.5	
Standard deviation						4.5	16.2	
Left hemisphere lesions								
V.M.	F, T, P	RH	N	0	0	69	90	22
W.M.	T, P	N	S	0	0	63	90	46
T.R.	T, P	RLQ	N	1	1	64	90	35
E.W.	T, P	N	N	0	0	67	86	34
A.S.	O, P	RLQ	S	0	0	67	107	55
G.M.	F, P, O	RH	S	3	0	65	98	35
Means for all left hemisphere cases						65.5	95.5	
Standard deviation						5.3	11.6	

O, P, T, F, refer to lesions involving occipital, parietal, temporal, and frontal lobes, respectively. FD = visual field defects; N none, LH left hemianopia, LUQ left upper quadrantanopia, RH right hemianopia, RLQ right lower quadrantanopia. E = epilepsy; N none, S slight. M = severity of motor defects, assessed on 0–3 scale. S = severity of somatosensory defects, assessed on 0–3 scale. A = age in years. MH = Mill Hill synonyms test IQ. PM = raw score on standard progressive matrices.

7

Face recognition and face imagery

Reprinted in slightly modified form from Young, A. W., Humphreys, G. W., Riddoch, J., Hellawell, D. J., and de Haan, E. H. F. (1994), Recognition impairments and face imagery, *Neuropsychologia*, **32**, 693–702. With kind permission of co-authors and Elsevier Science Ltd., The Boulevard, Langford Lane, Kidlington, Oxford OX5 1GB, UK.

Summary

Face imagery was investigated for HJA and PH, who experience profound difficulties in recognizing familiar faces. HJA's problems involve a perceptual impairment that compromises the integration of features into a coherent representation, and he does not show covert recognition of faces in indirect tests. In contrast, PH has shown extensive covert recognition effects, leading to the suggestion that his deficit occurs at a higher level of visual processing than HJA's. HJA and PH were given tasks intended to explore their ability to answer questions that depended on imaging single faces, and on configuration-based or feature-based comparisons of imaged sets of three faces. For all of these face imagery tasks, PH's overall performance was severely impaired. HJA, though, showed preserved face imagery when imaging single faces and when making feature-based comparisons between imaged faces. However, when configuration-based comparisons were demanded HJA also showed a severe and stable impairment of face imagery. These observations are inconsistent with the idea that face recognition impairments have a unitary underlying cause and vary only in severity. Instead, they imply multi-stage causation, with the nature of consequent impairments of face imagery being determined by the level at which the recognition deficit arises.

Introduction

In a classic report, Charcot and Bernard (1883) described the case of M. X..., who suffered a sudden loss of visual mental imagery and was no longer able to recognize faces and places. From Charcot's perspective, recognition was considered to involve matching a percept to a mental image, so that this parallel impairment of recognition and imagery was unsurprising.

Modern studies have also noted parallel impairments of imagery and recognition, though they tend to reverse the explanatory emphasis by arguing that the visual representations involved in recognition are also needed in forming mental images (Farah *et al.* 1989; Levine *et al.* 1985). However, the studies of parallel impairments of imagery and recognition emphasize that in such cases imagery is preserved for material that can still be recognized (Farah *et al.* 1989). It is therefore anomalous that Charcot's case M. X... should have lost *all* visual imagery, including that for objects he could apparently recognize without difficulty. In fact, later cases with loss of visual imagery without any noticeable impairment of visual recognition have been described (Brain 1954; Farah *et al.* 1988; Riddoch 1990).

To reconcile such observations, modern theories propose that some cognitive processes are specific to imagery whilst others are shared by imagery and perception. In particular, they distinguish the process of generating an image from accessing the stored material which may be needed to form a particular image of something familiar (Farah 1984; Riddoch 1990). From this perspective, the cases of generally impaired imagery and intact recognition involve deficits in image generation, whereas the cases of parallel deficits of imagery and recognition of particular materials (such as faces) involve damage or loss of access to a certain type of previously stored material. The important point here is that M. X... showed a combination of both types of deficit; he had lost the ability to generate visual images and he suffered a deficit affecting the recognition of faces and places, which can be considered to involve a form of prosopagnosia (Young and van de Wal 1996).

Powerful demonstrations of parallel impairments of imagery and recognition have come from cases where there are category-specific impairments affecting both imagery and recognition (Farah *et al.* 1989; Mehta *et al.* 1992), and these are clearly consistent with the view that the visual representations involved in recognition are also needed in forming mental images. For impairments of face recognition, this view has been cogently expressed by Levine and Calvanio (1989), who argued that 'prosopagnosics cannot identify objects whose critical distinguishing features have no independent identities', and claimed that this perceptual deficit and the loss of ability to image previously familiar faces that is often noted in cases of prosopagnosia (Bruyer *et al.* 1983; Habib 1986; Levine *et al.* 1985) are different aspects of the same problem.

A problem for this type of interpretation is that there are also cases of impaired visual recognition of objects in which visual imagery can be relatively preserved (Behrmann et al. 1992; Jankowiak et al. 1992). These form a double dissociation when set alongside the cases of impaired imagery and preserved recognition, suggesting the possibility that the relation between imagery and perception may not be as close as was thought. Similarly, some reports of face recognition impairments have described intact face imagery in prosopagnosic patients. In the first case, described by Bodamer (1947), the patient was noted to remain able to visualize and describe from memory faces he no longer recognized, and Pallis (1955) also observed that even though his patient had to wait for people to speak before he could recognize them, he claimed 'I can shut my eyes and can well remember what my wife looked like or the kids'. Information about face imagery has been included in some reviews of prosopagnosia (Blanc-Garin 1984; Ellis 1986; Hécaen and Angelergues 1962; Levine et al. 1985), which confirm that loss of imagery was noted in some cases and not in others. According to Hécaen and Angelergues (1962, p. 94), impairment in revisualization was only encountered in about half their cases, but Hécaen (1981, p. 41) later qualified this by remarking that those prosopagnosic patients who claimed to succeed in imaging faces did not give very adequate verbal descriptions of their images.

Cases of prosopagnosia with apparently preserved visual imagery were also discussed by Levine and Calvanio (1989, p. 164), who raised three questions concerning their validity. First, some reports have only noted preserved spatial imagery (e.g. descriptions of routes), but this is known to be dissociable from other aspects of visual imagery (Levine et al. 1985). Second, reports have generally relied upon the patient's introspective report that her or his imagery was intact, but they might not be aware of problems in this area. For example, Levine and Calvanio (1989) noted that their patient, LH, 'was not aware of his defective visual imagery until we tested it in the laboratory many years after the onset of his prosopagnosia'. Levine et al. (1985) had reported that when asked to describe faces from memory, LH (who was patient 1 in their report) knew that Abraham Lincoln had a beard, but described his face as short and round, and could not say anything at all about the appearance of Winston Churchill or John Kennedy. Third, Levine and Calvanio claimed that some of the commonly employed tests of visual imagery (such as drawing from memory) might not involve visual imagery per se (for example, they argued that drawing from memory might also tap spatio-motor skills). They maintained that 'there has been no case of prosopagnosia with allegedly preserved visual imagery where all of these pitfalls in the assessment of visual imagery were taken into account' (Levine and Calvanio 1989, p. 164).

It is clear, then, that the relation between face recognition impairments and face imagery remains poorly understood. We therefore investigated a person with severely impaired ability to recognize faces for whom there was likely to be evidence of preserved imagery, HJA (Humphreys et al. 1992a; Riddoch and Humphreys 1987), and contrasted his performance with that of PH, who has been found to have poor ability to recognize or image faces (de Haan et al. 1991). To deal with the methodological points raised by Levine and Calvanio (1989), each person was tested on tasks that demanded face imagery for successful performance. For example, tests required memory comparisons of the degree to which people's appearances differed along a particular dimension (whose hair was longest, whose glasses were round, etc.). These would not easily be achieved from verbal labelling of specific features. Quantitative comparisons were then made to the performances of matched control subjects.

Case descriptions

We investigated face imagery for HJA and PH, whose visual recognition abilities have been extensively described in the literature.

HJA (Humphreys et al. 1992a, b, 1993; Humphreys and Riddoch 1984, 1987; Riddoch and Humphreys 1986, 1987) has a dense object agnosia caused by a stroke after a routine operation in 1981, when he was aged 61 years. This has left him with profound difficulties in recognizing objects and faces both in everyday life and in formal clinical and laboratory tests. On tests of face recognition, he never recognizes anybody, and in everyday life he does not recognize people as familiar as his wife until she speaks.

PH (de Haan et al. 1987a, b, 1991; Young and de Haan 1988; Young et al. 1988) suffered a severe closed head injury in a motor cycle accident in 1982, when he was aged 19. In everyday life, he does not recognize familiar people from their faces, and in formal tests he is very impaired at recognizing faces and other visual stimuli which come from categories with a high degree of inter-item similarity [faces 0/60; cars 3/33; flowers 0/26 (de Haan et al. 1987a)]. Although PH does not show recognition problems for everyday objects in his daily life, he is poor at recognizing line drawings. His score on the Oldfield and Wingfield object naming test was 20/36, and his performance improved considerably when the objects were verbally described, indicating a degree of object agnosia (de Haan *et al.* 1987*a*), though his object recognition impairments are nothing like as severe as those experienced by HJA.

Although both HJA and PH are very severely impaired at recognizing familiar faces, previous studies have found that the reasons for the failure of overt recognition differ markedly in each case. HJA's problems with face recognition arise in the context of a perceptual impairment that compromises the integration of features into a coherent representation. Consistent with this relatively early deficit, he does not show covert recognition of faces in indirect tests involving face matching (familiar faces were matched no better than unfamiliar faces) or face–name learning (correct pairings of faces and names were no easier for HJA to learn than incorrect pairings) (Humphreys *et al.* 1992*a*). On the same tasks, PH has consistently shown covert recognition effects (de Haan *et al.* 1987*a*, 1991; Young and de Haan 1988). In addition, HJA performs at chance level when required to judge either the sex of the person or their emotional expression from static images of the face (Humphreys *et al.* 1993). PH is also poor at discriminating gender and expression, but his overall performance is well above chance level (de Haan *et al.* 1987*a*, 1991). These findings suggest that the principal locus of PH's deficit is at a higher level of visual processing than HJA's, and affects the output from otherwise well preserved face recognition units (Burton *et al.* 1991; Young and de Haan 1988). These well documented differences in the nature of the underlying recognition impairments for HJA and PH make it especially interesting to explore their ability to image faces they can no longer recognize.

Investigations of face imagery

When asked to describe the appearance of objects, PH gave reasonably fluent answers. For example, he described a bicycle as having 'two wheels, one at the front and one at the back. On top of the front wheels are the handlebars with two brakes. There is a crossbar going from the handlebars towards the back wheel, with a seat on top. A chain goes round from the pedals in the middle to the back wheel'. Hence PH did not seem to be suffering a generalized imagery deficit. However, de Haan *et al.* (1991) noted that PH could no longer form mental images of familiar faces. As he put it, 'I can't get a picture'. Even when he was asked about the appearance of celebrities with particularly striking facial features (e.g. Denis Healey: a British politician with prominent eyebrows), PH maintained that he no longer had any idea what they looked like. In addition, he had no image of personally familiar people, being unable to give even a remotely adequate description of members of the department where he has been seen regularly for several years.

HJA's face imagery has not previously been discussed in any detail, but Riddoch and Humphreys (1987; Humphreys and Riddoch 1987) noted that he was able to remember the appearances of objects he could no longer recognize; for example, he could describe from memory what they looked like, and he could make reasonably accurate drawings. When HJA was given the names of 20 famous people and asked to describe the appearance of each from memory, he was able to provide accurate descriptions in all cases. For example, he described Harold Wilson as having 'a round face with white or grey waved hair, round cheeks', Tony Benn as having 'a long face with quite a prominent chin', Denis Healey as having 'quite a fat face with a double chin, glasses, and noticeable eyebrows', Elvis Presley as having 'dark hair, side burns, with a slick smile', Prince Charles as having 'dark wavy hair, a long face, large ears'. These descriptions contrast markedly with Levine *et al.*'s (1985) observations with LH, who had claimed still to have imagery for faces but gave inaccurate descriptions. Instead, HJA's descriptions imply that he can accurately remember people's appearances, even though he no longer recognizes them.

There were therefore grounds to suggest that face imagery might be better preserved for HJA than for PH, and this is what we sought to document with formal testing. However, there are considerable differences in age and background between HJA and PH, which mean that the comparison has to be approached carefully. PH (aged 19 when he suffered his brain injury, and in his late 20s when the tests reported here were carried out) is much younger than HJA (now in his early 70s), and they each have quite different interests. The consequence of this is that faces of famous people that are well known to one person will often not be well known to the other. Obviously, it would be inappropriate to ask questions about the appearance of people who are unfamiliar, so we have adopted a procedure of screening items as suitable or unsuitable for each person and using separate age-matched groups of controls for HJA and PH, so that their performances can be compared to people who are likely to have similar experience of these faces.

HJA and PH were given tasks intended to explore their ability to answer questions that depended on imaging single faces, and on configuration-based or feature-based comparisons of imaged sets of three faces.

Imaging single faces

Four sets of 20 different famous people known to PH were created, in which 10 members of each set had a particular feature and 10 did not.

The features used were baldness (i.e. the set contained 10 balding people and 10 hirsute people), facial hair (10 people who usually have beards or moustaches, and 10 without), fair hair (10 people with fair hair, and 10 with dark hair), and glasses (10 people who usually wear spectacles, and 10 who do not). The names of the people in each set were arranged into a pseudo-random order, and then read out to PH one at a time. For each name, he was asked to image the person's appearance and then answer the relevant question (balding v. not balding, facial hair v. no facial hair, fair v. dark hair, or glasses v. no glasses, depending on the set being presented). Examples of items we used are: balding v. not balding, Bobby Charlton (correct answer 'yes'), Ronnie Barker ('no'); facial hair v. no facial hair, David Bellamy ('yes'), Cliff Richard ('no'); fair v. dark hair, Harold Wilson ('yes'), Elvis Presley ('no'); glasses v. no glasses, Ronnie Corbett ('yes'), John Cleese ('no').

For HJA, we assembled sets of 16 people familiar to him for the balding v. not balding question, 12 for facial hair v. no facial hair, 14 for fair v. dark hair, and 10 for glasses v. no glasses. HJA was asked the appropriate question about the appearances of these. To check that HJA was reliably able to image these faces, he was retested on the same items some six months later; this retest produced a closely similar performance to the original test session.

HJA's and PH's performances of these face imagery tasks with single faces are shown in Table 7.1, together with means, standard deviations, and ranges for the scores of six control subjects of comparable age and background to HJA, and six age-matched controls for PH.

Although the differences in ages and interests necessitated the use of different test items with HJA and PH, it is clear from the controls' data that each test was of comparable difficulty (controls scored 92 per cent correct overall on the test used with HJA, and 90 per cent for the test used with PH), so it is legitimate to compare HJA and PH's performance.

In comparison to controls, HJA's overall performance was unimpaired ($z = 0.60$, $p > 0.1$), whereas PH showed a severe impairment ($z = 4.10$, $p < 0.001$). HJA's overall performance (47/52 correct) was also significantly better than PH's (56/80 correct) for this task ($\chi^2 = 6.50$, d.f. $= 1$, two-tailed $p < 0.05$). This was also clear from the way each approached the task. HJA was confident and found the task reasonably easy. When asked to describe how he did it, he said that he formed images of the faces. In contrast, PH was hesitant, unconfident, and insistent that he could not form an image and was therefore having to guess. Despite his hesitancy and poor performance, PH's overall score was above chance level ($x = 56$, $N = 80$, $z = 3.47$, $p < 0.001$), but for some items he may have remembered some relevant

Table 7.1 Performance of HJA and PH on face imagery tasks with single faces, and means, standard deviations, and ranges for scores of control subjects of comparable age

	HJA and PH		Controls		
	First test	HJA retest	Mean	SD	Range
HJA					
Overall					
Total correct	47/52	47/52	48.00	1.67	45–49
Percentage correct	90%	90%	92%		
Performance for each question					
Balding?	14/16	14/16	14.67	1.03	13–16
Facial hair?	12/12	12/12	11.33	0.52	11–12
Fair hair?	11/14†**	12/14	12.83	0.75	12–14
Glasses	10/10	9/10	9/17	0.98	8–10
PH					
Overall					
Total correct	56/80†***		72.34	3.98	69–79
Percentage correct	70%		90%		
Performance for each question					
Balding?	16/20		17.17	1.17	16–19
Facial hair?	13/20†***		18.67	1.21	19–20
Fair hair?	10/20†***		18.17	1.47	16–20
Glasses	17/20		18.33	1.21	17–20

† Scores outside the range for control subjects.
Asterisked scores are significantly below the control mean: * $z > 1.65$, $p < 0.05$; ** $z > 2.33$, $p < 0.01$; *** $z > 3.10$, $p < 0.001$.

piece of semantic information on which to base a plausible guess. Certainly, he did not claim to use imagery at all.

In terms of their performance with each of the specific questions used, HJA was generally unimpaired, except on first testing with the fair v. dark hair question, when his score fell just outside the control range (HJA 11/14 correct, control range 12–14, $z = 2.44$, $p < 0.01$). On retest, however, he did slightly better (12/14 correct, $z = 1.11$, $p > 0.1$). For PH, severe impairments were found with the facial hair v. no facial hair and fair v. dark hair questions (facial hair v. no facial hair, PH 13/20 correct, control range 19–20, $z = 4.69$, $p < 0.001$; fair v. dark hair, PH 10/20 correct, control range 16–20, $z = 5.56$, $p < 0.001$), with his performance being no different from chance level in both cases (facial hair v. no facial hair, $x = 13$, $N = 20$, $z = 1.12$, $p > 0.1$; fair v. dark hair, $x = 10$, $N = 20$, $z = 0.22$, $p > 0.1$). For the other questions (balding v. not balding, glasses v. no glasses), PH was scoring at the bottom of the control range.

Configuration-based comparisons

This task was used with PH by de Haan *et al.* (1991), and their results are reproduced here in Table 7.2, together with control data. The version used with PH consisted of 20 trials, each involving three names of famous people. These people were chosen so that two were of similar appearance and one dissimilar. On each trial, PH was instructed to image the faces of all three celebrities, and to decide which looked most alike. This question was given in a two-choice format. For instance, 'Who looks more like Elizabeth Taylor; Joan Collins or Barbara Windsor?'. There was no time limit.

Nine normal people of comparable age to PH were used as control subjects. Of course, correct performance is defined simply as agreement with our own opinion of similarity in each case. From the results presented in Table 7.2 it is clear that PH was severely impaired on this task, performing significantly below the mean for control subjects ($z = 4.38$, $p < 0.001$), outside the control range (PH 10/20 correct, control range 14–19), and no better than chance level overall ($x = 10$, $N = 20$, $z = 0.22$, $p > 0.1$).

To test HJA, we assembled a set of eight trials by adapting the set used with PH; this adaptation was necessary because the presence of

Table 7.2 Performance of HJA and PH on face imagery tasks involving comparisons between three imaged faces, and means, standard deviations, and ranges for scores of control subjects of comparable age

	HJA and PH		Controls		
	First test	HJA retest	Mean	SD	Range
HJA					
Configuration test	2/8†***	3/8†***	7.17	0.75	6–8
Feature test	21/24		21.00	1.67	18–23
PH					
Configuration test	10/21†***		17.00	1.60	14–19
Feature test	10/24†***		20.33	1.63	18–22

† Scores outside the range for control subjects.
Asterisked scores are significantly below the control mean: * $z > 1.65$, $p < 0.05$; ** $z > 2.33$, $p < 0.01$; *** $z > 3.10$, $p < 0.001$.

three items in each trial means that a trial cannot be used if any one of these three people is unknown. For these eight trials, HJA experienced considerable difficulties and performed poorly in comparison to six age-matched controls, both in an initial test (HJA 2/8 correct, control range 6–8, $z = 6.89$, $p < 0.001$) and a retest some six months later (3/8 correct, $z = 5.56$, $p < 0.001$).

Although we were initially surprised at HJA's poor performance of this task, which was in marked contrast to his well preserved ability to answer questions about single faces, it seemed to be the fact that the question required an overall evaluation of appearance which was causing him difficulty, rather than the need to compare three faces *per se*. Of course, with hindsight, it can be seen that if imagery impairments really do directly mirror perceptual impairments, then comparisons based on each face's configuration would be impossible for HJA, since it is precisely the perception of configuration which is compromised by his visual problem.

To confirm that HJA's difficulties were being created by the need for configuration-based comparisons in this task, we devised an analogous task for HJA and PH that only required feature-based comparisons.

Feature-based comparisons

Sets of three famous people were collected separately for HJA and PH, in which one person possessed a particular feature more prominently than the others. In each case, we tried to use examples where the three faces differed continuously along the specified dimension, so that imagery would be required for a correct answer. These stimuli were presented as sets of three names. On each trial, HJA or PH was instructed to image the faces of all three celebrities, and to decide which had the most exaggerated feature in question. For example, 'Who has the longest hair: Bjorn Borg, Jimmy Connors, or John McEnroe?' (correct answer, Bjorn Borg), 'Who wore round glasses: Ernest Bevin, Jim Callaghan, or Roy Jenkins?' (correct answer, Ernest Bevin). There was no time limit.

Both HJA and PH were tested with 24 such trials, but in each case involving different items tailored to each person's age and interests. Results are presented in Table 7.2, together with data for six age-matched controls for each person. From the control data, it is clear that the tests used with HJA and PH were of equivalent difficulty (control mean for HJA's test = 21.00, SD = 1.67; control mean for PH's test = 20.33, SD = 1.63).

HJA performed normally on this feature-based comparison test

(21/24 correct, control range 18–23, $z = 0.00, p > 0.1$), whereas PH was severely impaired in comparison to controls (10/24 correct, control range 18–22, $z = 6.34, p < 0.001$) and at chance level overall ($x = 10$, $N = 24, z = 0.61, p > 0.1$).

Discussion

This study has confirmed previous findings that PH is unable to form mental images of familiar faces (de Haan *et al.* 1991). On all the tasks used, his overall performance was severely impaired, and often at chance level. HJA, however, showed relatively preserved face imagery. When imaging single faces, he performed as well as control subjects overall, and showed at most a transient impairment on one of the questions used. When feature-based comparisons between imaged faces were required, HJA also achieved a normal level of performance. It was only when configuration-based comparisons were demanded that HJA showed a severe and stable impairment of face imagery.

The principal interest of these findings lies in the fact that although HJA's imagery abilities are better preserved than PH's, it is HJA who has the more widespread and severe recognition impairment. We noted that HJA is unable to recognize many everyday objects as well as familiar faces, and that he has not shown any evidence of covert recognition of faces in indirect tests (Humphreys *et al.* 1992*a*). PH, however, does not experience any obvious recognition problems for most everyday objects in his daily life, and has been found to show extensive covert recognition effects with familiar faces (de Haan *et al.* 1987*a*; Young and de Haan 1992). Moreover, it has been possible to provoke a limited degree of overt recognition of some faces by presenting multiple exemplars drawn from the same semantic category to PH (de Haan *et al.* 1991). which also shows that his loss of recognition is not absolute.

These observations are important to the debate concerning whether prosopagnosia is a unitary or a multi-stage disorder. Many researchers have sought an account in terms of a single underlying deficit which is common to all cases of impaired recognition of familiar faces, in the form of impaired configural processing (Levine and Calvanio 1989), problems of contextual memory evocation with visually ambiguous stimuli (Damasio *et al.* 1982), and so on. These unitary accounts contrast with others which have emphasized that differences between the impairments shown by different patients suggest that the breakdown which creates problems in recognizing faces may arise at different levels of visual information processing (De Renzi *et al.* 1991; Ellis 1986; Hay and Young 1982; Hécaen 1981; Meadows 1974).

Unitary accounts of prosopagnosia explain these differences between cases by arguing that there is damage to a single mechanism, but this can vary in severity. For example, in Levine and Calvanio's (1989) account, all of the deficits found in cases of prosopagnosia are considered to reflect more or less severe impairments of visual configural processing. Phenomena such as covert recognition are then held to result from relatively mild impairments along this continuum, in which 'The prosopagnosic who is shown a familiar face may focus on a fragment or feature that is sufficiently familiar to unleash an autonomic response. However, he lacks the perceptual overview to identify the face immediately, and his subsequent sequential feature-by-feature analysis may yield insufficient information for accurate recognition or identification' (Levine and Calvanio 1989, p. 161). In the same way, Levine and Calvanio (1989) argue that recognition and imagery impairments in prosopagnosia 'are not distinct impairments in different stages of visual recognition but instead are two aspects of the same underlying disorder, which we call defective visual "configural processing"' (Levine and Calvanio 1989, p. 151).

An ingenious variant of this position has been developed by Farah (1991), who argues that there is a difference between the neural representations needed for the recognition of objects that cannot be decomposed into simpler but still recognizable parts and for objects which can be segregated in this way. Faces form an obvious example of the former type of object (non-decomposable, because it is very difficult to recognize a familiar nose or eyes in isolation), whereas words would be an example of the latter type (decomposable, because constituent letters are readily recognized in isolation). Mild impairments of the non-decomposable, whole-based representations would lead to a relatively pure prosopagnosia, but as these representations are increasingly impaired Farah (1991) claims that more and more everyday objects will also be affected, as is found in cases with co-occurring object agnosia and prosopagnosia (such as for HJA).

In terms of the hypotheses advanced by Farah (1991) and Levine and Calvanio (1989), it is therefore clear that HJA has the more severe visual recognition impairment than PH, since HJA's problems extend to everyday objects as well as faces and he does not show any evidence of covert recognition. If both patients' visual recognition difficulties are due to the same form of underlying problem (albeit differing in severity), and if imagery problems mirror the perceptual impairment, then one must predict that since HJA's visual recognition problems are more severe than PH's, his face imagery will also be the more severely impaired. This is the reverse of what we have found, so our results create severe problems for any account in terms of a single underlying deficit.

In contrast, our findings can be explained quite simply if it is accepted that impairments of face recognition can have different causes. One way to do this is to draw a distinction between the creation of an adequate structural description of a seen face and the brain's stored knowledge of the appearances of familiar faces; successful recognition depends on the integrity of both components. This distinction is often drawn by researchers who have distinguished perceptual from mnestic variants of prosopagnosia (De Renzi *et al.* 1991; Hécaen 1981); in the perceptual form, an adequate structural description suitable for recognition cannot be achieved, whereas in the mnestic form problems centre on damage or disconnection of stored knowledge of facial appearance.

To account for impairments of face imagery, one then needs only to adopt the widely held postulate that some processes are common to both imagery and perception. If access to stored knowledge of appearances is required for face imagery, people with mnestic prosopagnosias will (like PH) be impaired on all face imagery tasks, whereas people with perceptual prosopagnosias will (like HJA) be able to access these stored descriptions, and will therefore be successful in imagery tasks that do not demand sophisticated perceptual comparisons. The point has been made neatly by Ellis (1989), who first grasped the importance of impairments of face imagery for the unitary v. multi-stage debate, and had predicted just this pattern (Ellis 1989, p. 152):

One distinction that may be made between perceptual and mnestic prosopagnosics is that the former could have a preserved ability to image or revisualise a face whereas the latter may not be able to do so. This paradox arises if it is assumed that imagery relies upon preserved internal representations of faces. Mnestic prosopagnosics have either had these representations destroyed or have lost access to them; perceptual prosopagnosics should have them preserved but, because of perturbation at one of the input stages, the representations are not accessed by external stimuli but may be used to generate images.

Our findings are in accordance with Ellis's (1989) line of reasoning. Although HJA and PH are both very severely impaired at recognizing familiar faces, previous studies have indicated that the reasons for the failure of overt recognition differ markedly in each case. HJA's problems with face recognition arise in the context of a perceptual impairment that compromises the integration of features into a coherent representation; he is thus unable to achieve an adequate structural description for recognition. From our results, though, it seems that HJA's knowledge of the appearances of familiar faces remains relatively well preserved, as evidenced by his performance of face imagery tasks. It was only when the face imagery task we used directly paralleled his perceptual impairment (i.e. in the configuration-based task) that HJA experienced difficulties. Conversely, the extensive covert recognition effects documented for PH have led to the suggestion that his deficit is at a higher level of visual processing than HJA's, and affects the outputs from otherwise well preserved face recognition units which store descriptions of the appearances of known faces. One only needs to postulate that this impairment is bi-directional (i.e. that it is just as difficult for PH to access this previously stored knowledge of facial appearances) to explain his loss of face imagery. If this general position is correct, then impaired face imagery may be characteristic of prosopagnosic cases with relatively high-level impairment and covert recognition.

An alternative way to think about our results would be that they provide a further example of a dissociation between recognition and imagery, since HJA had severely impaired recognition yet relatively preserved imagery. However, the results from the configuration-based comparisons for HJA (Table 7.2) show that this is oversimple. Instead, HJA's face imagery *is* impaired, but only if it is tested in a way that directly parallels his perceptual problems in forming an integrated description. What we therefore have are findings which support the general view that imagery impairments mirror perceptual impairments, but show that this parallelism can be very close indeed, with the impairments of face imagery falling exactly into line with the problems creating the loss of face recognition.

References

Behrmann, M., Winocur, G., and Moscovitch, M. (1992). Dissociation between mental imagery and object recognition in a brain-damaged patient. *Nature*, **359**, 636–7.

Blanc-Garin, J. (1984). Perception des visages et reconnaissance de la physionomie dans l'agnosie des visages. *L'Année Psychologique*, **84**, 573–98.

Bodamer, J. (1947). Die Prosop-Agnosie. *Archiv für Psychiatrie und Nervenkrankheiten*, **179**, 6–53.

Brain, R. (1954). Loss of visualization. *Proceedings of the Royal Society of Medicine*, **47**, 288–90.

Bruyer, R., Laterre, C., Seron, X., Feyereisen, P., Strypstein, E., Pierrard, E., and Rectem, D. (1983). A case of prosopagnosia with some preserved covert remembrance of familiar faces. *Brain and Cognition*, **2**, 257–84.

Burton, A. M., Young, A. W., Bruce, V., Johnston, R., and Ellis, A. W. (1991). Understanding covert recognition. *Cognition*, **39**, 129–66.

Charcot, J.-M. and Bernard, D. (1883). Un cas de suppression brusque et isolée de la vision mentale des signes et des objets (formes et couleurs). *Le Progrès Médical*, **11**, 568–71.

Damasio, A. R., Damasio, H., and Van Hoesen, G. W. (1982). Prosopagnosia: anatomic basis and behavioral mechanisms. *Neurology*, **32**, 331–41.

de Haan, E. H. F., Young, A., and Newcombe, F. (1987*a*). Face recognition without awareness. *Cognitive Neuropsychology*, **4**, 385–415.

de Haan, E. H. F., Young, A., and Newcombe, F. (1987*b*). Faces interfere with name classification in a prosopagnosic patient. *Cortex*, **23**, 309–16.

de Haan, E. H. F., Young, A. W., and Newcombe, F. (1991). Covert and overt recognition in prosopagnosia. *Brain*, **114**, 2575–91.

De Renzi, E., Faglioni, P., Grossi, D., and Nichelli, P. (1991). Apperceptive and associative forms of prosopagnosia. *Cortex*, **27**, 213–21.

Ellis, H. D. (1986). Disorders of face recognition. In *Neurology*, (ed. K. Poeck, H. J. Freund, and H. Gänshirt), pp. 179–87. Springer, Berlin.

Ellis, H. D. (1989). Past and recent studies of prosopagnosia. In *Developments in clinical and experimental neuropsychology*, (ed. J. R. Crawford and D. M. Parker), pp. 151–66. Plenum, New York.

Farah, M. J. (1984). The neurological basis of mental imagery: a componential analysis. *Cognition*, **18**, 245–72.

Farah, M. J. (1991). Patterns of co-occurrence among the associative agnosias: implications for visual object representation. *Cognitive Neuropsychology*, **8**, 1–19.

Farah, M. J., Levine, D. N., and Calvanio, R. (1988). A case study of mental imagery deficit. *Brain and Cognition*, **8**, 147–64.

Farah, M., Hammond, K. H., Mehta, Z., and Ratcliff, G. (1989). Category-specificity and modality-specificity in semantic memory. *Neuropsychologia*, **27**, 193–200.

Habib, M. (1986). Visual hypoemotionality and prosopagnosia associated with right temporal lobe isolation. *Neuropsycholoigia*, **24**, 577–82.

Hay, D. C. and Young, A. W. (1982). The human face. In *Normality and pathology in cognitive functions*, (ed. A. W. Ellis), pp. 173–202. Academic Press, London.

Hécaen, H. (1981). The neuropsychology of face recognition. In *Perceiving and remembering faces*, (ed. G. Davies, H. Ellis, and J. Shepherd), pp. 39–54. Academic Press, London.

Hécaen, H. and Angelergues, R. (1962). Agnosia for faces (prosopagnosia). *Archives of Neurology*, **7**, 92–100.

Humphreys, G. W. and Riddoch, M. J. (1984). Routes to object constancy: implications from neurological impairments of object constancy. *Quarterly Journal of Experimental Psychology*, **36A**, 385–415.

Humphreys, G. W. and Riddoch, M. J. (1987). *To see but not to see: a case study of visual agnosia*. Lawrence Erlbaum, London.

Humphreys, G. W., Troscianko, T., Riddoch, M. J., Boucart, M., Donnelly, N., and Harding, G. F. A. (1992*a*). Covert processing in different visual recognition systems. In *The neuropsychology of consciousness*, (ed. A. D. Milner and M. D. Rugg), pp. 39–68. Academic Press, London.

Humphreys, G. W., Riddoch, M. J., Quinlan, P. T., Price, C. J., and Donnelly, N. (1992*b*). Parallel pattern processing and visual agnosia. *Canadian Journal of Psychology*, **46**, 377–416.

Humphreys, G. W., Donnelly, N., and Riddoch, M. J. (1993). Expression is computed separately from facial identity, and it is computed separately for moving and static faces: neuropsychological evidence. *Neuropsychologia*, **31**, 173–81.

Jankowiak, J., Kinsbourne, M., Shalev, R. S., and Bachman, D. L. (1992). Preserved visual imagery and categorization in a case of associative visual agnosia. *Journal of Cognitive Neuroscience*, **4**, 119–31.

Levine, D. N. and Calvanio, R. (1989). Prosopagnosia: a defect in visual configural processing. *Brain and Cognition*, **10**, 149–70.

Levine, D. N., Warach, J., and Farah, M. (1985). Two visual systems in mental imagery: dissociation of 'what' and 'where' in imagery disorders due to bilateral posterior cerebral lesions. *Neurology*, **35**, 1010–18.

Meadows, J. C. (1974). The anatomical basis of prosopagnosia. *Journal of Neurology, Neurosurgery, and Psychiatry*, **37**, 489–501.

Mehta, Z., Newcombe, F., and de Haan, E. (1992). Selective loss of imagery in a case of visual agnosia. *Neuropsychologia*, **30**, 645–55.

Pallis, C. A. (1955). Impaired identification of faces and places with agnosia for colours: report of a case due to cerebral embolism. *Journal of Neurology, Neurosurgery, and Psychiatry*, **18**, 218–24.

Riddoch, M. J. (1990). Loss of visual imagery: a generation deficit. *Cognitive Neuropsychology*, **7**, 249–73.

Riddoch, M. J. and Humphreys, G. W. (1986). Neurological impairments of object constancy: the effects of orientation and size disparities. *Cognitive Neuropsychology*, **3**, 207–24.

Riddoch, M. J. and Humphreys, G. W. (1987). A case of integrative visual agnosia. *Brain*, **110**, 1431–62.

Young, A. W. and de Haan, E. H. F. (1988). Boundaries of covert recognition in prosopagnosia. *Cognitive Neuropsychology*, **5**, 317–36.

Young, A. W. and de Haan, E. H. F. (1992). Face recognition and awareness after brain injury. In *The neuropsychology of consciousness*, (ed. A. D. Milner and M. D. Rugg), pp. 69–90. Academic Press, London.

Young, A. W. and van de Wal, C. (1996). Charcot's case of impaired imagery. In *Classic cases in neuropsychology*, (ed. C. Code, C.-W. Wallesch, Y. Joanette, and A. R. Lecours), pp. 31–44. Erlbaum (UK) Taylor & Francis, Hove, East Sussex.

Young, A. W., Hellawell, D. and de Haan, E. H. F. (1988). Cross-domain ꜱemantic priming in normal subjects and a prosopagnosic patient. *Quarterly Journal of Experimental Psychology*, **40A**, 561–80.

8

Accounting for delusional misidentifications

Reprinted in slightly modified form from Ellis, H. D. and Young, A. W.
(1990), Accounting for delusional misidentifications, *British Journal of
Psychiatry*, **157**, 239–48. With kind permission of Professor H. Ellis and
the Royal College of Psychiatrists.

Summary

Accounts of the major forms of delusional misidentification are given
using theoretical models of the functional components underlying
recognition of familiar people. Thus, Capgras syndrome is suggested to
involve impairment of processes that can support 'covert' recognition of
familiar faces in prosopagnosia. It therefore forms a potential 'mirror
image' of the impairments underlying prosopagnosia, and earlier
attempts to link the two conditions directly are questioned. Frégoli
syndrome and intermetamorphosis are explained as defects at different
stages of an information processing chain. Not only are these accounts
consistent with the association of different delusional misidentification
syndromes with different brain injuries, but they also offer both
suggestions for new inquiries and predictions about possible preserved
and impaired abilities.

Introduction

The delusional misidentification syndromes (DMSs) are psychiatric
disorders distinguished by the fact that they all involve some deviation
from normal processes of recognizing people. A collection of papers on
DMS (Christodoulou 1986) gives a good coverage of the history,
findings, and issues, and the papers in Young and Ellis (1989a) discuss
theoretical explanations for the way people process physiognomic

information. As yet, however, the theoretical insights gained from psychological and neurological studies have had little impact on the traditionally psychiatric field of DMS.

Before discussing three of the most prominent DMS disorders (Capgras, Frégoli, and intermetamorphosis), we first describe the model of face recognition by Bruce and Young (1986), which extends that by Hay and Young (1982) and is the best summary of available data. More extensive discussions of such models are available elsewhere (e.g. Bruce 1988; Young and Ellis, 1989a; Ellis 1989). Here, we simply focus on those parts of the model that are relevant for our attempts to provide theoretical explanations for DMS. Following this, we consider the neurological condition of prosopagnosia in order both to underline the conclusions of the face recognition model and to provide the specific hypothesis for our analysis of Capgras syndrome.

A model of face recognition

It is possible to attempt a theoretical explanation of DMSs within the kind of information processing model of face recognition put forward by Bruce and Young (1986). According to this model (Fig. 8.1) the recognition of a familiar face involves sequential stages. First, there is a stage (I) in which the information concerning the structure of the seen face is encoded using descriptions which are view-centred (i.e. represent the object as it is actually seen) and/or independent of expression. These descriptions provide raw data which are then analysed for expression, facial speech, and information about age, sex, race, and so on. Marr's (1982) model of vision was adapted for this stage. The second stage (II) is where the familiarity or otherwise of a face is signalled by the face recognition units (FRUs). Familiar faces then stimulate information held at the person identity node (PIN) level (III), where semantic or biographical information is stored. This third stage may also be accessed by voice or gait or other means of signalling identity. According to Hay and Young (1982), Bruce and Young (1986), and Ellis (1986a), other aspects of face processing, such as the perception of facial expression, are accomplished independently from and in parallel with the determination of individual identity. Furthermore, information about the person's name is stored and retrieved independent of his or her biographical details.

Support for the Bruce and Young (1986) model of face recognition comes from a diary study of everyday errors of identification (Young *et al.* 1985). This revealed problems including diarists recognizing a face as

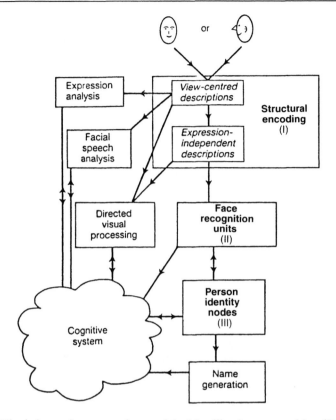

Fig. 8.1 The information processing model of familiar face recognition (Bruce and Young 1986).

being familiar but being unable to access biographical information concerning the person, and, more often, them knowing not only that the face is familiar but also all sorts of biographical details, yet not being able to locate the individual's name. Such experiences are consistent with the idea that the recognition process can become 'blocked' at each of the successive stages shown in Fig. 8.1.

Other experiments using reaction-time techniques have also produced data consistent with a sequential series of stages, each of which takes a finite time to complete in a prescribed order (see Bruce 1988; Sergent 1986). The existence of independent modules for analysing other aspects of faces than identity (age, sex, race, etc., and facial expression) is also supported by latency data (see Bruce 1986; Young *et al.* 1986; Bruce *et al.* 1988).

Much of the strongest evidence for this model, however, comes from neurological case histories of patients suffering from prosopagnosia, the inability to recognize previously familiar faces (Bodamer 1947) which usually follows bilateral occipital-inferotemporal damage (Meadows 1974). This condition produces a more or less complete breakdown of overt face recognition ability in which even the most familiar faces – friends, relatives, family, and the patient's own face when seen in a mirror – are not consciously recognized. (For a history of the disorder, see Ellis 1989.) Typically, prosopagnosic patients fall into one of two or more groups depending on whether their symptoms are primarily perceptual, whereby they see faces as blobs, caricatures, all alike, and so on, or more memory based, whereby faces look normal enough but evoke no sense of familiarity (Hécaen 1981; De Renzi 1986).

The majority of prosopagnosics have suffered strokes and are middle-aged to elderly men (Mazzuchi and Biber 1983). Usually, bilateral areas of occipito-temporal cortex are involved (Meadows 1974; Damasio *et al.* 1982), but in some cases neuroimaging techniques have revealed occipito-temporal lesions involving only the right cerebral hemisphere (De Renzi 1986; Landis *et al.* 1986). Most prosopagnosic patients manage to identify familiar people on the basis of voice, gait, and clothing which suggests that the damage occurs before the PIN stage of processing. Some display problems in identifying facial expression (Shuttleworth *et al.* 1982) but a number of prosopagnosics can interpret the moods of others based upon physiognomic cues (Bruyer *et al.* 1983). Face recognition and expression interpretation, however, are doubly dissociable, implying separate mechanisms (Kurucz and Feldmar 1979). By the same token, face recognition and the ability to make use of lip-reading to aid normal communication also show double dissociation (Campbell *et al.* 1986). As Ellis (1986*b*) has argued, these different cases lend support to the various stages of the model shown in Fig. 8.1.

Theoretical approach to understanding DMS

Our aim in this paper is to advance explanations for the major DMSs based on the current understanding of normal face recognition processes and the ways in which they can be impaired. In doing this, our explicit intention is to extend the cognitive neuropsychological approach to the study of conditions that have been traditionally defined as being psychiatric in nature.

Recent developments in cognitive neuropsychology have leant heavily on the view that complex mental functions involve the interaction of a number of modular subcomponents (Fodor 1983; Ellis and Young 1988; Shallice 1988). The neurological and neurophysiological literature now provides abundant evidence for such modular organization, which would make sense in terms of the important 'design principles' of keeping essential neural interconnections as short as possible and allowing part of a complex system to be modified by experience or evolution without adversely affecting the performance of the rest of the system (Marr 1982; Cowey 1985).

Studies of the different types of breakdown that can affect performance of any complex cognitive capacity can thus provide insight into the underlying organization of the responsible functional components. More importantly, an adequate theoretical model should be able to account for the types of impairment that can occur and in turn, should itself be modified if inconsistent forms of impairment are actually observed (Ellis and Young 1988).

Here we try to demonstrate that this approach, which has been successful in understanding the breakdown of normal performance, both in terms of everyday slips and errors and the deleterious effects of brain injury, can also be of benefit in understanding delusional misidentifications. In doing so, we do not entirely take a leap into the dark, since much recent evidence has begun to suggest some organic involvement in DMS, and parallels to neurological conditions have already been drawn. Furthermore, such an approach, carried out systematically, has advantages in allowing a more theoretical understanding of the conditions, in suggesting aspects worthy of further investigation, and in predicting certain patterns of co-occurring symptoms.

The last point leads us to an important caveat. It is traditional to refer to delusional misidentification *syndromes*, but in fact, unlike when they were first introduced, each of these is now actually defined by a single particular symptom, rather than a symptom constellation. We would thus prefer to speak of Capgras *symptom*, and so on, but have retained the conventional 'syndrome' terminology here because it has become so thoroughly entrenched in the literature.

The major DMSs

Capgras syndrome

In 1923 Capgras and Reboul-Lachaux reported the case of a 53-year-old woman who displayed what they called 'l'illusion des sosies', a delusional belief that people who she knew had been replaced by identical doubles [see Berson (1983) for an explanation of 'sosies' and Christodoulou (1986) for the historical/mythological background]. In addition to believing that her husband and children had been replaced

by doubles, the woman later claimed that police and neighbours had
been similarly duplicated. She also believed that there existed doubles
of herself.

Berson (1983) reports a computer search which located 133 similar
case reports in English, as well as reports in French, Italian, Russian,
Dutch, German, Spanish, and Japanese; and Signer (1987) found
reports of 315 patients in the English and French literature. In most
cases the diagnosis was of schizophrenia. Many cases also appeared to
involve organic disorders, but, regardless of the cause of Capgras
syndrome, the symptoms of most patients are dominated by a marked
paranoid component (Berson 1983). It is also worth noting that the
people believed to have been duplicated are generally those close to the
patients. These are the kind of people for whom the patient has strongly
positive or negative affective responses. Sometimes patients believe that
there is more than a single impersonator (Todd *et al.* 1981).

Capgras patients tend to be paranoid, or, at least, rather suspicious by
nature, and the doubles are usually thought of as evil or dangerous in
some way. Capgras patients also tend to suffer from depersonalization–
derealization. Patients sometimes report that everything looks strange,
for example, things may look painted or not natural and faces may look
like masks or wax models or seem to have been changed by plastic
surgery. The incidence of Capgras among females is generally thought
to be rather higher than it is among males (Sims and White 1973).

Organic v. functional aetiology of Capgras syndrome: Although labelling
Capgras syndrome as a manifestation of paranoid schizophrenia has
constituted an explanation of the disorder for some commentators, it is
a rather unsatisfactory and incomplete one. Merrin and Silberfarb
(1976), whose ideas were more impressive, saw a connection between
depersonalization–derealization and Capgras syndrome symptoms when
they wrote 'a number of cases began with reduced feelings of unreality
or depersonalization, (were) followed by indiscriminate misidentification and finally by the establishment of the Capgras delusion'.
However, as Todd *et al.* (1981), point out, this in itself does not fully
explain the development of Capgras syndrome, because patients
afflicted by feelings of depersonalization or derealization have insight
and appreciate the illusory nature of the phenomenon, whereas those
with Capgras delusion generally don't.

In the main, Capgras syndrome has been treated as a functional
disorder. A number of investigators have noted, however, that Capgras
patients often have associated brain lesions, or that their symptoms may
have resulted from some form of poisoning or other exogenous factor.

In his review of focal abnormalities of the central nervous system in patients with a DMS, Joseph (1986) discovered that the majority of patients have clear computerized tomography (CT) scan evidence of brain abnormalities. Of the 23 patients studies by him, approximately two-thirds had signs of cortical atrophy. In all cases the signs were bilateral; in some they were largely frontal, in others parietal or temporal. Unfortunately, Joseph did not break down his group by specific DMS so there is no way of attributing specific sites of brain damage to particular types of DMS. It may be noted that Kiriakos and Ananth (1980) found obvious evidence of organic damage in only four out of 13 Capgras patients, but they employed X-ray and electro-encephalography (EEG) measures – rather gross forms of imaging – whereas many lesions require CT scan or magnetic resonance imaging (MRI) to become evident. Joseph (personal communication, 1989) claims that all DMS patients given full evaluation have revealed some CNS abnormality.

Fishbain and Rosomoff (1986) reported the case of someone displaying Capgras syndrome following metrizanide myelography. The patient, a 67-year-old male, had been admitted to hospital following pain in his left calf. Twenty hours after myelography, the patient developed the following symptoms; severe vomiting, severe headache, confusion, disorientation to time and place (he thought he was in his son's home), and a delusional belief that his doctor was a duplicate of the original. After treatment with prochlorperazine, symptoms gradually remitted.

MacCallum (1973) also reported Capgras syndrome following medical intervention; in this case it appeared to be due to the patient inhaling an overdose of a bronchial dilator containing adrenaline and adropine-methonitrate. In another of MacCallum's cases, Capgras syndrome appeared to be related to the patient's diabetes. A patient described by Hay et al. (1974) showed Capgras-like symptoms following electro-convulsive therapy (ECT). All of these instances cast doubt on Enoch's (1963) suggestion that the title 'Capgras syndrome' should be reserved for the delusional misidentification and replacement for an identical double in a clear sensorium, and this *without organic basis* (i.e. in a setting of functional illness with a psychodynamic interpretation).

Explaining Capgras syndrome: As we have indicated earlier, a number of researchers now take the view that Capgras syndrome may be the result of underlying organic brain damage. Although the evidence for this is not yet conclusive, modern brain-imaging techniques have shown that in a large number of cases of Capgras syndrome there is clear evidence of brain lesions. None the less, some commentators, such as Berson (1983), argue that 'organic factors in themselves, however, seem neither necessary nor sufficient to explain the particular and peculiar content of the delusion'. This view is perhaps overstated.

One of the most interesting suggestions put forward by those who favour an organic basis for Capgras syndrome is that the condition is related to one long recognized in the neurological literature, known as reduplicative paramnesia (Alexander *et al.* 1979). Such paramnesias often involve reduplication of places, with the patient maintaining that he/she is in a place which is an almost exact copy of the actual location. There is a clear parallel with the Capgras delusion, which involves reduplication of people, and Alexander *et al.* (1979) demonstrated that a combination of bilateral frontal and right hemisphere damage seemed to be present for patients of both types. The link between the two conditions is supported by Anderson (1988), who drew attention to a number of cases in which Capgras patients were observed to reduplicate more than just people. Interestingly, Kapur *et al.* (1988) reported the case of a 71-year-old man who developed reduplicative paramnesia for places but not faces following right frontal vascular lesion, indicating the dissociable nature of reduplicative paramnesia.

A link between prosopagnosia and Capgras syndrome has also been suggested, but never successfully forged. Lewis (1987) in his study of a single case of transient Capgras syndrome, for example, provided MRI data demonstrating the presence of bilateral occipito-temporal lesions as well as smaller bilateral frontal lesions. The frontal lesions are consistent with the findings of Alexander *et al.* (1979) but occipito-temporal lesions are the usual anatomical correlate of prosopagnosia (Meadows 1974; Damasio *et al.* 1982). As we have said, the occipito-temporal lesions underlying prosopagnosia are often bilateral, but in some cases (based only on evidence from brain imaging) are apparently located exclusively in the right cerebral hemisphere (De Renzi 1986; Landis *et al.* 1986).

The patient studied by Lewis (1987) had actually shown signs of mild prosopagnosia during childhood, and this prompted him to suggest some sort of connection between the two syndromes. According to Lewis there seems to be a parallel between prosopagnosia and Capgras syndrome. In the latter case there would appear to be a disconnection between the percept of a face and its evocation of affective memories.

Joseph (1986) also posited a disconnection explanation. 'It may be that in misidentification syndromes in particular and reduplicative phenomena in general, brain disease causes a disconnection between the right and left hemisphere cortical areas, that decode afferent sensory information and maintain the normal functions of orientation to person, place, time and object relationship that we describe as "orientation".' In Joseph's view each cerebral hemisphere forms a representation of a face separately. Normally, these images are 'fused' by interhemispheric transfer, and thus are presented on a conscious level as a fully integrated representation of the external world. 'In patients with misidentification syndromes . . . each hemispheric 'image' is presented separately leading to an awareness at the conscious level of two simultaneously separate but physically identifiable or similar persons, places, objects, times or object relationships. Depending upon which hemispheric connections are most impaired, the clinical syndromes of misidentification, re-duplication, or disorientation will result.' Although there is as yet no very compelling empirical evidence to support Joseph's view, it merits further investigation and is not necessarily inconsistent with the theoretical ideas which we present shortly.

Face processing impairments in Capgras patients: There seem little doubt that face processing impairments can be found in Capgras patients. Tzavaras *et al.* (1986) found that on face-matching tests (Tzavaras *et al.* 1970) DMS patients were significantly poorer than pathological and normal controls. They deemed this 'an infra-clinical prosopagnosic symptom' which may imply some organic factor in DMS. Shraberg and Weitzel (1979) studied two Capgras patients by giving them the Benton face-matching test (Benton *et al.* 1983) which they claimed was particularly sensitive to prosopagnosia. Finding that their Capgras patients also performed poorly on this test they then argued that a parallel existed between the two syndromes. However, as Benton (1980) has emphasized, the face-matching test is not sensitive to proso-pagnosia; many, if not most, prosopagnosics can perform the test adequately (Bauer 1984; Young and Ellis 1989*b*), although they may rely on unusual strategies (Newcombe 1979). Instead, it is often patients with right parietal lesions who perform such tasks especially poorly; yet these are not prosopagnosic (i.e. they remain able to recognize familiar faces). In the same way, it should be emphasized that patients who experience the Capgras delusion are not prosopagnosic; they continue to recognize without apparent difficulty the dummies and impostors that they say have replaced their relatives. So if there is any connection between DMS and prosopagnosia it is unlikely to be a direct one.

Other misconceptions of the nature of prosopagnosia have also been introduced into the literature on Capgras syndrome. For example, Todd *et al.* (1981) maintain that in order for an organic aetiology for Capgras syndrome to be established, it is necessary to show a clear cause and effect relationship between prosopagnosia and Capgras syndrome. They even add that the association is particularly doubtful in view of the fact that there are usually no signs of any visual field defects in Capgras patients. Here they appear to believe, erroneously, that visual field defects are a necessary concomitant of prosopagnosia. This is not the case. Prosopagnosia can exist in the absence of visual field defects, although they frequently accompany the condition but not, it would seem, in any causally connected way (Meadows 1974).

If there is a connection between prosopagnosia and Capgras syndrome, then it operates in a rather more subtle way. In order to develop this argument, it is necessary to consider evidence for different recognition routes, derived from the phenomena of 'covert recognition' of faces by prosopagnosics. Bauer (1984) studied a prosopagnosic patient, LF, who had suffered bilateral occipito-temporal brain damage following a motorcycle accident. He was profoundly prosopagnosic, and yet when shown pictures of previously familiar faces (famous or personally known), along with five names drawn from the same semantic category, which were read out to him, LF displayed significantly greater autonomic responses to the correct name compared with the four incorrect names. This technique, known as the guilty knowledge test, is widely used by American police forces as a method for detecting lying by criminal suspects. Bauer's data mainly concern the skin conductance response (SCR). LF showed a discriminatory SCR to some 62.5 per cent of the known faces – well above chance level of performance (which would be 20 per cent). Tranel and Damasio (1985) confirmed Bauer's observations using a modified technique in which a series of randomly arranged known and unknown faces were presented to two prosopagnosic patients. They also showed increased autonomic reactions to the previously known faces.

Bauer (1984, 1986) advanced the view that there are two routes to facial recognition. The main route runs from visual cortex to temporal lobes via the inferior longitudinal fasciculus. Following Bear (1983), he termed this the 'ventral route'; it corresponds to the system responsible for overt or conscious recognition, and it is the route which typically is damaged in cases of prosopagnosia. The other, described as the 'dorsal route', runs between the visual cortex and the limbic system, via the inferior parietal lobule, and is sometimes intact in prosopagnosic patients. It is this latter route which, Bauer claims, gives the face its emotional significance and hence, when the ventral route is selectively damaged, can give rise to covert recognition (i.e. recognition at an unconscious level).

If we accept Bauer's dual recognition route (and from the work of de Haan *et al.* 1987, it may be that we should be looking for more than two routes), we can try to apply the notion towards an understanding of Capgras syndrome. Here, we begin to explore the phenomenon of Capgras syndrome by suggesting that it is a mirror image of prosopagnosia. In other words, patients with Capgras syndrome seem to have an intact primary or ventral route to face recognition, but may have a disconnection along or damage within the secondary or dorsal route. This would mean that they receive a veridical image of the person they are looking at, which stimulates all the appropriate overt semantic data held about that person, but they lack another, possibly confirming, set of information which, as Lewis (1987) and Bauer (1986) have independently suggested, may carry some sort of affective tone. When patients find themselves in such a conflict (that is, receiving some information which indicates that the face in front of them belongs to X, but not receiving confirmation of this), they may adopt some sort of rationalization strategy in which the individual before them is deemed to be an impostor, a dummy, a robot, or whatever extant technology may suggest.

Derombies (1935) also attached great importance to the affective state of Capgras patients. He suggested that Capgras syndrome results from a simultaneous intellectual recognition and affectively engendered non-recognition of faces; at one level the patient recognizes the face but at another level he or she does not recognize it. More recently (and also independently) Anderson (1988) made a similar suggestion when he argued 'that the Capgras delusion results from lesions of the pathway for visual recognition at a stage where visual images are imbued with affective familiarity'. Anderson's ideas (1988) (and those of Derombies) are similar to the ones presented above although he is not able to be more specific about the mechanism by which 'affective familiarity' may operate. Indeed, one difference is that our hypothesis rests on the view that more than one recognition pathway is involved, and makes the clear prediction that Capgras patients will *not* show the normally appropriate skin conductance responses to familiar faces, despite the fact that these will be overtly recognized.

The explanation, however, is still incomplete. Berson (1983) pointed out that in Capgras syndrome, not all faces seem to be duplicated, only those of people close to the patient. A possible answer to this is that it is only in these instances that one expects more than the basic information about a face. Only certain faces normally have associated with them a particularly strong affective component, and therefore only these are vulnerable in the case of any disconnection between the visual areas and the cerebral structures involved in Bauer's dorsal recognition pathway.

One may extend this argument to other reduplicative paramnesias. Places, objects, and so on are not affectively neutral and so the absence of an emotionally charged input could produce the feeling of recognition, but it not being quite right. Again this would be particularly true for those places and objects with which the patient is most familiar.

Frégoli syndrome

In 1927 Courbon and Fail reported another form of DMS. Their patient was a 27-year-old labourer's daughter who had worked variously as a domestic servant, in a factory, in a restaurant, and so on. She was paid by the day and slept in Salvation Army type refuges. Her abiding passion was the theatre; she preferred to go without food in order to attend a performance. Admitted to hospital following an attack on an employer, she reported to Courbon and Fail that she was the victim of enemies; in particular of the actresses Robine and Sarah Bernhardt whom she had often seen in the theatre. She insisted that these actresses had followed her about for many years, taking the form of people she knew or met, overpowering her thoughts, making her do this instead of that and stroking her or forcing her to masturbate. The patient reported often being interfered with or attacked by people who particularly took the form of Robine.

Courbon and Fail adopted the term 'Frégoli syndrome' after the Italian actor and mimic, Leopoldo Frégoli, famous for his ability to impersonate people on the stage. The hallmark of the Frégoli syndrome is the delusional misidentification of familiar persons disguised as others. De Pauw et al. (1987) classified the Frégoli delusion as hyper-identification. They contrast this with Capgras syndrome, which was classified as hypo-identification. They reported the case of Mrs C, a 66-year-old widow, who believed that she was being persecuted by her cousin and his female friend. She described in detail how the couple disguised themselves with make-up, wigs, dark glasses, false beards, and different clothes, and repeatedly accosted her when she was out. She confronted strangers in public demanding that they reveal their true identity; she took complicated routes on her way home to shake off her persecutors; and she often reported their activities to the local police. 'They keep changing their clothes and their hairstyles, but I know it's them. He can look like an old man. They want a medal for doing that. It's like an actor and actress preparing for different scenes', she said.

Mrs C had a history of brain damage; she suffered haematoma over the left frontal area after a fall in 1982. A CT scan also showed a right-sided posterior temporo-parietal infarct together with some general cortical atrophy. She had earlier been treated for hypertension and she had also been diagnosed as having right-sided temporal arteritis. Although she recovered from her initial symptoms of speech slurring and memory problems as well as her orientation difficulties, she then developed the delusional belief just described. Her Frégoli syndrome seemed to be controllable with trifluoperazine.

As in cases of Capgras syndrome, Frégoli may be associated with some degree of objective face processing impairment. De Pauw *et al.* (1987) found that Mrs C scored poorly on the Warrington face-recognition test. More detailed investigation of such impairments would be worthwhile.

Frégoli syndrome bears some relation to a type of error that all of us make in everyday life (Young *et al.* 1985). When we expect to meet a particular person, occasionally and transiently we will misidentify a stranger as that person. However, we usually quickly correct this mistake when inconsistent evidence is picked up. In the Frégoli syndrome, on the other hand, such inconsistencies are also noted, but attributed to the effects of disguise. The syndrome can thus be characterized as involving impaired decision mechanisms. In Bruce and Young's terms, the impairment is in the cognitive system itself, which places an inappropriate evaluation on the evidence it receives. Such decision mechanisms can also malfunction for normal people, as other everyday errors collected by Young *et al.* (1985) showed.

The PIN stage and associated cognitive system would therefore be the likely site for malfunction leading to Frégoli syndrome (see Fig. 8.2). Specifically, either the PIN system becomes driven by a deranged cognitive system or hyperexcitable nodes representing particular people appear to become engaged, sometimes almost regardless of whatever output from the previous FRU stage occurs, and impaired decision mechanisms accept this evidence. Since strangers' faces are often the source of the patients' delusions it is clear that it would be of interest to study whether any degree of resemblance to the misidentified person is necessary.

Intermetamorphosis

First described by Courbon and Tusques (1932), intermetamorphosis refers to cases where, for the patient, the physical appearance of some people may change radically to correspond with the appearance of someone else. Courbon and Tusques described a 49-year-old depressive

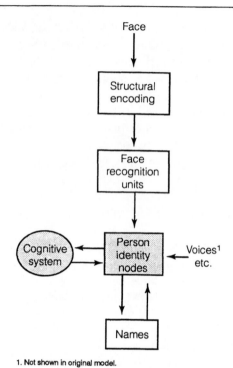

1. Not shown in original model.

Fig. 8.2 Simplified face recognition model indicating the level at which it is proposed the Frégoli delusion occurs.

patient who reported that animals and objects she owned took the form of another animal or object. She also experienced changes in her husband's appearance, which could become exactly like that of a neighbour or could rapidly transform to look larger or smaller or younger. Various people in rapid succession also took on the guise of her son, but she used the particularly large size of his feet to discount these delusions.

Courbon and Tusques (1932) pointed out that intermetamorphosis involves a false recognition of both appearance and associated identity, whereas in the illusion of Frégoli the patient is not confused about physical appearance. Intermetamorphosis is relatively rare; Bick (1986) reviewed two cases reported after Courbon and Tusques' (Christodoulou 1975; Malliaras *et al.* 1978) and presented another, a 42-year-old woman who had had a long history of epilepsy and paranoid schizophrenia. During a period in hospital, she became suddenly agitated and declared that her doctor was her dead uncle.

According to Bick (1986), three of the four cases reviewed by him had temporal lobe epilepsy. Joseph (1987) has subsequently described a

49-year-old patient who displayed both Capgras syndrome (believing her husband had been replaced by an identical impostor) and inter-metamorphosis (stating that several other patients looked like her father and that her son's physical appearance had altered). In this case a CT scan was performed and it revealed mild atrophy of the frontal lobe, severe bilateral atrophy of the temporal lobe, moderate atrophy of the occipital lobe and a mildly enlarged ventricular system. The *prima facie* evidence for a possible organic component in intermetamorphosis, as for other DMS disorders, is thus quite strong.

In order to establish an explanation for intermetamorphosis within the Bruce and Young (1986) model of normal face recognition pro-cesses, it is necessary to focus on the second stage, the FRU stage, highlighted in Fig. 8.3. Representations for known faces are posited to exist, each of which is somehow excited or triggered by the appearance of the particular person. The FRUs then signal familiarity and, in turn, communicate with appropriate PINs in the semantic memory system where the person's biographical details are stored.

Intermetamorphosis may be construed as an inappropriate excitation

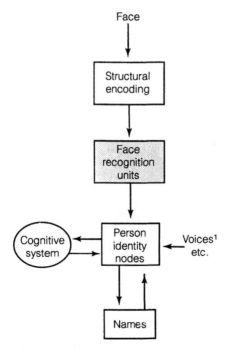

1. Not shown in original model.

Fig. 8.3 Simplified face recognition model indicating the level at which it is proposed that intermetamorphosis occurs.

of an FRU which could occur, for example, if the particular FRU had a considerably lowered triggering threshold. A corollary to this suggestion is that it is more likely that faces similar to the misidentified person will cause the unit to fire inappropriately, and, as with the Frégoli symptom, more systematic investigation of the resemblance between the appearance of the actual and delusionally substitued people would be useful. A clear prediction from our account of these conditions is that physical resemblance will be important in triggering episodes of intermetamorphosis but much less important to the Frégoli delusion.

At this stage it is not possible to establish why and how such threshold shifts occur, but notice that once an FRU has fired it will automatically then cause the corresponding and equally inappropriate PIN to become excited. Unfortunately, none of the case histories of patients' behaviour during such an instance of misidentification has reported how the patients responded to voices. According to the model shown in Fig. 8.3, voices input from a different recognition system but employ the same PINs. Joseph and O'Leary (1987) indeed reported a Frégoli patient who claimed that a Mr B had been replaced by another acquaintance. While the physical appearance of Mr B was unchanged he appeared to have the other person's voice. Thus, whereas Frégoli patients may mis-perceive voices, those with intermetamorphosis syndrome could make an incorrect facial identification but should not produce the same error on the voice. This should produce discrepancies at times which would, perhaps, be resolved because of the primacy of visual over aural perception but could, none the less, be elicited during clinical interview.

Conclusion

The advantages in attempting to explain various DMS states within the theoretical constructs derived from studies of normal and pathological face recognition are numerous. Chief among them, of course, is the hope that it may lead both to a complete understanding of DMSs and, in turn, assist clinicians in diagnosis and treatment.

Secondly, the opportunity to bring together a seemingly disparate set of phenomena, for some time effectively dealt with as being largely unrelated, carries with it many advantages. For example, the ideas that have been posited regarding Capgras syndrome allow us to perceive a very obvious deficit in the model outlined in Fig. 8.1, that is, it only depicts the 'overt' route to face recognition. Experiments on proso-pagnosic patients, together with the theoretical ideas we have presented here, strongly suggest that the model is incomplete in that it only displays a single route to recognition and fails to accommodate what, perhaps, may turn out to be a sort of emotional recognition of faces (and indeed other routes, as well).

The third aspect of our endeavours to which we wish to draw attention is its potential value in organizing clinical observations of DMS patients. We have suggested various types of evidence that should be collected routinely in such cases. It is, for instance, clearly important to note patients' responses to voices as well as faces, because by doing so we may refine our ideas concerning the level of impairment. Some assessment of the similarity between people mistakenly perceived in intermetamorphosis and wrongly categorized in Frégoli syndrome would also be of theoretical benefit.

The final point we wish to stress is that discussing DMS in relation to prosopagnosia reinforces the suggestions made by Joseph (1986) and others that DMS may originate primarily from organic bases. The next step must surely be to derive routinely, in cases of DMS, high-quality brain images that should assist in classification. In time it should be possible to correlate particular DMSs with damage to specific brain areas.

References

Alexander, M. P., Stuss, D. T. and Benson, D. F. (1979). Capgras syndrome: a reduplicative phenomenon. *Neurology*, **29**, 334–9.

Anderson, D. N. (1988). The delusion of inanimate doubles: implications for understanding the Capgras phenomenon. *British Journal of Psychiatry*, **153**, 694–9. -

Bauer, R. M. (1984). Autonomic recognition of names and faces: a neuropsychological application of the guilty knowledge test. *Neuropsychologia*, **22**, 457–69.

Bauer, R. M. (1986). The cognitive psychophysiology of prosopagnosia. In *Aspects of face processing*, (ed. H. Ellis, M. Jeeves, F. Newcombe, and A. Young). Martinus Nijhoff, Dordrecht.

Bear, D. M. (1983). Hemispheric specialization and the neurology of emotion. *Archives of Neurology*, **40**, 195–202.

Benton, A. L. (1980). The neuropsychology of facial recognition. *American Psychologist*, **35**, 176–86.

Benton, A. L., Hamsher, K., Varney, N. R., and Spreen, O. (1983). *Contributions to neuropsychological assessment*. Oxford University Press.

Berson, R. J. (1983). Capgras syndrome. *American Journal of Psychiatry*, **140**, 8.

Bick, P. A. (1986). The syndrome of intermetamorphosis. *Bibliotheca Psychiatrica*, **164**, 131–5.

Bodamer, J. (1947). Die Prosop-Agnosie. *Archiv für Psychiatrie und Nervenkrankheiten*, **179**, 6–54.

Bruce, V. (1986). Recognising familiar faces. In *Aspects of face processing*, (ed. H. Ellis, M. Jeeves, F. Newcombe, and A. Young). Martinus Nijhoff, Dordrecht.

Bruce, V. (1988). *Recognizing faces*. Lawrence Erlbaum, Hillsdale, NJ.

Bruce, V. and Young, A. (1986). Understanding face recognition. *British Journal of Psychology*, **77**, 305–27.

Bruce, V., Ellis, H., Gibling, F., and Young, A. W. (1988). Parallel processing of the sex and familiarity of faces. *Canadian Journal of Psychology*, **41**, 510–20.

Bruyer, R., Laterre, C., Seron, X., Feyereisen, P., Strypstein, E., Pierrard, E., and Rectem, D. (1983). A case of prosopagnosia with some preserved covert remembrance of familiar faces. *Brain and Cognition*, **2**, 257–84.

Campbell, R., Landis, T., and Regard, M. (1986). Face recognition and lip reading: a neurological dissociation. *Brain*, **109**, 509–21.

Capgras, J. and Reboul-Lachaux, J. (1923). L'illusion des 'sosies' dans un délire systématise chronique. *Bulletin de la Société Clinique de Médecine Mentale*, **2**, 6–16.

Christodoulou, G. N. (1975). Reported in Bick (1986).

Christodoulou, G. W. (1986). Role of depersonalization-derealization phenomena in the delusional misidentification syndromes. *Bibliotheca Psychiatrica*, **164**, 99–104.

Courbon, P. and Fail, G. (1927). Syndrome d'illusion de Frégoli et schizophrénie. *Bulletin de la Société Clinique de Medicine Mentale*, **15**, 121–5.

Courbon, P. and Tusques, J. (1932). Illusions d'intermetamorphose et de charme. *Annales Médico-Psychologiques*, **14**, 401–6.

Cowey, A. (1985). Aspects of cortical organization related to selective attention and selective impairments of visual perception: a tutorial review. In *Attention and performance, XI*, (ed. M. Posner and O. Marin). Erlbaum, New Jersey.

Damasio, A. R., Damasio, H. and Van Hoesen, G. W. (1982). Prosopagnosia: anatomical basis and behavioral mechanisms. *Neurology*, **32**, 331–41.

De Haan, E., Young, A., and Newcombe, F. (1987). Face recognition without awareness. *Cognitive Neuropsychology*, **4**, 385–415.

De Pauw, K. W., Szulecka, T. K., and Poltock, T. L. (1987). Frégoli syndrome after cerebral infaction. *Journal of Nervous and Mental Diseases*, **175**, 433–8.

De Renzi, E. (1986). Current issues in prosopagnosia. In *Aspects of face processing*, (ed. H. Ellis, M. Jeeves, F. Newcombe, and A. Young). Martinus Nijhoff, Dordrecht.

Derombies, M. (1935). L'illusion de sosies, forme particulière de la méconnaissance systématique (Thèse de Paris: quoted by A. Brochado, *Annales Médico-Psychologiques*, **94**, 706–17).

Ellis, H. D. (1986a). Processes underlying face recognition. In *The neuropsychology of face perception and facial expression*, (ed. R. Bruyer). Lawrence Erlbaum, Hillsdale, NJ.

Ellis, H. D. (1986b). Disorders of face recognition. In *Neurology*, (ed. K. Poek, H. J. Freund, and H. Ganshirt). Springer, Heidelberg.

Ellis, H. D. (1989). Past and recent studies of prosopagnosia. In *Developments in clinical and experimental neuropsychology* (ed. J. R. Crawford and D. M. Parker). Plenum, New York.

Ellis, A. W. and Young, A. W. (1988). *Human cognitive neuropsychology.* Erlbaum, London.

Enoch, M. (1963). The Capgras syndrome. *Acta Psychiatrica Scandinavica*, **39**, 437–62.

Fishbain, D. A. and Rosomoff, H. (1986). Capgras syndrome associated with metrizamide myelography. *International Journal of Psychiatry in Medicine*, **16**, 131–6.

Fodor, J. (1983). *The modularity of mind.* MIT Press, Cambridge, MA.

Hay, D. C. and Young, A. W. (1982). The human face. In *Normality and pathology in cognitive functions*, (ed. A. Ellis). Academic Press, New York.

Hay, G. G., Jolley, D. J., and Jones, R. G. (1974). A case of Capgras syndrome in association with pseudo-hypoparathyroidism. *Acta Psychiatrica Scandinavica*, **50**, 73–7.

Hécaen, H. (1981). The neuropsychology of face recognition. In *perceiving and remembering faces*, (ed. G. Davies, H. Ellis, and J. Shepherd). Academic Press, London.

Joseph, A. B. (1986). Focal central nervous system abnormalities in patients with misidentification syndromes. *Bibliotheca Psychiatrica*, **164**, 68–79.

Joseph, A. B. (1987). Delusional misidentification of the Capgras and inter-metamorphosis types responding to clorazepate. *Acta Psychiatrica Scandinavica*, **75**, 330–2.

Joseph, A. B. and O'Leary, D. H. (1987). Anterior cortical atrophy in Frégoli syndrome. *Journal of Clinical Psychiatry*, **48**, 409–11.

Kapur, N., Turner, A., and King, C. (1988). Reduplicative paramnesia: possible anatomical and neuropsychological mechanisms. *Journal of Neurology, Neurosurgery, and Psychiatry*, **51**, 579–81.

Kiriakos, R. and Ananth, J. (1980). Review of 13 cases of Capgras syndrome. *American Journal of Psychiatry*, **137**, 1605–7.

Kurucz, J. and Feldmar, G. (1979). Proso-affective agnosia as a symptom of cerebral organic disease. *Journal of the American Geriatrics Society*, **27**, 225–30.

Landis, T., Cummings, J. G., Christen, L., Bogen, J. E. and Imhof, H.-G. (1986). Are unilateral right posterior cerebral lesions sufficient to cause prosopagnosia? Clinical and radiological findings in six additional patients. *Cortex*, **22**, 243–52.

Lewis, S. W. (1987). Brain imaging in a case of Capgras syndrome. *British Journal of Psychiatry*, **150**, 117–21.

MacCallum, W. A. G. (1963). Capgras symptoms with an organic basis. *British Journal of Psychiatry*, **123**, 639–42.

Malliaras, D. E., Kossovitsa, Y. T. and Christodoulou, G. N. (1978). Organic contributors to the intermetamorphosis syndrome. *American Journal of Psychiatry*, **135**, 985–7.

Marr, D. (1982). *Vision.* Freeman, San Francisco.

Mazzuchi, A. and Biber, C. (1983). Is prosopagnosia more frequent in males than females? *Cortex*, **19**, 509–16.

Meadows, J. C. (1974). The anatomical basis of prosopagnosia. *Journal of Neurology, Neurosurgery, and Psychiatry*, **37**, 489–501.

Merrin, E. L. and Silberfarb, P. M. (1976). The Capgras phenomenon. *Archives of General Psychiatry*, **33**, 965–8.

Newcombe, F. (1979). The processing of visual information in prosopagnosia and acquired dyslexia: functional versus physiological interpretation. In *Research in psychology and medicine I* (ed. D. Osborne, M. Gruneberg and J. Eiser). Academic Press, London.

Sergent, J. (1986). Methodological constraints on neuropsychological studies of face perception in normals. In *The neuropsychology of face perception and facial expression*, (ed. R. Bruyer). Erlbaum, Hillsdale, NJ.

Shallice, T. (1988). *From neuropsychology to mental structure*. Cambridge University Press.

Shraberg, D. and Weitzel, W. D. (1979). Prosopagnosia and the Capgras syndrome. *Journal of Clinical Psychiatry*, **40**, 313–16.

Shuttleworth, E. C., Syring, V. and Allen, N. (1982). Further observations on the nature of prosopagnosia. *Brain and Cognition*, **1**, 307–22.

Signer, S. F. (1987). Capgras syndrome: the delusion of substitution. *Journal of Clinical Psychiatry*, **48**, 147–150.

Sims, A. and White. (1973). Coexistence of the Capgras and de Clérambault syndromes: a case history. *British Journal of Psychiatry*, **123**, 635–7.

Todd, J., Dewhurst, K., and Wallis, D. (1981). The syndrome of Capgras. *British Journal of Psychiatry*, **139**, 319–27.

Tranel, D. and Damasio, A. R. (1985). Knowledge without awareness: an autonomic index of facial recognition by prosopagnosics. *Science*, **228**, 1453–4.

Tzavaras, A., Hécaen, H., and LeBras, H. (1970). Le problème de la specificité du déficit de la reconnaissance du visage humain lors des lésions hemisphériques unilatérales. *Neuropsychologia*, **8**, 403–18.

Tzavaras, A., Luate, J., and Didault, E. (1986). Face recognition dysfunction and delusional misidentification syndromes. In *Aspects of face processing*, (ed. H. Ellis, M. Jeeves, F. Newcombe, and A. Young). Martinus Nijhoff, Dordrecht.

Young, A. W. and Ellis, H. D. (1989a). *Handbook of research on face processing*. North-Holland, Amsterdam.

Young, A. W. and Ellis, H. D. (1989b). Childhood prosopagnosia. *Brain and Cognition*, **9**, 16–47.

Young, A. W., Hay, D. C., and Ellis, A. W. (1985). The faces that launched a thousand slips: everyday difficulties and errors in recognizing people. *British Journal of Psychology*, **76**, 495–523.

Young, A. W., McWeeny, Hay, D. C., *et al.* (1986). Matching familiar and unfamiliar faces on identity and expression. *Psychological Research*, **48**, 63–8.

9

Reduplication of visual stimuli

Reprinted in slightly modified form from Young, A. W., Hellawell, D. J., Wright, S., and Ellis, H. D. (1994), Reduplication of visual stimuli, *Behavioural Neurology*, **7**, 135–42. With kind permission of co-authors and Professor H. Sagar (Editor, *Behavioural Neurology*).

Summary

Investigation of P.T., a man who experienced reduplicative delusions, revealed significant impairments on tests of recognition memory for faces and understanding of emotional facial expressions. On formal tests of his recognition abilities, P.T. showed reduplication to familiar faces, buildings, and written names, but not to familiar voices. Reduplication may therefore have been a genuinely visual problem in P.T.'s case, since it was not found to auditory stimuli. This is consistent with hypotheses which propose that the basis of reduplication can lie in part in malfunction of the visual system.

Introduction

Reduplication is a curious phenomenon in which patients are convinced that people or things have exact or nearly exact duplicates (Weinstein and Burnham 1991). Cases have been described involving reduplication of people [such as the Capgras delusion (Capgras and Reboul-Lachaux 1923)], places [reduplicative paramnesia (Pick 1903)], and everyday objects [e.g. the belief that one's possessions have been replaced (Anderson 1988)]. For many years, accounts of reduplication of people, and especially the Capgras delusion, appeared mainly in the psychiatric literature whereas reduplicative paramnesia was considered a neurological problem, despite the fact that Pick's (1903) original report included a patient who reduplicated both people and places. However, studies showing the presence of brain disease in Capgras cases (Förstl *et al.* 1991) have led to the recognition of an underlying similarity between these different forms of reduplication (Alexander *et al.* 1979; Weinstein and Burnham 1991).

Although the now frequent observation of brain disease in patients who show reduplication is obviously important, it does not in itself explain the strange content of these delusions. One promising approach is to argue that they reflect an interaction of impairments, in which some form of anomalous experience created by a cognitive or perceptual deficit it itself misinterpreted, thus giving rise to the delusion (Fleminger 1992; Fleminger and Burns 1993; Young *et al.* 1993; Ellis and de Pauw 1994).

In fact, a number of researchers take the view that reduplication is based on a combination of perceptual, memory, and cognitive deficits (Benson *et al.* 1976; Patterson and Mack 1985; Kapur *et al.* 1988). Since these may interact to create reduplicative delusions, the roles of different hypothesized causal factors need not necessarily be mutually exclusive; it is conceivable that some factors are more important than others in particular cases (Fleminger and Burns 1993). However, it should still be possible to tease out their relative contributions.

A number of possible bases for the impairment underlying reduplication have been proposed. Here, we will distinguish six hypotheses which have been advanced.

1. The *psychodynamic* hypothesis (Berson 1983; Enoch and Trethowan 1991) proposes that conflicting or ambivalent feelings of love and hate are resolved by the delusion (the 'double' can be hated without guilt).

2. The *cerebral hemisphere disconnection* hypothesis (Joseph 1986) proposes that each cerebral hemisphere independently processes visual information, and that reduplicative delusions arise when the two processes fail to integrate.

3. The *categorization failure* hypothesis (Cutting 1991) suggests that reduplicative delusions reflect a disturbance in the judgement of identity or uniqueness, owing to a breakdown of the normal structure of semantic categories.

4. The *memory deficit* hypothesis (Staton *et al.* 1982) maintains that there is a failure in the updating of the patient's mental representations of familiar visual stimuli, and that reduplicative delusions result from the consequent mismatch between what is seen and its outdated representation.

5. The Capgras delusion has been said to represent a state of *pathological unfamiliarity*, resembling a state of selective persisting *jamais*

vu (Feinberg and Shapiro, 1989). Ellis and de Pauw (1994) have extended this by using Mandler's (1980) idea that recognition of a stimulus (in the sense of assigning it an identity learnt in previous encounters) is separate from the processing of familiarity, and suggesting that patients may lose the latter and retain the former.

6. The *affective response* hypothesis argues that the basis of the Capgras and other reduplicative delusions lies in damage to neuroanatomical pathways responsible for appropriate emotional reactions to familiar visual stimuli, and that the delusions represent the patients' attempts to make sense of the fact that these visual stimuli no longer have appropriate effective significance. This conception can be traced back to Brochado's (1936) description of a thesis by Derombies (1935), and has recently been emphasized by several authors (Lewis 1987; Anderson 1988; Ellis and Young, 1990; Weinstein and Burnham, 1991).

These hypotheses obviously differ in a number of ways, and are couched at different levels of description. For example, hypotheses 5 and 6 are more closely related than the others, since they can each be seen as variants of a more general proposal of impaired processing of affective familiarity.

The available evidence suggests that hypotheses 1 and 2 are unlikely to provide adequate accounts of reduplication. The cerebral hemisphere disconnection hypothesis (hypothesis 2) has not been supported by empirical work (Ellis *et al.* 1993). The psychodynamic hypothesis (hypothesis 1) does not imply a direct role for brain disease, and hence has difficulty in accommodating the now frequent finding of an organic contribution. It is also difficult to see how reduplication of objects fits the psychodynamic view, even though the duplicate objects are often those with personal significance (Anderson 1988), since it seems unlikely that objects would evoke the strongly ambivalent feelings required by the psychodynamic account. Furthermore, the attitudes of patients with the Capgras delusion to the 'doubles' often fail to show the overt hostility which would be expected on the psychodynamic view (Wallis 1986). In making these points we are not trying to deny that *psychological* factors may play a role in some or all cases of reduplication; we only seek to point out that the psychodynamic account is insufficient as a sole explanation.

The remaining hypotheses (hypotheses 3–6) differ in the postulated mechanisms, and these differences predict differences in the patterns of cognitive impairment which should accompany reduplicative delusions; detailed testing of different cognitive abilities may thus prove useful in understanding them (Ellis and Young 1990). A particularly striking difference of this type is that some hypotheses (primarily hypotheses 4–6) treat reduplication as a malfunction of the visual recognition system, whereas on the categorization failure hypothesis (hypothesis 3) the problem should arise regardless of input domain.

We report here a patient with reduplicative delusions in whom we investigated recognition of faces, names, objects, and buildings to determine what defects there were in visual recognition, and also tested voice recognition to determine the extent to which reduplication might reflect a specific malfunction of the visual recognition system or a more general problem.

Case description

P.T. was a 41 year old single man who lived with his parents. He was first admitted in 1983 (when he was 33 years old) after becoming increasingly withdrawn, preoccupied with religion and with a belief that there was a conspiracy between several ex-workmates and the DHSS offices against him. He believed his thoughts were being controlled, that they were broadcast to other people, and that he heard the voices of others talking to him. At this time he also believed that John the Baptist had visited him, being sent by God in the guise of a charge nurse.

A diagnosis of paranoid schizophrenia was made, and P.T. responded well to neuroleptic medication. He was maintained in the community in a day centre until 1988, when he re-presented after decreasing his medication. He became deluded that the staff at the day centre were abusing the patients, and that his house was bugged. On this admission he described how he now believed that there were two distinct consultants looking after him. The first (named John Smith) was 'a nice bloke', whereas the second (a Dr J. Smith) was someone who was 'distant and aloof'. P.T. was insistent that these were two separate individuals, both psychiatrists who could be 'brothers or cousins'.

He was again readmitted in late 1990, once again paranoid, self-neglectful, and suspicious. He claimed that 'poisonous gas' was being pumped into his house. He also claimed that furniture in his house had been 'replaced' by exact replicas, consistent with an inanimate Capgras-like delusion. At times during this admission P.T. frequently claimed to know unfamiliar people from many years ago. For example, he thought that two student nurses whom he had not seen before were in fact cousins of his, this belief once again probably reflecting a delusional misidentification.

During this latest admission P.T. was investigated more fully. A computed tomography (CT) head scan was reported as normal. An electro-encephalogram (EEG) showed almost continuous fairly rhythmic 2–6 Hz activity, bilaterally represented, and fairly frequent short bursts of rhythmic delta activity maximal in the mid and anterior temporal regions with a slight right hemisphere preponderance. Both features were enhanced by overbreathing, and the EEG was thought to contain more slow activity than is commonly found in schizophrenia. A later investigation by single photon emission tomography (SPECT) using a ^{99m}Tc PAO tracer was carried out when P.T.'s delusions had been controlled by medication. This showed reduced uptake anteriorly, more marked on the left side, with extension to include the temporal area on that side. These SPECT findings are consistent with other studies of blood flow in schizophrenia (Devous 1989).

P.T. responded slowly to treatment with high-dose pimozide, no longer voicing his delusional ideas, and was eventually discharged back to the community.

Investigation of recognition abilities

We were able to test P.T. whilst he was still making delusional misidentifications involving reduplication. These investigations were carried out in the first two months of his latest admission, during which there were several reported incidents.

During this period, P.T. was correctly oriented in time and place, and there was no evidence of impairment of basic visual functions, with normal spatial contrast sensitivity function on the Vistech VCTS6000 chart. He was initially suspicious about our purposes, however, thinking that we might be acting on behalf of the police to collect evidence against him. Despite this suspicion, he took part willingly when appropriate assurances were given.

The large number of tasks used can be divided into three types for convenience of exposition. These examined

(1) face processing, and recognition memory for faces and words;

(2) person recognition from face, name, or voice; and

(3) recognition of everyday objects and recognition of buildings.

For all of these tasks, P.T.'s performance was compared with that of 20 control subjects (10 men, 10 women) aged 30–49 years. This control group was well matched to P.T. on age (P.T. = 41 years; control mean =

40.30 years, SD = 7.16), and on predicted IQ using the revised version of the National adult reading test (Nelson 1991; P.T. = 110; control mean = 115.05, SD = 10.03).

Face processing and recognition memory for faces and words

Tasks using unfamiliar faces were given, to examine P.T.'s ability to determine facial expression and to match unfamiliar faces. He was also given a standard test involving recognition memory for faces and words (Warrington 1984), and a variant of this test which we produced to assess recognition memory for pronounceable non-words. The results are summarized in Table 9.1.

Facial expressions: Ability to recognize emotional facial expressions was tested with 24 photographs from the Ekman and Friesen (1976) series, presented one at a time with a list of six possible emotion labels printed below each face (Young *et al.* 1990). The task required P.T. to choose the correct label describing the facial expression. He performed very poorly, both on initial testing (12/24 correct, shown in Table 9.1) and on retesting two months later (15/24 correct, still below control mean at *p* < 0.001).

Unfamiliar face matching: The Benton Test of Facial Recognition (Benton *et al.* 1983) was given. In this test, subjects have to choose which of six photographs of unfamiliar faces are pictures of the same person as a simultaneously presented target face photograph. The test includes

Table 9.1 P.T.'s performance on tests of facial expression labelling, unfamiliar face matching, and recognition memory for faces, words, and pronounceable non-words

	P.T.	Controls	
		Mean	SD
Facial expressions			
Labelling	12/24***	22.05	1.99
Unfamiliar face matching			
Benton test	49/54	49.00	3.63
Disguise test	19/24	22.65	2.52
Recognition memory			
Warrington RMT: faces	35/50***	45.65	3.22
Warrington RMT: words	47/50	47.40	3.47
Recognition memory for non-words	42/50	44.20	3.52

Significantly impaired in comparison with the performance of controls: ***z > 3.10, *p* < 0.001.

items involving choice of identical photographs, as well as transformations of orientation or lighting, which are pooled to form an overall composite score. P.T.'s overall score (49/54 correct) was unimpaired both in terms of the test's norms and our own control data.

A second unfamiliar face matching test examined ability to match disguised faces. Two separate test sheets were used, each showing a 4×4 matrix of faces in which each of the four faces in the top row appeared three times in disguised or undisguised forms elsewhere on the sheet (Young *et al*. 1990). P.T.'s accuracy was not significantly impaired at matching these faces ($z = 1.44, 0.1 > p > 0.05$), but his performance of the task was slow and unusual in that all his errors involved refusals to accept that some of the faces appeared more than once or twice.

Recognition memory: The Warrington Recognition Memory Test (Warrington 1984) was given. In this test, recognition memory is tested separately for faces and words. In the 'faces' part of the test, 50 faces are shown at the rate of one every 3 s for a 'pleasant or unpleasant' decision, and recognition memory is then tested immediately by pressing each of the faces paired with a distractor, with the subject having to choose which has been seen before. A similar procedure is used with words. P.T.'s score of 35/50 correct for the faces part of the test was impaired in terms of the test's norms and our own control data (shown in Table 9.1), and markedly different from his score of 47/50 correct on recognition memory for words (significant faces discrepancy score on the test's norms). A retest given two months later (not shown in Table 9.1) produced no change in performance (faces 33/50 correct; words 46/50 correct).

To assess further P.T.'s recognition memory, we developed an equivalent test using pronounceable non-words, in which 50 non-words were shown at the rate of every 3 s for a 'pleasant or unpleasant' decision, and then recognition memory was tested by presenting each of the non-words paired with a distractor, with the subject having to choose which had been seen before. The reasoning behind this was that we wanted to explore recognition memory for unfamiliar verbal stimuli. P.T.'s performance (42/50 correct, see Table 9.1) was unimpaired.

Person recognition

Tests were used to assess P.T.'s ability to recognize familiar people from face, name or voice. Results of these are summarized in Table 9.2.

Table 9.2 P.T.'s ability to recognize familiar people from face, name, or voice

	P.T.	Controls	
		Mean	SD
Identification of familiar faces			
High familiarity faces			
Familiarity	20/20[1]	18.16	1.42
Occupation	18/20[1]	17.68	1.80
Name	17/20[1]	15.53	3.29
Unfamiliar faces			
Correct rejections	9/20***	19.11	1.15
Identification of familiar names			
High familiarity names			
Familiarity	19/20	19.16	1.01
Occupation	19/20	19.05	0.97
Unfamiliar names			
Correct rejections	18/20	19.05	2.30
Identification of familiar voices			
Familiar voices			
Familiarity	21/30	22.45	4.27
Occupation	21/30	18.25	5.32
Name	17/30	14.35	6.60
Unfamiliar voices			
Correct rejections	10/10	9.20	0.83

[1]P.T. recognized most of the faces correctly, but made spontaneous comments about duplicates, e.g. "It's one of them Jimmy Saviles".
Significantly impaired in comparison with the performance of controls: ***$z > 3.10, p < 0.001$.

Identification of familiar faces: Twenty highly familiar faces, 20 moderately familiar, and 20 unfamiliar faces were presented one at a time in random order. For each face P.T. was asked whether or not it was a familiar person and, if so, his or her occupation and name. The data of interest concern P.T.'s ability to recognize as familiar and give correct occupations and names to the 20 highly familiar faces, and the rate at which the 20 unfamiliar faces were misidentified. Data for the moderately familiar faces are not included in Table 9.2, because the control subjects showed high variance in their responses to these items.

P.T. was as accurate as control subjects at recognizing and identifying the highly familiar faces, but he made spontaneous comments about duplicates to some of the stimuli (2/20 highly familiar faces; 2/20 of the moderately familiar faces). For example, 'It's one of them Jimmy Saviles'. When asked what he meant by this, P.T. added that 'It could be one of his brothers – there's lots of them'. Similar comments to the effect that this was only one of a number of otherwise near-identical people with the same name were made to photographs of Marilyn Monroe, Anna Ford, and Diana Dors. In addition, P.T. showed a pronounced tendency to think that the unfamiliar faces were people he knew, with only 9/20 correct rejections of unfamiliar faces.

Because of his comments, P.T. was interviewed about the 'doubles'. He commented that 'Some of them are bad – there's good ones and bad ones. They can switch from good to bad but it's not always the same person. You just think it is. There's more than one of them. You can just tell they're different, but you've got to be careful. Some people wouldn't notice'. In line with his remarks, we observed that he continued to be very suspicious of many people, but he was no more noticeably so toward the duplicates.

Identification of familiar names: A parallel test to the familiar face recognition test was given, using written names of the 20 highly familiar people and 20 moderately familiar people from the face recognition test, interspersed with 20 unfamiliar names. For each name P.T. was asked whether or not it was a familiar person and, if so, his or her occupation. His performance was unimpaired, both in terms of recognition of highly familiar faces and rejection of unfamiliar names. There were a further two comments about duplicates, though both of these may have referred back to remarks he had made previously about the faces (Diana Dors and Anna Ford – in each case from the moderately familiar set).

Identification of familiar voices: It was not possible immediately to get recordings of the voices of all the people used in the face and name recognition tests. P.T. was therefore tested on a set of voices already available to us, which included 30 voices of famous people and 10 unfamiliar voices, recorded in clips of about 5 s duration each, with few useful cues to identity from the content of what they were saying. P.T. was asked whether or not each voice was familiar and, if so, to give the person's occupation and his or her name. He achieved a normal level of performance at recognizing the familiar voices, and made no comments about duplicates. All of the unfamiliar voices were correctly rejected.

These formal test results were backed up by several informal observations that P.T. did not make comments about duplicates to recordings of people's voices, whereas he made them to several photographs of faces.

Object recognition

As well as testing his ability to recognize familiar people, we examined P.T.'s ability to recognize objects and buildings. Data from these tasks are summarized in Table 9.3.

Identification of familiar objects: P.T. showed no problems in recognizing line drawings of objects. He correctly identified 19/20 drawings of living objects and 20/20 non-living objects from the set used by Young and Ellis (1989), and made no comments about duplicates. Of course, object recognition tests generally require only that an object is assigned to a general category (a horse, a hammer, etc.) rather than given a specific, individual identity. Hence, comments about an object being 'one of them horses' or 'one of them hammers' would in any case be less unusual.

Identification of familiar buildings: To test P.T.'s ability to assign individual identities in tests of object recognition, we used buildings. He was shown 20 photographs of familiar buildings (the White House, Sydney Opera House, etc.) and 10 photographs of grand but largely unfamiliar buildings, in random order, and asked whether each was familiar and, if so, what it was. Although P.T. had no problems in correctly recognizing or naming the famous buildings, there were again comments about duplicates for 6/20 famous buildings; 'the White House – but not as we know it – there are a few of them', 'the Post Office Tower

Table 9.3 P.T.'s ability to identify objects and buildings

	P.T.	Controls	
		Mean	SD
Identification of familiar objects			
Living	19/20	19.20	0.83
Non-living	20/20	19.55	0.76
Identification of familiar buildings			
Familiar buildings			
Recognized	16/20[1]	17.60	2.66
Named	15/20[1]	14.90	4.32
Unfamiliar buildings			
Correct rejections	10/10	9.45	0.60

[1]P.T. recognized most of the buildings correctly, but made spontaneous comments about duplicates, e.g. "The White House – but not as we know it – there are a few of them", "The Post Office Tower – but a different version of it", etc.

– but a different version of it', and so on. All of the unfamiliar buildings were correctly rejected.

Discussion

P.T.'s clinical history included a number of incidents involving delusional misidentification. The most striking of these were of a reduplicative form, including the two consultants and the replica furniture in his house. The claim of duplicate consultants seems closely related to the Capgras delusion, but P.T. maintained that these consultants were two separate people, rather than that one was an impostor. However, there were also less easily classified incidents, including the charge nurse/John the Baptist, claims to know people from years ago, and the student nurses/cousins. Some of these inhabit the grey area between more general delusions and delusional misidentification, but others probably did reflect genuine misidentification.

On formal testing, P.T. showed reduplication of familiar faces and buildings, and some evidence of reduplication from written names (though we suspect that this might refer back to previous incidents with the same people's faces), but he did not reduplicate voices at all. Hence it appears that reduplication was a genuinely visual problem for P.T., since it was not found to auditory stimuli. Of course, we cannot prove that P.T. *never* reduplicated auditory stimuli; we can only note that he did not do so under any circumstances we observed, whereas he regularly reduplicated visual stimuli. Further studies of reduplication of visual and auditory stimuli in other cases should therefore be of interest.

The florid reduplications produced by P.T. in tests of recognition of buildings and faces are consistent with the idea that there is a parallel between reduplication of people and reduplication of places (Alexander *et al.* 1979). This is particularly interesting because P.T. had not shown any clinical evidence of reduplication of places. The reduplicative delusions noted in his case history were primarily for people, with some relating to everyday objects.

Reduplication was found in visual tests for which P.T. had to assign a unique identity to visual stimuli (the White House, Jimmy Savile, etc.). In contrast, no problems were evident in tests of recognition of everyday objects, which only required recognition of the general category to which an object belongs (a cup, a guitar, etc.). However, it was clear from P.T.'s case history that he did reduplicate objects in everyday life when correspondingly required to assign them individual identities (he thought that his furniture had been replaced, etc.).

This finding that reduplication was only evident in tasks that required the assignment of a unique identity is reminiscent of the categorization failure hypotheses (hypothesis 3). The fact that this only held for visual stimuli, however, is inconsistent with a strong form of this hypothesis, because models of semantic memory usually assume that visual and auditory stimuli access the same semantic representations. Any degradation of the semantic representations themselves should therefore affect both input modalities, rather than creating the specifically visual problem noted for P.T.

A deficit in assigning a unique identity to visual stimuli belonging to a common superordinate category has been considered by some authorities to be the cardinal feature of the neurological condition prosopagnosia (Damasio et al. 1982). This is of interest because there have been attempts to draw parallels between prosopagnosia and one of the most widely recognized forms of reduplication, the Capgras delusion (Hayman and Abrams 1977). The parallel has been bolstered by reports of face processing impairments in Capgras patients (Shraberg and Weitzel 1979; Tzavaras et al 1986), but in our view it needs to be treated cautiously. P.T. certainly did not show the inability to recognize familiar faces which is characteristic of prosopagnosia. Instead, he recognized just as many familiar faces as control subjects, but made comments about their being duplicates, and showed a pronounced tendency to produce false recognitions of unfamiliar faces.

The visual basis for P.T.'s reduplication fits most easily with those hypotheses (hypotheses 4, 5, and 6) that propose a specific role for visual dysfunction. Additional support comes from the fact that P.T. showed a deficit in facial expression processing and impaired recognition memory for faces. However, a key issue relating to findings of face processing impairments or other visual problems in cases of reduplication concerns whether these deficits are instrumental in the production of reduplicative delusions, or arise coincidentally because of the nature of the underlying cerebral dysfunction. These problems of interpretation of associated deficits are widely recognized in neuropsychology.

Lewis (1987), Anderson (1988), and Ellis and Young (1990) have independently suggested that the basis of the Capgras and related reduplicative delusions lies in damage to neuroanatomical pathways responsible for appropriate emotional reactions to familiar visual stimuli (hypothesis 6). Since substantial parts of these pathways which imbue visual stimuli with affective significance are in close proximity to those involved in visual recognition (Bauer 1984), one would expect that few brain disorders will compromise emotional reactions to visual stimuli without also affecting other visual functions to some extent, and this would be consistent with our observations of defective face processing abilities for P.T. On this hypothesis, P.T. showed defective face processing abilities because these are, for neuroanatomical reasons, likely to co-occur with the fundamental problem in affective reactions.

As would be expected on the hypothesis that reduplication is based on an interaction of deficits, it is possible that this dysfunction is coupled with another problem in forming correct judgements and attributions. P.T.'s SPECT scan revealed anterior as well as temporal blood flow abnormalities, which are consistent with Benson and Stuss's (1990) view that reduplicative phenomena implicate prefrontal areas involved in reality testing and self-analysis.

Our investigation of P.T., then, demonstrated a visual basis for reduplication which would fit most easily with those hypotheses (hypotheses 4, 5, and 6) that propose a specific role for visual dysfunction. Of course, we do not claim that it is anything other than an empirical question whether this will prove to be so for all other cases involving reduplication. We suspect not from some of the other reports in the literature. For example, reports of the Capgras delusion in blind patients show that it cannot have an exclusively visual basis (Signer *et al.* 1990; Rojo *et al.* 1991; Reid *et al.* 1993). Hence it may well turn out that there are parallel forms of impairment affecting other sensory modalities, or that ideas such as the categorization failure hypothesis (hypothesis 3) are more appropriate in some cases than others.

To date, the classification of reduplicative delusions has largely been based on the type of material affected (people, places, etc.). Our findings suggest that, with the development of appropriate methods of investigation, it may eventually become possible to arrive at a more sophisticated classification of these delusions in terms of their functional basis. More generally, these findings further strengthen the view that significant advances in the understanding of delusional beliefs can be achieved by careful testing of underlying cognitive deficits (Ellis and de Pauw 1994; Young 1994; Young *et al.* 1994).

References

Alexander, M. P., Stuss, D. T., and Benson, D. F. (1979). Capgras syndrome: a reduplicative phenomenon. *Neurology*, **29**, 334–9.

Anderson, D. N. (1988). The delusion of inanimate doubles. Implications for understanding the Capgras phenomenon. *British Journal of Psychiatry*, **153**, 694–9.

Bauer, R. M. (1984). Autonomic recognition of names and faces in prosopagnosia: a neuropsychological application of the guilty knowledge test. *Neuropsychologia*, **22**, 457–69.

Benson, D. F., and Stuss, D. T. (1990). Frontal lobe influences on delusions: a clinical perspective. *Schizophrenia Bulletin*, **16**, 403–11.

Benson, D. F., Gardner, H., and Meadows, J. C. (1976). Reduplicative paramnesia. *Neurology*, **26**, 147–51.

Benton, A. L., Hamsher, K. de S., Varney, N., and Spreen, O. (1983). *Contributions to neuropsychological assessment: a clinical manual.* Oxford University Press.

Benson, R. J. (1983). Capgras syndrome. *American Journal of Psychiatry*, **140**, 969–78.

Brochado, A. (1936). Le syndrome de Capgras. *Annales Médico-Psychologiques*, **15**, 706–17.

Capgras, J., and Reboul-Lachaux, J. (1923). L'illusion des 'sosies' dans un délire systématisé chronique. *Bulletin de la Société Clinique de Médicine Mentale*, **11**, 6–16.

Cutting, J. (1991). Delusional misidentification and the role of the right hemisphere in the appreciation of identity. *British Journal of Psychiatry*, **159**, 70–5.

Damasio, A. R., Damasio, H., and Van Hoesen, G. W. (1982). Prosopagnosia: anatomic basis and behavioural mechanisms. *Neurology*, **32**, 331–41.

Derombies, M. (1935). L'illusion de sosies, forme particulière de la méconnaissance systématique. Thèse de Paris, Paris.

Devous, M. D. (1989). Blood flow in schizophrenia. In *Brain imaging: applications in psychiatry*, (ed. N. C. Andreasen), pp. 195–204. American Psychiatric Press,

Ekman, P., and Friesen, W. V. (1976). *Pictures of facial affect.* Consulting Psychologists Press, Palo Alto, CA.

Ellis, H. D. and de Pauw, K. W. (1994). The cognitive neuropsychiatric origins of the Capgras delusion. In *The neuropsychology of schizophrenia*, (ed. A. S. David and J. C. Cutting), pp. 317–35. Lawrence Erlbaum, Hove.

Ellis, H. D., and Young, A. W. (1990). Accounting for delusional misidentifications. *British Journal of Psychiatry*, **157**, 239–48.

Ellis, H. D., de Pauw K. W., Christodoulou, G. N., Papageorgiou, L., Milne, A. B., and Joseph, A. B. (1993). Responses to facial and non-facial stimuli presented tachistoscopically in either or both visual fields by patients with the Capgras delusion and paranoid schizophrenics. *Journal of Neurology, Neurosurgery, and Psychiatry*, **56**, 215–19.

Enoch, M. D., and Trethowan, W. H. (1991). *Uncommon psychiatric syndromes*, 3rd edn. Butterworth-Heinemann, Oxford.

Feinberg, T. E., and Shapiro, R. M. (1989). Misidentification–reduplication and the right hemisphere. *Neuropsychiatry, Neuropsychology and Behavioral Neurology*, **2**, 39–48.

Fleminger, S. (1992). Seeing is believing: the role of 'preconscious' perceptual processing in delusional misidentification. *British Journal of Psychiatry*, **160**, 293–303.

Fleminger, S., and Burns, A. (1993). The delusional misidentification syndromes in patients with and without evidence of organic cerebral' disorder: a structured review of case reports. *Biological Psychiatry*, **33**, 22–32.

Förstl. H., Almeida, O. P., Owen, A. M., Burns, A., and Howard R. (1991). Psychiatric, neurological and medical aspects of misidentification syndromes: a review of 260 cases. *Psychological Medicine*, **21**, 905–10.

Hayman, M. A., and Abrams, R. (1977). Capgras syndrome and cerebral dysfunction. *British Journal of Psychiatry*, **130**, 68–71.

Joseph, A. B. (1986). Focal central nervous system abnormalities in patients with misidentification syndromes. *Bibliotheca Psychiatrica*, **164**, 68–79.

Kapur, N., Turner, A., and King, C. (1988). Reduplicative paramnesia: possible anatomical and neuropsychological mechanisms. *Journal of Neurology, Neurosurgery, and Psychiatry*, **51**, 579–81.

Lewis, S. W. (1987). Brain imaging in a case of Capgras syndrome. *British Journal of Psychiatry*, **150**, 117–21.

Mandler, G. (1980). Recognizing: the judgment of previous occurrence. *Psychological Review*, **87**, 252–71.

Nelson, H. E. (1991). *National adult reading test (NART): test manual* (revised). NFER-Nelson, Windsor.

Patterson, M. B. and Mack, J. L. (1985). Neuropsychological analysis of a case of reduplicative paramnesia. *Journal of Clinical and Experimental Neuropsychology*, **7**, 111–21.

Pick, A. (1903). Clinical studies: III. On reduplicative paramnesia. *Brain*, **26**, 260–7.

Reid, I., Young, A. W., and Hellawell, D. J. (1993). Voice recognition impairment in a blind Capgras patient. *Behavioural Neurology*, **6**, 225–8.

Rojo, V. I., Caballero, L., Iruela, L. M., and Baca, E. (1991). Capras syndrome in a blind patient. *American Journal of Psychiatry*, **148**, 1272.

Shraberg, D., and Weitzel, W. D. (1979). Prosopagnosia and the Capgras syndrome. *Journal of Clinical Psychiatry*, **40**, 313–16.

Signer, S. F., Van Ness, P. C., and Davis, R. J. (1990). Capgras's syndrome associated with sensory loss. *Western Journal of Medicine*, **152**, 719–20.

Staton, R. D., Brumback, R. A., and Wilson, H. (1982). Reduplicative paramnesia: a disconnection syndrome of memory. *Cortex*, **18**, 23–6.

Tzavaras, A., Luauté, J. P., and Bidault, E. (1986). Face recognition dysfunction and delusional misidentification syndromes (DMS). In *Aspects of face processing*, (ed. H. D. Ellis, M. A. Jeeves, F. Newcombe, and A. Young), pp. 310–16. Martinus Nijhoff, Dordrecht.

Wallis, G. (1986). Nature of the misidentified in the Capgras syndrome. *Bibliotheca Psychiatrica*, **164**, 40–8.

Warrington, E. K. (1984). *Recognition memory test*. NFER-Nelson, Windsor.

Weinstein, E. A., and Burnham, D. L. (1991). Reduplication and the syndrome of Capgras. *Psychiatry*, **54**, 78–88.

Young, A. W. (1994). Recognition and reality. In *The neurological boundaries of reality*, (ed. E. M. R. Critchley), pp. 83–100. Farrand, London.

Young, A. W., and Ellis, H. D. (1989). Childhood prosopagnosia. *Brain and Cognition*, **9**. 16–47.

Young, A. W., Ellis, H. D., Szulecka, T. K., and de Pauw, K. W. (1990). Face processing impairments and delusional misidentification. *Behavioural Neurology*, **3**, 153–68.

Young, A. W., Reid, I., Wright, S., and Hellawell, D. J. (1993). Face-processing impairments and the Capgras delusion. *British Journal of Psychiatry*, **162**, 695–8.

Young, A. W., Leafhead, K., and Szulecka, T. K. (1994). The Capgras and Cotard delusions. *Psychopathology*, **27**, 226–31.

10

Recognition and reality

Reprinted in slightly modified form from Young, A. W. (1994), Recognition and reality, in *The neurological boundaries of reality*, (ed. E. M. R. Critchley), pp. 83–100, Farrand Press, London. With kind permission of Farrand Press.

Introduction

All of us know that if we are very ill, or under the influence of drink or drugs, we may lose our grip on reality and start to misperceive or imagine things, and even to act on them. Conversely, we know, too, that we can daydream when awake, or have 'lucid' dreams whilst asleep, without mistaking these imaginings as real.

How can we so easily see one group of phenomena as unreal, yet accept other imaginings as real? Wherein lies the difference? The question is seldom raised, because we so much take for granted our experience of the reality of the external world. Yet it is central to everyday conceptions of insanity, in which loss of touch with reality is a central feature. Moreover, the discoveries of modern science do not reveal that the world is exactly as it is presented to us by our senses.

Striking examples of failures of reality discrimination arise in hallucinations. Slade and Bentall (1988) have marshalled impressive evidence pointing to the conclusion that hallucinators mistake internally generated phenomena for external events, and have shown that they suffer more widespread difficulties in distinguishing between internal and external states. Much the same point arises in confabulation, which can also be seen as a disturbance of reality testing (Benson and Stuss 1990). Some patients can provide vivid accounts of memories and events which are entirely fictitious, yet they do not seem to be deliberately lying. These confabulations occur in people who have suffered damage to the frontal lobes (Stuss *et al.* 1978). In the absence of any easy way of distinguishing fantasy from reality, the confabulator may take her or his imaginings as real.

One of the ways in which we establish the 'reality' of things and events is by recognizing them as meaningful and appropriate to the context in which we are located. If you saw a herd of elephants enter your living room, you might well be disconcerted if you did not recognize the source of the image as a television screen. In fact, studies of mental illness have shown that some patients will treat television images as real (Förstl *et al.* 1991*a*) or, conversely, react to everyday events as if they were part of an elaborate film production (Shubsachs and Young 1988; Vié 1944).

More specific misidentifications can also be caused by brain disease, where they may arise as part of a confusional state or in an otherwise clear sensorium (Geschwind 1982). Like confabulations, these delusional misidentifications imply a failure of reality testing (Benson and Stuss 1990), and they can lead to extraordinary statements about the misidentified objects, such as that relatives have been replaced by impostors, or that the patient is in a hospital which is an exact duplicate of the original but in a different geographical location.

This chapter examines how visual recognition mechanisms support our experience of reality by looking at some of the consequences of recognition impairments, and especially those caused by brain injury. This will involve considering how our emotional reactions to visual stimuli relate to our ability to recognize them, and examining preserved non-conscious aspects of recognition in cases of face recognition impairment after brain injury (prosopagnosia), everyday recognition errors, and delusional misidentifications in psychiatric and neuropsychiatric patients.

Preference and overt recognition

It is tempting to equate recognition with the ability to recognize things overtly and make an explicit identification. However, evidence suggests that overt recognition is only part of a much more complex process. In particular, studies following from the seminal work of Zajonc and his colleagues have found that certain types of affective reaction to familiar visual stimuli need not depend on overt recognition (Bornstein 1989; Kunst-Wilson and Zajonc 1980; Zajonc 1980).

In a now famous experiment, Kunst-Wilson and Zajonc (1980) showed people some eight-sided random shapes. Five exposures of each shape were given, but these were all for only 1 ms so that the shapes could not be seen consciously. Afterwards, each of the shapes was paired with a new (unseen) shape, and subjects were asked which they had seen before, which they preferred, and how certain they were of each judgement. Although recognition of previously seen shapes was at chance level, people did tend to prefer them.

In experiments on preference, people often prefer things that are familiar to things that are novel. However, Kunst-Wilson and Zajonc's (1980) findings show that this preference for familiarity can extend to stimuli whose familiarity need not be consciously recognized at all. It is therefore clear that preference need not depend on overt recognition. As Zajonc (1980) explains, such findings contradict the commonly held assumption that affect is postcognitive. Instead, he suggests that 'affective judgements may be fairly independent of, and precede in time, the sorts of perceptual and cognitive operations commonly assumed to be the basis of these affective judgements. Affective reactions to stimuli are often the very first reactions of the organism, and for lower organisms they are the dominant reaction'. (Zajonc 1980, p. 151).

Surprising though they may be, similar findings have been reported in other studies (Bornstein 1989). Of course, there is a sense in which the familiarity of the briefly presented stimuli must have been registered somewhere in the visual system in order for subjects to show any preference. But the important point is that this is independent of consciously experienced recognition that the preferred stimuli have been seen before. Some form of non-conscious recognition is involved.

Covert recognition in prosopagnosia

A dramatic demonstration that recognition mechanisms can operate automatically and non-consciously has come from studies of proso-pagnosia, a neurological impairment characterized by an apparent inability to recognize familiar faces (Meadows 1974).

Prosopagnosic patients usually fail all tests of overt recognition of familiar faces. They cannot name the face, give the person's occupation or other biographical details, or even state whether or not a face belongs to a familiar person. Even the most well known faces may not be recognized, including famous people, friends, family, and the patient's own face when looking in a mirror. The patients know when they are looking at a face, and can often describe and identify facial features, or even use facial information to determine age, sex, and expression, but appear not to experience any sense of recognizing to whom the face might belong. In order to recognize familiar people, they must thus rely on non-facial cues, such as voice, name, and sometimes even clothing or gait.

The brain lesions that cause prosopagnosia involve inferior and mesial occipitotemporal cortex and underlying white matter, especially in the region of the lingual, fusiform and parahippocampal gyri (Damasio *et al.* 1982; Meadows 1974). Often, the cerebral damage is more extensive in, or, macroscopically confined to the right cerebral hemisphere (De Renzi 1986; Landis *et al.* 1986; Meadows 1974; Sergent and Villemure 1989).

Although prosopagnosic patients no longer recognize familiar faces overtly, there is substantial evidence of covert, non-conscious recognition from physiological and behavioural measures (Bruyer 1991; Young and de Haan 1992).

Bauer (1984) used the guilty knowledge test, a technique sometimes used in criminal investigations, which is based on the view that a guilty person will show some involuntary physiological response to stimuli related to the crime. He measured skin conductance whilst a prosopagnosic patient, LF, viewed a familiar face and listened to a list of names. When the name belonged to the face LF was looking at, there was a greater skin conductance change than when someone else's name was read out. Yet if LF was asked to choose which name in the list was correct for the face, his performance was at chance level. Comparable findings have been reported with a different technique in which the patients simply looked at a series of familiar and unfamiliar faces (Tranel and Damasio 1985, 1988). Skin conductance changes were greater to familiar than unfamiliar faces, even though the patients experienced no sense of familiarity.

Behavioural indices of covert recognition complement these electrophysiological measures. Eye movement scan-paths differ to familiar and unfamiliar faces, despite the absence of overt recognition (Rizzo *et al.* 1987). The patients are better at matching photographs of familiar faces than photographs of unfamiliar faces across transformations of orientation or age (de Haan *et al.* 1987; Sergent and Poncet 1990). In name classification tasks, they show interference from simultaneously presented face distractors (de Haan *et al.* 1987) and priming from previously presented face primes (Young *et al.* 1988). When looking at a face, they are better at learning correct information than incorrect information about that person (de Haan *et al.* 1987, 1991*a*; Sergent and Poncet 1990). This superior learning of correct over incorrect information is found even for faces of people who have been known only since the patient's illness (de Haan *et al.* 1987). All of these findings imply that faces can be recognized to some degree, even though the prosopagnosic patient is not aware of this.

A question which naturally arises concern whether or not such findings will hold for all patients with severely impaired overt face recognition ability. In fact, although covert recognition has been demonstrated for some patients with a number of techniques, several patients who failed to show covert recognition have also been reported in the literature (see Young and de Haan 1992, for a review). As clinicians have long suspected, there is more than one form of prosopagnosia (De Renzi *et al.* 1991; Meadows 1974); the presence or absence of covert recognition may thus provide an important pointer to the nature of the functional impairment in each case.

For cases with covert recognition, what seem to be preserved are those aspects of recognition whose operation is relatively automatic and does not require conscious initiation (Young 1988). We might therefore expect that the Zajonc 'preference' effect would be among those shown by such patients, and this has been demonstrated by Greve and Bauer (1990). They showed faces to the prosopagnosic patient LF for 500 ms each, and then paired each of these faces with a completely novel face. LF tended to choose the faces shown to him previously as being 'more likeable' than the faces he had not seen before, whereas, when he was told that he had seen one of the faces before and asked which it was he performed at chance level. This is equivalent to the findings of preference without overt recognition in normal subjects.

Such findings profoundly alter our conception of the nature of prosopagnosia, since they show that it is inadequate to think of it as simply involving loss of recognition mechanisms. Instead, at least some degree of recognition does take place; what the patient has lost is *awareness of recognition.*

Bauer (1984, 1986) offered an intriguing hypothesis concerning the neuroanatomical pathways involved in this phenomenon. He suggested that overt recognition depends on a ventral visual system–limbic system pathway involving ventromedial occipitotemporal cortex, whereas a more dorsal visual–limbic pathway through the superior temporal sulcus and the inferior parietal lobule subserves processes of emotional arousal. In prosopagnosia, the ventral pathway is impaired, whereas the dorsal pathway may remain intact, leading to covert recognition of familiar faces that cannot be recognized overtly.

It is worth spending a little more time on the properties Bauer attributed to the dorsal pathway. He suggested that it 'subserves processes of selective attention and tonic emotional arousal, and is implicated in the process whereby "relevance" is attached to an attended object' (Bauer 1984, p. 466). Thus it has multiple functions encompassing automatic emotional responses to stimuli which have personal relevance; these have been widely implicated as putative specialized functions of the right cerebral hemisphere (Bear 1983; Van Lancker 1991).

Everyday errors

Prosopagnosia involves a dense and often permanent impairment of overt recognition, but there are also transitory errors which all of us make from time to time. Studies of these everyday difficulties and errors show that many of them reflect breakdown at different levels of overt recognition (Young et al. 1985). For example:

1. We may completely fail to recognize a familiar face, and mistakenly think that the person is unfamiliar.
2. We may recognize the face as familiar, but be unable to bring to mind any other details about the person, such as her or his occupation or name.
3. We may recognize the face as familiar and remember appropriate semantic information about the person, whilst failing to remember her or his name.

The orderliness of these types of everyday error suggests that overt recognition involves some form of sequential access to different types of information, in the order familiarity, then semantics, then name retrieval, and other studies of normal subjects have given strong support to this suggestion (Ellis 1992).

Each of these types of error can also arise after neurological impairment. In such cases, a brain-injured patient will make her or his characteristic error to many or almost all seen faces. In prosopagnosia, for example, known faces seem unfamiliar, which corresponds to error type 1. My colleagues and I have recently reported a case in which known faces were familiar only (de Haan et al. 1991b), corresponding to error type 2. In anomia (a defect in the ability to name objects), name retrieval to known faces may become problematic even though semantic information can be properly accessed (Flude et al. 1989), as in error type 3.

We thus have converging evidence from studies of normal people and people with brain injuries indicating that the functional organization of the face recognition system involves sequential access to different types of information. Recent work has therefore concentrated on how this might be achieved, and Burton and his colleagues have offered plausible computer simulations (Burton et al. 1990; Bruce et al. 1992).

The basic structure of Burton et al.'s (1990) model consists of active units connected to each other by modifiable links which can be excitatory or inhibitory. Their model is able to simulate known properties of the face recognition system derived from experimental studies and, surprisingly, it provides a simple account of some aspects of covert recognition in prosopagnosia. This is because preserved priming and interference effects without explicit classification of face inputs, which are functionally equivalent to effects found in cases of prosopagnosia, can be demonstrated with the Burton *et al.* (1990) model by halving the connection strengths between two of its pools of units (Burton *et al.* 1991). This makes the finding of this pattern in some cases of prosopagnosia much less mysterious, though it does not provide a complete account of covert recognition effects; for example, the simulation does not offer any detailed explanation of the skin conductance findings, for which a neurological model such as Bauer's (1984; 1986) may well be more useful.

Bauer's (1984) model is also important in that it highlights the interplay of cognitive and affective aspects of recognition. This interplay may be important in generating anomalous experiences that all of us have from time to time, and which can also arise in pathological states, such as *déjà vu* (Fleminger 1991; Sno and Linszen 1990).

Delusional misidentification

Delusional misidentification is a problem which used to be considered to be purely 'psychodynamic', but modern neuroimaging techniques have revealed evidence of brain injury in many cases. Recent reviews have therefore emphasized the importance of organic factors in delusional misidentification (Cutting 1991; Förstl *et al.* 1991*b*), and modern psychiatric opinion is that a thorough search for organic factors should always be made when such delusions are present (Collins *et al.* 1990).

Different types of delusional misidentification have been identified by clinicians (Vié 1944). Joseph (1986) gives a list of 11 specific variants, which are usually considered as distinct syndromes, but we can question the wider appropriateness of the syndrome concept since each of the types of delusional misidentification is really only defined by a single symptom (the delusion itself) and they can quite often occur in combination with each other (Cutting 1991; Förstl *et al.* 1991*b*).

Here, I will concentrate on two of the most widely discussed forms of delusional misidentification; the Capgras delusion (Capgras and Reboul-Lachaux 1923), in which patients claim that relatives have been replaced by 'doubles' or impostors, and reduplicative paramnesia (Pick 1903), in which patients claim to be in a 'duplicate' hospital.

The Capgras delusion

The Capgras delusion used to be considered very rare, perhaps because it is often unrecognized, and its prevalence is probably rather higher than was once thought (Förstl *et al.* 1991*a,b*). The patient's belief that relatives (and sometimes non-relatives) have been replaced by impostors usually seems to be genuinely and strongly held, but can have some curious features. The impostors are usually considered to be almost exact replicas of the originals, but the patients tend to claim that they differ in some way which is difficult to put into words. A case we investigated, ML, expressed it like this: 'There's been someone like my son's double which isn't my son . . . I can tell my son because my son is different . . . but you have got to be quick to notice it'. (Young *et al.* 1993).

Most Capgras patients do not show too much concern about what has happened to their 'real' relatives, and some of them accept the substitutes with a compliant equanimity; Wallis (1986) pointed out that a substantial proportion (around 30 per cent) were friendly toward the duplicates. However, there are also cases where there is verbal abuse of the 'impostor'; for example, Vogel's (1974) case I commented that 'I call him Earl but he answers to ass-hole too', and there is an appreciable overall risk of (sometimes extreme) physical violence (de Pauw and Szulecka 1988). A review of 260 cases of delusional misidentification by Förstl *et al.* (1991*a*) found that physical violence had been noted in 46 cases (18 per cent).

There can be insight into the absurdity of the delusion, even when it is subjectively convincing. The following dialogue comes from a case reported by Alexander *et al.* (1979):

E. Isn't that [duplicate families] unusual?
S. It was unbelievable!
E. How do you account for it?
S. I don't know. I try to understand it myself, and it was virtually impossible.

Work on the Capgras delusion was initially dominated by psycho-dynamic accounts (Berson 1983; Capgras and Carrette 1924; Vogel 1974), most of which proposed that conflicting or ambivalent feelings of love and hate are resolved by the delusion, so that the double can be hated without guilt. However, psychodynamic hypotheses do not imply a direct role for brain disease, and hence have difficulty in accommodating the now frequent finding of an organic contribution. Furthermore, we have noted that Capgras patients' attitudes to the doubles often fail to show the overt hostility which would be expected on the psychodynamic view (Wallis 1986). In making these points I am not trying to deny that *psychological* factors may play a role in some or all cases of reduplication; only that the psychodynamic account is insufficient as a sole explanation.

In Capgras cases with clear neurological damage, there are usually occipitotemporal or temporoparietal lesions, often of the right hemisphere only, and frontal lesions which can be bilateral (Alexander *et al.* 1979; Feinberg and Shapiro 1989; Förstl *et al.* 1991a,b; Joseph 1986; Lewis 1987). However, although such observations of brain disease in patients who experience the Capgras delusion are obviously important, they do not in themselves explain the peculiar content of the delusion. One needs a theory that can link the observed brain disease to the disturbed psychological functions that create the delusion. Our studies of cases of Capgras delusion have convinced us that a principled account can be achieved by integrating neuropsychological investigations with recent findings on delusions derived from work in clinical psychology and psychiatry.

Our working hypothesis is that the Capgras delusion may be due in part to impairment of the visual system. In effect, the patient's beliefs change because the evidence on which they are based has altered. If correct, this emphasizes the fundamental importance of vision as a source of evidence about the world.

To examine this further, a simple schematic model of how delusional misidentifications might arise is shown in Fig. 10.1. This proposes that we can only know the world through our senses, but beliefs are created through (among other things) the interpretation of sense data. Once formed, beliefs will affect both how we interpret the data available and what kind of information we seek; we become predisposed to see what we expect, and Fleminger (1992) has given a compelling analysis of how such expectations contribute to delusional misidentification.

In the model shown in Fig. 10.1, delusional misidentification is taken to reflect an interaction of impairments at two levels. One set of contributory factors involves perceptual impairment, or anomalous perceptual experience, and the other factors lead to an incorrect interpretation of this. Incorrect interpretation might happen for various reasons. In Fig. 10.1, I have drawn attention to two of these; incorrect attribution of the perceptual changes, and an inadequate search for alternatives to the delusional explanation. The influence of both of

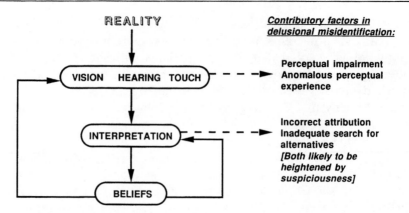

Fig. 10.1 Schematic model of delusional misidentification.

these factors would be heightened by the suspiciousness which is often noted in Capgras patients.

The suggestion of an inadequate search for alternatives to the delusional explanation is based on the work of Huq *et al.* (1988), who found that people with delusions were more confident and requested less information than non-deluded people before reaching a decision in a probability judgement task. This is an important finding because, superficially, probability judgements would seem to have nothing to do with the patients' delusions. The other factor favouring mis-interpretation, incorrect attributions, has been noted in suspicious patients by Kaney and Bentall (1989) and Candido and Romney (1990), who found that people with persecutory delusions were inclined to attribute hypothetical negative events to *external* causes, whereas depressed people attributed them to *internal* causes. The persecutory delusions and suspiciousness that are often noted in Capgras cases may therefore contribute to the fundamental misinterpretation in which the patients mistake a change in themselves for a change in others.

It is thus plausible that the Capgras delusion is caused by the misinterpretation of unusual perceptual experiences. But what kind of unusual experiences? The presence of right occipitotemporal lesions in Capgras cases is reminiscent of the brain lesions that cause proso-pagnosia, and the possibility of a link between prosopagnosia and the Capgras delusion is strengthened by observations that Capgras patients perform poorly on face processing tests (Morrison and Tarter 1984; Shraberg and Weitzel 1979; Tzavaras *et al.* 1986; Wilcox and Waziri 1983; Young *et al.* 1993). However, it is necessary to treat this possible link carefully (Ellis and Young 1990; Lewis 1987). It seems unlikely that there is any direct and sufficient causal connection. Prosopagnosic patients do not usually experience the Capgras delusion and, conversely, although their ability to recognize familiar faces may be impaired (Young *et al.* 1993), Capgras patients still can recognize a number of highly familiar people; for example, they still recognize that the 'double' looks like their husband, wife, or whoever. Hence any link to prosopagnosia must be more subtle.

Lewis (1987) and Ellis and Young (1990) have suggested that the basis of the Capgras delusion lies in damage to neuroanatomical pathways responsible for appropriate emotional reactions to familiar visual stimuli, such as Bauer's (1984) dorsal visual–limbic route. The delusion would then represent the patient's attempt to make sense of this puzzling change; it typically involves close relatives because these would normally produce the strongest reactions, and hence suffer the greatest discrepancy. On this hypothesis, the Capgras delusion represents a mirror-image of prosopagnosia, in which Bauer's (1984) dorsal route is more severely affected than the ventral route. Since substantial parts of the pathways which imbue visual stimuli with affective significance are in close proximity to those involved in visual recognition, one would expect that few brain lesions will compromise emotional reactions to visual stimuli without also affecting other visual functions involved in recognition to some extent. Most Capgras patients will thus show defective face processing abilities because these are, for neuroanatomical reasons, likely to co-occur with the fundamental problem in affective reactions.

The proposal that defective emotional reactions to familiar visual stimuli are implicated in the Capgras delusion was one which often found favour in early descriptions (Brochado 1936), but other accounts of the impairment that underlies the Capgras delusion have also been suggested. Joseph (1986) proposed a cerebral hemisphere disconnection hypothesis, in which each cerebral hemisphere independently processes facial information, and the Capgras delusion arises when the two processes fail to integrate. Cutting (1991) argued against a perceptual account, and thought that the delusion is due to a breakdown of the normal structure of semantic categories, leading to a disturbance in the judgement of identity or uniqueness. Staton *et al.* (1982) drew attention to the possibility of a memory deficit, in which the Capgras patient compares a present percept with an old representation of the face, and notes the mismatch. Feinberg and Shapiro (1989) noted a failure to register familiarity, and suggested that the Capgras delusion resembles a state of selective persisting *jamais vu*.

Some of these hypotheses are clearly incompatible with the model presented here, whereas others can be regarded as variants with a different emphasis; for example, Feinberg and Shapiro's (1989) proposal can be accommodated by suggesting that the pervasive sense of strangeness resulting from the malfunction of the dorsal visual–limbic route is described by the patient as a lack of familiarity. The important point, however, is that all of the accounts lead to testable predictions which can be investigated in future cases.

The Capgras delusion is one of the most striking neuropsychiatric problems, but the use of tests to determine whether or not measurable cognitive deficits play any role in the creation and maintenance of the delusion is still at an early stage. However, it is clear that this approach has promise for uncovering the basis of this bizarre phenomenon.

Capgras and Cotard delusions

In the 1880s, Cotard described a syndrome of nihilistic delusions (*le délire de négation*) in which everything seems so unreal that the patient thinks she or he has died (Cotard 1880, 1882). This was recognized as of sufficient importance to justify a monograph by Séglas (1897), who adopted Regis's suggestion that it should be known by the eponym Cotard's syndrome. Although a key feature of this syndrome was the delusion of being dead, Cotard had noted that there could be differing and fluctuating degrees of severity. Other florid symptoms associated with the Cotard syndrome included thinking that the entire world had ceased to exist, feelings of putrefaction of internal bodily organs, self-mutilating or (paradoxically) suicidal urges, and beliefs in the absence or (conversely) enormity of parts of the body. However, the 11 patients reported in Cotard's (1882) key paper did not invariably display all of these accompanying features, which again brings into question the utility of the syndrome concept in cases presenting with the delusion of being dead, if by syndrome is meant a pattern of symptoms which will inevitably co-occur. For this reason, we have preferred to refer to the specific symptom of believing that you are dead as the Cotard delusion.

At first sight, the Cotard and Capgras delusions would seem to have little to do with each other, except that they both involve bizarre claims about existence (for self or others). On closer examination, however, there are other parallels. Both delusions can be produced by broadly similar types of brain injury (Drake 1988; Young *et al.* 1992). For example, in a case we investigated, patient WI, the Cotard delusion followed contusions affecting temporoparietal areas of the right cerebral hemisphere and some bilateral frontal lobe damage (Young *et al.* 1992). Moreover, there are similarities in the cognitive impairments. WI not only became convinced that he was dead, but he also experienced difficulties in recognizing familiar faces, buildings, and places, as well as feelings of derealization; all of which are often noted in Capgras cases. In fact, people suffering the Cotard delusion commonly report that they must be dead because they 'feel nothing inside', which presses the parallel with the hypothesized lack of affective reactions in Capgras cases still further. Young *et al.* (1992) therefore suggested that the underlying pathophysiology and neuropsychology of the Cotard and Capgras delusions may be related. We think that, although these delusions are phenomenally distinct, they may represent the patients' attempts to make sense of fundamentally similar experiences.

Young *et al.* (1992) noted that this suggestion of a link between the Capgras and Cotard delusions is strengthened by the fact that cases of coexistent or sequential Capgras and Cotard delusions have been described in the literature. The underlying basis of both delusions could therefore lie in a delusional interpretation of altered perception (especially loss of affective familiarity).

A clue to how this could happen comes from the studies which have shown that people with persecutory delusions tend to attribute negative events to external rather than internal causes, whereas depressed people tend to attribute them to internal causes (Candido and Romney 1990; Kaney and Kentall 1989). The relevance of these findings is that it is quite common for the Cotard delusion to arise in the setting of a depressive illness and for the Capgras delusion to be accompanied by persecutory delusions and suspiciousness (Enoch and Trethowan 1991; Wright *et al.* 1993). Hence, whilst the persecutory delusions and suspiciousness that are often noted in Capgras cases contribute to the patients mistaking a change in themselves for a change in others ('they must be impostors'), people who are depressed might exaggerate the negative effects of a similar change whilst correctly attributing it to themselves ('I must be dead').

These points were in fact made or anticipated by Cotard, but many of them seem to have got lost in the intervening century. Cotard's 1882 paper ends with a very thorough table listing the parallels and differences between delusions of negation and delusions of persecution. This table gives a version of the attribution hypothesis, in which Cotard points out that in delusions of persecution 'Le malade s'en prend au monde extérieur', whereas in delusions of negation 'Le malade s'accuse lui-même'. Even the combination of the specific delusions of being dead oneself and having one's relatives replaced by impostors is hinted at in this report; as well as experiencing nihilistic delusions, case 4 in Cotard's (1882) series had claimed that her daughter was a devil in disguise, and did not recognize her husband and children when they visited (though

Cotard implied that she may not have recognized her husband and children because she no longer believed in their existence). Moreover, in his 1880 paper, Cotard commented that there was a kind of logic to the delusions, and in 1884 he noted the presence of a loss of visual imagery in his patients (Cotard 1884). Loss of visual imagery is a frequent concomitant of visual recognition impairments, and Cotard's mentor, Charcot, had recently described such a case (Charcot and Bernard 1883; Young and van de Wal 1996). Considering this to be more than a coincidence, Cotard (1884) suggested that the delusions reflected a misinterpretation of this change. Plus ça change . . .

Reduplicative paramnesias

Patients with reduplicative paramnesias assert 'the presence of two or more places with nearly identical attributes, while only one exists in reality' (Patterson and Mack 1985). The term comes from Pick (1903), who described two cases; patient 1 'asserted that there were two clinics exactly alike in which he had been, two professors of the same name were at the head of these clinics, &c', whereas patient 2, who was in a clinic in Prague, 'imagined she was in K., and in reply to the assistant's question how it was that he was in K. also, she said that she was very pleased to see him *here too*'. Both of Pick's cases were similar in that they thought there were duplicate hospitals; they differed in that for patient 1 the hospital staff and patients had been duplicated as well, whilst when patient 2 was asked how the same staff and patients would be in both clinics she replied that 'They come from one place to the other'.

The parallels between reduplicative paramnesia and the Capgras delusion have been widely recognized (Alexander *et al.* 1979; Feinberg and Shapiro 1989; Staton *et al.* 1982; Weinstein and Burnham 1991). Not only is there a parallel in the phenomenon of reduplication itself, but the brain lesions responsible for reduplicative paramnesias often involve bilateral frontal atrophy and a more discrete lesion in the region of the temporo-parieto-occipital junction of the right hemisphere (Benson *et al.* 1976; Hakim *et al.* 1988; Staton *et al.* 1982). In addition, as is suggested by Pick's (1903) patient 1, the Capgras delusion and reduplicative paramnesia can be found together (Alexander *et al.* 1979; Staton *et al.* 1982). For example, Staton *et al.*'s (1982) patient stated that 'everything is so different' [from before the accident]. 'Friends and relatives, including his parents and siblings, were not "real" – but were slightly different "look-alikes", or doubles – not the real people he had known before the accident. This was also true of places, including the family farm and the city where he was hospitalized.' (Staton *et al.* 1982, p. 24). In a particularly expansive case, a patient thought that there were eight entire duplicate cities, each an exact replica of his home city, and each peopled with duplicates of his family members; he knew these were impostors 'because they did not "feel" like the real people to him' (Thompson *et al.* 1980).

If reduplicative paramnesia involves fundamentally similar mechanisms to those which create the Capgras delusion, and if the Cotard and Capgras delusions are also closely related, we might expect to find cases showing the Cotard delusion and reduplicative paramnesia; yet there seems to have been only one historic report to date (Förstl and Beats 1992). The rarity of this combination of delusions may, however, be in part explained by suggesting that reduplicative paramnesias would be masked in cases where the Cotard delusion led the patient to question the reality of his or her surroundings.

Recently, a further variant of delusional misidentification has been recognized, involving the duplication of inanimate objects (Anderson 1988). Anderson's 1988 patient, Mr B, was a 74-year-old man with a pituitary tumour. He believed that his wife and nephew had been plotting across 10 years to ruin him by stealing his belongings, and had kept a typewritten record of over 300 items they had 'stolen'; these were predominantly household items (screws, nails, paint brushes, screwdrivers) or personal belongings (shirts, underpants, wellingtons, electric razor). According to Mr B, some of these items had been replaced by inferior doubles identical in size, shape, colour, and manufacturer's name. Mr B agreed that this story was incredible and would be difficult to believe, but he sincerely believed it himself, and he made his wife sleep on the kitchen floor because of his persecutory delusions.

Anderson (1988) suggested that this is a variant of the Capgras delusion, and that 'the reason why Mr B presented the delusion of doubles for objects rather than people lies in understanding his character and interests. Mr B was a private and solitary man who made few friends, and obtained pleasure in life from his pastimes of repairing and using his tools, areas in which he had developed some expertise and spent many hours' (Anderson 1988, p. 698). Anderson went on to propose an account of such delusions which is very similar to that given here, suggesting that they are due to 'lesions of the pathway for visual recognition at a stage where visual images are imbued with affective familiarity. This results in familiar images evoking unfamiliar and incongruous affective responses and such inconsistency is then rationalized by the interpretation that the image cannot be that which it physically resembles.' (Anderson 1988, p. 698).

Conclusions

Studies of recognition impairments offer an interesting insight into one facet of the complex neurological mechanisms that sustain our experience of the world as real. The Capgras and Cotard delusions seem to contravene quite basic assumptions we generally make about our own existence and that of other people. Both delusions may hinge on powerful perceptual experiences in which things do not seem to be the way they should; even when recognized, they feel strange and unfamiliar. Yet more severe recognition impairments, such as prosopagnosia, are not generally linked to delusions. This points to the idea that delusional misidentifications result from interactions between different impairments, but it also underlines the complexity of the processes involved in recognition. In particular, I have emphasized the interplay of cognitive and emotional aspects in normal recognition, and shown how the breakdown of this interplay may provide a pointer to understanding how brain injuries can sometimes lead to bizarre delusions.

Investigations of these issues have also served to highlight areas in which our models of recognition need refinement. One of these is the notion of 'familiarity'. As we have noted, a striking form of recognition error, which occurs both in everyday life and after certain types of brain injury, involves knowing that a face is familiar but having no idea *who* it is, and such observations have led us to model familiarity as if it were a relatively basic piece of cognitive information (Young *et al.* 1985; Bruce and Young 1986). This has been a useful tactic, but studies of the Capgras delusion and related conditions show that familiarity is more complex. We will now need to pay more attention to distinguishing different kinds of familiarity (Critchley 1989; Mandler 1980), and integrating these into an overall model which can encompass cognitive and affective reactions to people, things, and events which have personal relevance (Van Lancker 1991).

References

Alexander, M. P., Stuss, D. T., and Benson, D. F. (1979). Capgras syndrome: a reduplicative phenomenon. *Neurology*, **29**, 334–9.

Anderson, D. N. (1988). The delusion of inanimate doubles. *British Journal of Psychiatry*, **153**, 694–9.

Bauer, R. M. (1984). Autonomic recognition of names and faces in prosopagnosia: a neuropsychological application of the guilty knowledge test. *Neuropsychologia*, **22**, 457–69.

Bauer, R. M. (1986). The cognitive psychophysiology of prosopagnosia. In *Aspects of face Processing*, (ed. H. D. Ellis, M. A. Jeeves, F. Newcombe, and A. Young), pp. 253–67. Martinus Nijhoff, Dordrecht.

Bear, D. M. (1983). Hemispheric specialization and the neurology of emotion. *Archives of Neurology*, **40**, 195–202.

Benson, D. F. and Stuss, D. T. (1990). Frontal lobe influences on delusions: a clinical perspective. *Schizophrenia Bulletin*, **16**, 403–11.

Benson, D. F., Gardner, H., and Meadows, J. C. (1976). Reduplicative paramnesia. *Neurology*, **26**, 147–51.

Berson, R. J. (1983). Capgras syndrome. *American Journal of Psychiatry*, **140**, 969–78.

Bornstein, R. F. (1989). Exposure and affect: overview and meta-analysis of research, 1968–1987. *Psychological Bulletin*, **106**, 265–89.

Brochado, A. (1936). Le syndrome de Capgras. *Annales Médico-Psychologiques*, **15**, 706–17.

Bruce, V. and Young, A. (1986). Understanding face recognition. *British Journal of Psychology*, **77**, 305–27.

Bruce, V., Burton, A. M., and Craw, I. (1992). Modelling face recognition. *Philosophical Transactions of the Royal Society, London*, **B335**, 121–8.

Bruyer, R. (1991). Covert face recognition in prosopagnosia: a review. *Brain and Cognition*, **15**, 223–35.

Burton, A. M., Bruce, V., and Johnston, R. A. (1990). Understanding face recognition with an interactive activation model. *British Journal of Psychology*, **81**, 361–80.

Burton, A. M., Young, A. W., Bruce, V., Johnston, R., and Ellis, A. W. (1991). Understanding covert recognition. *Cognition*, **39**, 129–66.

Candido, C. L. and Romney, D. M. (1990). Attributional style in paranoid vs. depressed patients. *British Journal of Medical Psychology*, **63**, 355–63.

Capgras, J. and Carrette, P. (1924). l'Illusion des sosies et complexe d'Oedipe. *Annales Médico-Psychologiques*, **82**, 48–68.

Capgras, J. and Reboul-Lachaux, J. (1923). l'Illusion des 'sosies' dans un délire systématisé chronique. *Bulletin de la Société Clinique de Médecine Mentale*, **11**, 6–16.

Charcot, J.-M. and Bernard, D. (1883). Un cas de suppression brusque et isolée de la vision mentale des signes et des objets (formes et couleurs). *Le Progres Médical*, **11**, 568–71.

Collins, M. N., Hawthorne, M. E., Gribbin, N., and Jacobson, R. (1990). Capgras syndrome with organic disorders. *Postgraduate Medical Journal*, **66**, 1064–7.

Cotard, J. (1880). Du delire hypocondriaque dans une forme grave de la mélancolie anxieuse. *Annales Médico Psychologiques*, **38**, 168–70.

Cotard, J. (1882). Du délire des négations. *Archives de Neurologie*, **4**, 150–70, 282–95.

Cotard, J. (1884). Perte de la vision mentale dans la mélancolie anxieuse. *Archives de Neurologie*, **7**, 289–95.

Critchley, E. M. R. (1989). The neurology of familiarity. *Behavioural Neurology*, **2**, 195–200.

Cutting, J. (1991). Delusional misidentification and the role of the right hemisphere in the appreciation of identity. *British Journal of Psychiatry*, **159**, 70–5.

Damasio, A. R., Damasio, H., and Van Hoesen, G. W. (1982). Prosopagnosia: anatomic basis and behavioral mechanisms. *Neurology*, **32**, 331–41.

de Haan, E. H. F., Young, A., and Newcombe, F. (1987). Face recognition without awareness. *Cognitive Neuropsychology*, **4**, 385–415.

de Haan, E. H. F., Young, A. W., and Newcombe, F. (1991a). Covert and overt recognition in prosopagnosia. *Brain*, **114**, 2575–91.

de Haan, E. H. F., Young, A. W., and Newcombe, F. (1991b). A dissociation between the sense of familiarity and access to semantic information concerning familiar people. *European Journal of Cognitive Psychology*, **3**, 51–67.

de Pauw, K. W. and Szulecka, T. K. (1988). Dangerous delusions: violence and the misidentification syndromes. *British Journal of Psychiatry*, **152**, 91–7.

De Renzi, E. (1986). Prosopagnosia in two patients with CT scan evidence of damage confined to the right hemisphere. *Neuropsychologia*, **24**, 385–9.

De Renzi, E., Faglioni, P., Grossi, D., and Nichelli, P. (1991). Apperceptive and associative forms of prosopagnosia. *Cortex*, **27**, 213–21.

Drake, M. E. J. (1988). Cotard's syndrome and temporal lobe epilepsy. *Psychiatric Journal of the University of Ottawa*, **13**, 36–9.

Ellis, A. W. (1992). Cognitive mechanisms of face processing. *Philosophical Transactions of the Royal Society, London*, **B335**, 113–19.

Ellis, H. D. and Young, A. W. (1990). Accounting for delusional misidentifications. *British Journal of Psychiatry*, **157**, 239–48.

Enoch, M. D. and Trethowan, W. H. (1991). *Uncommon psychiatric syndromes*, 3rd edn. John Wright, Bristol.

Feinberg, T. E. and Shapiro, R. M. (1989). Misidentification–reduplication and the right hemisphere. *Neuropsychiatry, Neuropsychology, and Behavioral Neurology*, **2**, 39–48.

Fleminger, S. (1991). Déjà vu phenomena. *American Journal of Psychiatry*, **148**, 1418–19.

Fleminger, S. (1992). Seeing is believing: the role of 'preconscious' perceptual processing in delusional misidentification. *British Journal of Psychiatry*, **160**, 293–303.

Flude, B. M., Ellis, A. W., and Kay, J. (1989). Face processing and name retrieval in an anomic aphasic: names are stored separately from semantic information about familiar people. *Brain and Cognition*, **11**, 60–72.

Förstl, H. and Beats, B. (1992). Charles Bonnet's description of Cotard's delusion and reduplicative paramnesia in an elderly patient (1788). *British Journal of Psychiatry*, **160**, 416–18.

Förstl, H., Burns, A., Jacoby, R., and Levy, R. (1991a). Neuroanatomical correlates of clinical misidentification and misperception in senile dementia of the Alzheimer type. *Journal of Clinical Psychiatry*, **52**, 268–71.

Förstl, H., Almeida, O. P., Owen, A. M., Burns, A., and Howard, R. (1991b). Psychiatric, neurological and medical aspects of misidentification syndromes: a review of 260 cases. *Psychological Medicine*, **21**, 905–10.

Geschwind, N. (1982). Disorders of attention: a frontier in neuropsychology. *Philosophical Transactions of the Royal Society, London*, **B298**, 173–85.

Greve, K. W. and Bauer, R. M. (1990). Implicit learning of new faces in prosopagnosia: an application of the mere-exposure paradigm. *Neuropsychologia*, **28**, 1035–41.

Hakim, H., Verma, N. P., and Greiffenstein, M. F. (1988). Pathogenesis of reduplicative paramnesia. *Journal of Neurology, Neurosurgery, and Psychiatry*, **51**, 839–41.

Huq, S. F., Garety, P. A., and Hemsley, D. R. (1988). Probabilistic judgements in deluded and non-deluded subjects. *Quarterly Journal of Experimental Psychology*, **40A**, 801–12.

Joseph, A. B. (1986). Focal central nervous system abnormalities in patients with misidentification syndromes. *Bibliotheca Psychiatrica*, **164**, 68–79.

Kaney, S. and Bentall, R. P. (1989). Persecutory delusions and attributional style. *British Journal of Medical Psychology*, **62**, 191–8.

Kunst-Wilson, W. R. and Zajonc, R. B. (1980). Affective discrimination of stimuli that cannot be recognized. *Science*, **207**, 557–8.

Landis, T., Cummings, J. L., Christen, L., Bogen, J. E. and Imhof, H. G. (1986). Are unilateral right posteror cerebral lesions sufficient to cause prosopagnosia? Clinical and radiological findings in six additional patients. *Cortex*, **22**, 243–52.

Lewis, S. W. (1987). Brain imaging in a case of Capgras syndrome. *British Journal of Psychiatry*, **150**, 117–21.

Mandler, G. (1980). Recognizing: the judgement of previous occurrence. *Psychological Review*, **87**, 252–71.

Meadows, J. C. 91974). The anatomical basis of prosopagnosia. *Journal of Neurology, Neurosurgery, and Psychiatry*, **37**, 489–501.

Morrison, R. L. and Tarter, R. E. (1984). Neuropsychological findings relating to Capgras syndrome. *Biological Psychiatry*, **19**, 1119–28.

Patterson, M. B. and Mack, J. L. (1985). Neuropsychological analysis of a case of reduplicative paramnesia. *Journal of Clinical and Experimental Neuropsychology*, **7**, 111–21.

Pick, A. (1903). Clinical studies: III. On reduplicative paramnesia. *Brain*, **26**, 260–7.

Rizzo, M., Hurtig, R., and Damasio, A. R. (1987). The role of scanpaths in facial recognition and learning. *Annals of Neurology*, **22**, 41–5.

Séglas, J. (1897). *Le délire des négations: séméiologie et diagnostic*. Masson, Gauthier-Villars, Paris.

Sergent, J. and Poncet, M. (1990). From covert to overt recognition of faces in a prosopagnosic patient. *Brain*, **113**, 989–1004.

Sergent, J. and Villemure, J.-G. (1989). Prosopagnosia in a right hemispherectomized patient. *Brain*, **112**, 975–95.

Shraberg, D. and Weitzel, W. D. (1979). Prosopagnosia and the Capgras syndrome. *Journal of Clinical Psychiatry*, **40**, 313–16.

Shubsachs, A. P. W. and Young, A. (1988). Dangerous delusions: the 'Hollywood' phenomenon. *British Journal of Psychiatry*, **152**, 722.

Slade, P. and Bentall, R. P. (1988). *Sensory deception: a scientific analysis of hallucinations*. Croom-Helm, London.

Sno, H. N. and Linszen, D. H. (1990). The déjà vu experience: remembrance of things past? *American Journal of Psychiatry*, **147**, 1587–95.

Staton, R. D., Brumback, R. A., and Wilson, H. (1982). Reduplicative paramnesia: a disconnection syndrome of memory. *Cortex*, **18**, 23–6.

Stuss, D. T., Alexander, M. P., Lieberman, A., and Levine, H. (1978). An extraordinary form of confabulation. *Neurology*, **28**, 1166–72.

Thompson, M. I., Silk, K. R., and Hover, G. L. (1980). Misidentification of a city: delimiting criteria for Capgras syndrome. *American Journal of Psychiatry*, **137**, 1270–2.

Tranel, D. and Damasio, A. R. (1985). Knowledge without awareness: an autonomic index of facial recognition by prosopagnosics. *Science*, **228**, 1453–4.

Tranel, D. and Damasio, A. R. (1988). Non-conscious face recognition in patients with face agnosia. *Behavioural Brain Research*, **30**, 235–49.

Tzavaras, A., Luauté, J. P., and Bidault, E. (1986). Face recognition dysfunction and delusional misidentification syndromes (DMS). In *Aspects of face processing*, (ed. H. D. Ellis, M. A. Jeeves, F. Newcombe, and A. Young), pp. 310–16. Martinus Nijhoff, Dordrecht.

Van Lancker, D. (1991). Personal relevance and the human right hemisphere. *Brain and Cognition*, **17**, 64–92.

Vié, J. (1944). Les méconnaissances systèmatiques: étude séméiologique. *Annales Médico-Psychologiques*, **102**, 229–52.

Vogel, B. F. (1974). The Capgras syndrome and its psychopathology. *American Journal of Psychiatry*, **131**, 922–4.

Wallis, G. (1986). Nature of the misidentified in the Capgras syndrome. *Bibliotheca Psychiatrica*, **164**, 40–8.

Weinstein, E. A. and Burnham, D. L. (1991). Reduplication and the syndrome of Capgras. *Psychiatry*, **54**, 78–88.

Wilcox, J. and Waziri, R. (1983). The Capgras symptom and nondominant cerebral dysfunction. *Journal of Clinical Psychiatry*, **44**, 70–2.

Wright, S., Young, A. W., and Hellawell, D. J. (1993). Sequential Cotard and Capgras delusions. *British Journal of Clinical Psychology*, **32**, 345–9.

Young, A. W. (1988). Functional organization of visual recognition. In *Thought without language*, (ed. L. Weiskrantz), pp. 78–107. Oxford University Press.

Young, A. W. and de Haan, E. H. F. (1992). Face recognition and awareness after brain injury. In *The neuropsychology of consciousness*, (ed. A. D. Milner and M. D. Rugg), pp. 69–90. Academic Press, London.

Young, A. W. and van de Wal, C. (1996). Charcot's case of impaired imagery. In *Clasic cases in neuropsychology*, (ed. C. Code, C.-W. Wallesch, A. R. Lecours, and Y. Joanette), pp. 31–44. Lawrence Erlbaum, London.

Young, A. W., Hay, D. C., and Ellis, A. W. (1985). The faces that launched a thousand slips: everyday difficulties and errors in recognizing people. *British Journal of Psychology*, **76**, 495–523.

Young, A. W., Hellawell, D., and de Haan, E. H. F. (1988). Cross-domain semantic priming in normal subjects and a prosopagnosic patient. *Quarterly Journal of Experimental Psychology*, **40A**, 561–80.

Young, A. W., Robertson, I. H., Hellawell, D. J., de Pauw, K. W., and Pentland, B. (1992). Cotard delusion after brain injury. *Psychological Medicine*, **22**, 799–804.

Young, A. W., Reid, I., Wright, S., and Hellawell, D. (1993). Face processing impairments and the Capgras delusion. *British Journal of Psychiatry*, **162**, 695–8.

Zajonc, R. B. (1980). Feeling and thinking: preferences need no inferences. *American Psychologist.* **35**, 151–75.

11

Covert face recognition in prosopagnosia

Reprinted in slightly modified form from Young, A. W. (1994), Covert recognition, in *The neuropsychology of high-level vision: collected tutorial essays*, (ed. M. J. Farah and G. Ratcliff), pp. 331–58, Lawrence Erlbaum, Hillsdale, New Jersey. With kind permission of Lawrence Erlbaum Associates, Inc.

Summary

One of the most remarkable findings to arise from investigations of visual recognition impairments due to brain injury has been that patients who do not seem to show normal, overt recognition of things they see may none the less demonstrate a form of non-conscious, covert recognition if appropriate tests are used. These patients do not seem to suffer any general alteration of consciousness, but one specific aspect, awareness of recognition, is lost.

If correct, this finding fundamentally changes the way in which we think about recognition impairments, and has implications for our understanding of awareness itself. It is therefore appropriate to give it careful scrutiny. In this chapter, I provide a tutorial review of findings of covert recognition, concentrating on those arising in cases of prosopagnosia, but sketching their relation to other neuropsychological phenomena. I then consider some of the issues which arise and accounts of the phenomena that have been attempted, in the context of recent findings.

Background

In order to understand work on covert recognition, it is necessary to have some background information concerning prosopagnosia, to examine the findings obtained with electrophysiological and behavioural measures, and to consider the extent to which these hold across faces familiar before and after the patients' illnesses. I also draw attention to the fact that not all prosopagnosic patients show covert recognition, and explore briefly the relation of covert recognition in prosopagnosia to other forms of neuropsychological impairment.

Prosopagnosia

Most of the work on covert recognition after brain injury has arisen from studies of prosopagnosia. Prosopagnosic patients are unable to identify familiar faces overtly, and rely on voice, context, name, or sometimes clothing or gait to achieve recognition of people they know. A review of the clinical findings is given by Hécaen and Angelergues (1962). The patients know when they are looking at a face, and can describe its features, but the loss of any sense of overt recognition is often complete, with no feeling of familiarity to even the most well known faces.

Prosopagnosia was first identified as a distinct neuropsychological problem by Bodamer (1947). The underlying pathology involves lesions affecting occipito-temporal regions of cerebral cortex. Usually these are bilateral lesions (Damasio *et al.* 1982; Meadows 1974), but several cases apparently involving unilateral lesions of the right cerebral hemisphere have been reported (e.g. De Renzi 1986*a*; Landis *et al.* 1986; Sergent and Villemure 1989; see Benton 1990, for a review). The neuro-anatomical correlates are discussed in detail by Damasio *et al.* (1983, 1990).

Covert recognition from electrophysiological responses

Bauer (1984) measured skin conductance (galvanic skin responses or GSRs) while a prosopagnosic patient, LF, viewed a familiar face for 90 s and listened to a list of five names being read out. When the name belonging to the face being viewed was read out, there was a greater skin conductance change than when someone else's name was read out. yet if LF was asked to choose which name in the list went with the face, his performance was at chance level. These findings are summarized in Table 11.1, which makes it clear that the same effect was found to personally known faces (LF's family) and famous faces he would only have encountered in the mass media.

Bauer's (1984) study showed compellingly a difference between overt recognition, which was at chance level for LF, and some form of preserved covert recognition, as evidenced by his skin conductance responses. In a subsequent study, Bauer and Verfaellie (1988) demon-

Table 11.1 Percentages of famous faces and family faces for which LF showed spontaneous naming, selection of the correct name from five alternatives, and maximum GSR to the correct name in the list of five alternatives (Bauer 1984)

	Spontaneous naming	Name selection	Maximum GSR to correct name
Famous faces	0%	20%	60%
Family faces	0%	25%	63%

strated that it is the correspondence between the specific identity of the face and name that is crucial, rather than the mere presence of some kind of match, because differential GSR was not found for a matching task with unfamiliar faces.

Bauer's (1984; Bauer and Verfaellie 1988) findings profoundly affect our conception of the nature of prosopagnosia, because they show that it is inadequate to think of it as simply involving loss of recognition mechanisms. Instead, at least some degree of recognition does take place; what has been lost is *awareness of recognition*.

Comparable findings were reported by Tranel and Damasio (1985, 1988), using a different technique in which the patients simply looked at a series of familiar and unfamiliar faces. GSR changes were greater to familiar than unfamiliar faces. This shows that it is possible to demonstrate a preserved electrophysiological response to the familiarity of the face alone (i.e., without any accompanying name), which is a useful adjunct to Bauer's (1984) procedure.

A further electrophysiological demonstration of covert recognition in prosopagnosia comes from Renault *et al.*'s (1989) work on evoked potentials.

Behavioural indices of covert recognition

Findings of covert recognition are not restricted to electrophysiological measures. Bruyer *et al.* (1983) asked their prosopagnosic patient, Mr W, to learn names to sets of five faces. Some of the data from this study are shown in Table 11.2, which summarizes the condition in which famous faces were used. On each trial, Mr W was given a written name for each of five famous faces, and allowed 30 s to examine them. The faces were then removed, and he was asked to pair them up with the names, which were reordered at random. As can be seen, Mr W seemed better able to learn 'true' names to the faces (i.e. the person's actual name) than

Table 11.2 Mr W's learning of different types of name to sets of five famous faces (Bruyer *et al.* 1983)

Visual stimuli	Verbal stimuli	Trials					Overall percentage correct
		1	2	3	4	5	
Famous male faces	True names	3	5	5	5	5	92%
Famous male faces	Untrue names	1	3	3	5	3	60%
Famous male faces	Male first names	1	1	3	3	3	44%

'untrue' names, which were the names of other people in the set of faces. As Bruyer *et al.* noted, this superior learning of true than untrue pairings demonstrates some form of preserved recognition of the faces, even though Mr W was not able to access this overtly.

Bruyer *et al.* (1983) must be given credit for introducing this conveniently simple learning technique, which has been adapted for use in several subsequent demonstrations of covert recognition of familiar faces (e.g. de Haan *et al.* 1987*a*; Sergent and Poncet 1990; Young and de Haan 1988), and has been extended to examine covert recognition of stimuli from other visual categories (de Haan *et al.* 1991).

Covert recognition has also been demonstrated with a number of other behavioural indices including eye movement scan paths (Rizzo *et al.* 1987), reaction times for face matching across transformations of orientation or age (faster to familiar than unfamiliar faces: de Haan *et al.* 1987*a*, task 1; Sergent and Poncet, 1990), matching of internal and external facial features (faster for familiar than unfamiliar faces with internal features only; de Haan *et al.* 1987*a*, task 2), and interference from distractor faces belonging to the 'wrong' semantic category in a name classification task (politician's name versus non-politician's name; de Haan *et al.* 1987*a*, *b*). Figure 11.1 shows an example taken from de Haan *et al.* (1987*a*, task 4), which illustrates that interference was found even when each of the photographs of the faces in a particular category was matched quite closely in appearance to one of the photographs of the faces in the opposite category.

A very useful procedure has been to examine associative priming from face or name primes onto name targets. Associative priming tasks (also known as semantic priming in the research literature) examine the influence of one stimulus on the recognition of a related stimulus; for instance, the effect of seeing John Lennon's face on recognition of Paul McCartney's name. Recognition of a target stimulus is facilitated by an immediately preceding prime stimulus that is a close associate of the target (Bruce and Valentine 1986).

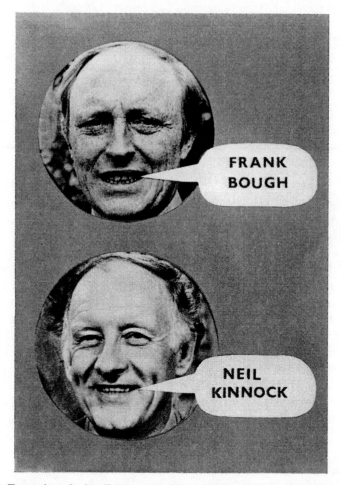

Fig. 11.1 Examples of stimuli from a condition of de Haan *et al.*'s (1987*a*, task 4) study in which there was significant interference of the distractor face on classification of the name as being that of a politician or non-politician. The non-politician Frank Bough's name is combined with the face of politician Neil Kinnock, and vice versa. As can be seen, the two faces are of similar appearance. Copyright 1987 by Lawrence Erlbaum Associates. Reprinted by permission.

Using this technique, we were able to demonstrate that the proso-pagnosic patient PH shows associative priming from faces he does not recognize. Table 11.3 shows PH's mean correct reaction times for classification of target names as familiar when they were preceded by face or name primes (reaction times to unfamiliar names are not shown). The data are taken from Young *et al.* (1988), who presented primes to PH for 450 ms each, with a 50 ms interstimulus interval before

Table 11.3 Reaction times (ms) for correct responses to target names of familiar people preceded by related, neutral, or unrelated face or name primes for PH (Young *et al.* 1988) and MS (Newcombe *et al.* 1989)

	Related	Neutral	Unrelated
PH			
Face primes	1016	1080	1117
Name primes	945	1032	1048
MS			
Face primes	1260	1276	1264
Name primes	1178	1370	1439

onset of the target name. Three types of prime were used; related (e.g. John Lennon as a prime for the target name 'Paul McCartney'), neutral (an unfamiliar prime with a familiar target name), or unrelated (e.g. Ronald Reagan as a prime for the target name 'Paul McCartney').

As the data in Table 11.3 show, PH recognized familiar target names more quickly when they were preceded by related face primes than when they were preceded by neutral or by unrelated face primes. Hence he showed associative priming from faces he did not recognize overtly. Lack of overt recognition was confirmed by a separate post test given immediately after the experiment, in which PH could only recognize two of the 20 familiar faces used (shown to him with unlimited exposure duration), despite the fact that these faces had all been presented many times in the course of the experiment. The associative priming effect was measured (and statistically tested) across all the primes used, so there is no question of the result simply being due to these two faces that could be recognized overtly after the experiment.

It is possible to compare the size of the priming effect across face primes (which PH mostly did not recognize overtly) and printed name primes (which he could recognize). These are exactly equivalent; the possibility of overt recognition of name primes made no additional contribution to the associative priming effect.

In absolute terms, PH's response latencies (Table 11.3) were quite long for this type of task. However, slow responding is a common consequence of certain types of brain injury (van Zomeren and Deelman 1978). The important point is that the pattern of PH's reaction times across conditions is the same as that found for normal people, with faster reaction times in the related condition regardless of whether face or name primes are employed.

Learning new faces

The findings I have presented thus far mostly involve tasks in which prosopagnosic patients are shown faces of people who would have been familiar to them before their illnesses. But what about people who have only been encountered since the patient's illness? Would there be covert recognition effects for these as well?

One of the patients studied by Tranel and Damasio (1985, case 2) could recognize overtly the faces of people familiar to her before her illness, but did not recognize overtly faces of people she had only met since her illness. This clinical pattern is somewhat different to prosopagnosia, which involves both a retrograde recognition deficit (faces known before the patient's illness) and an anterograde deficit (faces met since the illness). Tranel and Damasio (1985, 1988) referred to their patient as having an 'anterograde prosopagnosia', and other authors have described similar cases in which old but not new faces can be recognized (Hanley *et al.* 1990; Ross 1980, case 2).

Tranel and Damasio (1985, case 2) found that their patient showed larger electrodermal responses to faces she could only have encountered since her illness than to unfamiliar faces, which implies that the face processing system is able to continue to create representations of people even when they are not consciously recognized. A similar case was reported by Tranel and Damasio (1988, case 2), with equivalent findings.

Covert recognition of the faces of people who have only been met since the patient's illness has also been found in patients with anterograde and retrograde face recognition defects, both with GSR (Tranel and Damasio 1988, cases 3 and 4) and learning tasks (de Haan *et al.* 1987a; Sergent and Poncet 1990). Again, it is clear that some form of representation of newly encountered faces is still being created despite the absence of normal, conscious identification.

Prosopagnosia without covert recognition

Although covert recognition of familiar faces can be demonstrated with a range of behavioural and electrophysiological indices, not all prosopagnosic patients show covert recognition effects.

For example, Table 11.3 contains data from the associative priming task for patient MS (Newcombe *et al.* 1989) as well as PH (Young *et al.* 1988). Notice that MS showed associative priming from name primes (which he can recognize overtly), but that there was no difference between his reaction times in the related, neutral, and unrelated conditions when face primes were used. The priming effect was only found with name primes for MS, not faces.

Comparable findings of lack of covert recognition by some patients have been reported with GSR (Bauer 1986; Etcoff *et al.* 1991) and learning tasks (Etcoff *et al.* 1991; Humphreys *et al.* 1992; McNeil and Warrington 1991; Newcombe *et al.* 1989; Sergent and Villemure 1989; Young and Ellis 1989).

The finding that some prosopagnosic patients show covert recognition and some do not makes it clear that, as clinicians have long suspected (e.g. De Renzi 1985*b*; Meadows 1974), there is more than one form of prosopagnosia. Presence or absence of covert recognition may thus provide an important pointer to the nature of the functional impairment in each case.

Relation of covert recognition in prosopagnosia to other forms of neuropsychological impairment

We have seen that prosopagnosic patients can show quite a wide range of phenomena indicating covert recognition of faces they do not recognize overtly. But are covert effects unique to prosopagnosia?

The answer is clearly 'no'. It is better to consider prosopagnosia to be one of a group of neuropsychological impairments in which covert effects can be found (Schacter *et al.* 1988; Young and de Haan 1990). For example, there are reports of preserved ability to give the location of visual stimuli presented to perimetrically blind areas of the visual field (Pöppel *et al.* 1973; Weiskrantz 1986; Weiskrantz *et al.* 1974), covert processing of 'neglected' or 'extinguished' stimuli (Marshall and Halligan 1988; Volpe *et al.* 1979), responses to words that cannot be overtly read in alexia (Coslett and Saffran 1989; Shallice and Saffran 1986), priming effects in patients with semantic memory impairments (Nebes *et al.* 1984; Young *et al.* 1989), and priming of fragment completion tasks in amnesia (Warrington and Weiskrantz 1968, 1970).

Schacter *et al.* (1988) characterized these impairments as involving failures of 'access to consciousness'. In each case there is no general alteration of consciousness. but specific types of information seem to be no longer able to enter awareness.

Summary and implications

Before turning to consider issues, accounts, and more recent findings, I try now to summarize the key points that emerge from this tutorial review, and their implications.

The main point is that patients who do not recognize familiar faces when they are asked directly who the person is can none the less show evidence of recognition on a variety of measures including GSR, evoked potentials, eye movement scan paths, learning of true and untrue information, and reaction times in matching, interference, and associative priming tasks. Covert recognition effects can be found not only to faces of people who had long been familiar to the patient, but also for faces of people who have only been encountered since the patient's illness.

In many of these tasks the information that is accessed covertly is none the less dependent on precise visual discriminations, and must reflect the operation of sophisticated visual recognition mechanisms. For example, interference on name classification from the semantic category of an 'unrecognized' face is found even when the faces used are matched for overall appearance (de Haan *et al.* 1987*a*; see Fig. 11.1). Even more strikingly, the results from associative priming tasks indicate covert processing of the identity of a face that has been presented quite briefly. Bauer's (1984) and Bauer and Verfaellie's (1988) GSR results also involved covert processing of identity, and so did Sergent and Poncet's (1990) finding of preserved ability to match photographs of the same person's face across a 30-year age difference (using photographs of the people taken in 1955 and 1985). By 'processing of identity' I mean that the visual system can narrow down the possibilities to the face of a specific person from all the thousands it has encountered in the past, and that it is still capable of using this information in certain ways (as reflected in associative priming, interference, etc.). I do not seek to claim that this means there is also covert retrieval of any very detailed semantic information about the individual.

For prosopagnosic patients with covert recognition, we can consider their impairment as involving a loss of awareness of recognition. This changes our conception of prosopagnosia, which had previously been considered an absolute recognition defect, with no distinction between conscious and non-conscious forms of recognition.

However, not all patients show covert recognition. There are also cases where there does seem to be a loss of both overt and covert recognition ability. It is thus useful to use tests of covert recognition to distinguish different forms of prosopagnosia due to varying underlying causes.

This would be interesting even if it were thought that these measures simply pick up the residual abilities of a recognition system that has suffered widespread general damage. But the fact that covert recognition effects involve the face's identity suggests that thinking in terms of a generally damaged recognition system is inadequate. What we find fits more easily with the idea that a substantial part of the face recognition system is intact, but its *outputs* have been damaged or disconnected (Young and de Haan 1988), and this allows us to see covert recognition as one of a group of neuropsychological impairments characterized by selective failures of access to consciousness for certain types of information (Schacter *et al.* 1988).

Issues, accounts, and recent findings

Having examined the background of findings on covert recognition, I now turn to consider in more depth some of the issues that arise, accounts that have been given, and recent findings.

Extent of the loss of overt recognition in prosopagnosia

It is worth considering more carefully the extent of the loss of overt recognition in prosopagnosia, because this is obviously central to any claims of covert recognition. Reports of non conscious recognition by neurologically normal people have been greeted with considerable scepticism, and great care is needed in conducting and interpreting such studies. Some of the same considerations apply to studies of covert recognition after brain injury.

The first possibility that needs to be considered is response bias. When looking at a face, prosopagnosic patients typically state that it does not seem familiar, and they have no idea who it is. However, it might be thought that they are simply very uncertain as to who it might be, and thus unwilling to venture any hypothesis about the face's identity or its familiarity to them. For example, if prosopagnosic patients are shown a series of faces one at a time, and asked to pick out those that are familiar, it is usual to find chance-level performance because all of the faces are considered unfamiliar. It is thus desirable to eliminate the effects of what might be merely a very pronounced response bias. This can be done by means of forced-choice tasks (McNicol 1972).

Table 11.4 shows results for forced-choice familiarity decision to faces and names by patients MS (Newcombe *et al.* 1989) and PH (Young and De Haan 1988). On each trial, they were presented with a familiar face and an unfamiliar face, or with a familiar name and an unfamiliar name, and asked to choose the familiar member of each pair. The rationale behind this task is that the sense of familiarity is considered the most

Table 11.4 Forced-choice familiarity decision to faces and names by PH (Young and de Haan 1988), MS (Newcombe *et al.* 1989), and age-matched controls

	Faces	Names
PH	65/128	118/128
MS	67/128	116/128
Controls		
Mean	125.50	127.50
SD	3.33	0.84

basic evidence of overt recognition (e.g. a common everyday error is to know that a face is familiar, but not who it is; Young *et al.* 1985).

As Table 11.4 indicates, both MS and PH show chance-level performance of forced-choice familiarity decisions to faces, but are well above chance with names (though still impaired in comparison to age-matched controls). The chance-level forced-choice performance to faces makes it clear that their inability to respond to face familiarity is not just a response bias; yet as we have seen, PH has been found to show a variety of covert recognition effects. In fact, de Haan *et al.* (1987*a*, task 1) had shown that PH matched photographs of familiar faces more quickly than he matched photographs of unfamiliar faces using exactly the same photographs as were employed in this forced-choice familiarity decision task by Young and de Haan (1988).

So far, so good. We also need, though, to know that patients who are thought to show covert recognition are not gaining some degree of overt access to the specific information required by the test used to demonstrate covert recognition.

Again, there are grounds for being reasonably confident. For example, notice that in Bauer's (1984) study (Table 11.1) he included a condition in which his patient, LF, was asked to select the correct name for each face from the five alternatives used in the GSR test. LF performed very poorly in this task (choice of correct name for famous faces = 20 per cent correct; family faces = 25 per cent correct; chance = 20 per cent correct), yet his GSR presented quite a different picture (maximum GSR to correct name for famous faces = 60 per cent; family faces = 63 per cent; chance = 20 per cent). Hence LF could not perform successfully on an exactly equivalent test of his overt knowledge of the information he accessed covertly.

We have also examined the same point in our interference tasks with PH (de Haan *et al.* 1987*a, b*). In these tasks, PH was asked to classify familiar names as those of politicians or non-politicians, and the names could be accompanied by a distractor face belonging to the same or the opposite semantic category (see Fig. 11.1). Like normal subjects, PH showed interference from the face distractors if they belonged to the opposite category to the name.

Although PH could not give any indication that he recognized the specific, personal identity of the faces we used in these tasks, it is obviously important to know how reliably he could assign them to 'politician' or 'non-politician' categories, because it was interference at this semantic category level that was investigated. In each of the three interference experiments we have reported for PH, he was therefore also given a test that required him to assign the faces (presented without accompanying names) to politician or non-politician categories.

In one experiment (de Haan et al. 1987a, task 3) we used pop stars as the non-politicians, partly because we could then conveniently compare PH's performance to that of normal subjects (Young et al. 1986), but also because we were curious as to whether the possibility of arriving at the politician versus non-politician discrimination using relatively superficial features would prove important (age and hairstyle will distinguish most politicians from most pop stars). As expected, PH could achieve quite accurate classification of these faces as politicians or pop stars (only 4.2 per cent errors), but he was very slow at doing this, with a mean reaction time for face categorization that was more than 200 ms longer than his slowest mean reaction time for any of the name categorization conditions used in the interference task. In another experiment (de Haan et al. 1987b), the non-politicians (television and film personalities) were chosen to be of comparable age to the politicians. This considerably reduced PH's ability to classify the faces overtly (30 of 48 correct), though he tried to deploy strategies such as thinking that the politicians would probably be less likely to be smiling. These may have been partially successful, because as Farah (1990) pointed out, his overt classification ability fell in a range that was close to being above chance level (62.5 per cent correct; score 30/48, $z = 1.59$, $p = 0.06$). Finally, in the third experiment we have reported (de Haan et al. 1987a, task 4) faces from the politician and non-politician categories were matched to each other on the appearance of the specific photographs used (with television personalities as the non-politicians; see Fig. 11.1), so that a purely visually based classification could not be successful. PH then performed at chance level (55.5 per cent correct; score 40/72, $z = 0.83$, $p = 0.20$). However, in all three tasks he showed interference from the face distractors, regardless of the ease with which he could or could not assign them to the appropriate category when asked directly to do this. Hence the possibility of successfully achieving overt classification is not necessary in the production of the interference effects. There is interference even when overt classification of the faces is at chance level.

This impairment of PH's overt ability to assign faces to semantic categories was stable and consistent. De Haan *et al.* (1991) tested him on 20 repetitions of a politician versus non-politician decision task, using a set of five politicians and five non-politicians (all repeated 20 times). Across the 200 trials involved, PH made 104 correct choices (52 per cent correct; chance = 50 per cent correct), with no indication of any improvement in his performance. This contrasts markedly with cases involving semantic access impairment, where continuous exposure to the same stimuli with the same task requirement can 'warm up' previously inaccessible representations (Shallice 1987, 1988).

Also striking is the extent to which covert recognition effects can be task specific. A good example comes from one of our learning tasks in which we taught PH to pair true and untrue names to photographs of our own faces (de Haan *et al.* 1987*a*, task 8; untrue names were our own names, but paired to the wrong faces). Despite the fact that PH had never met any of us before his accident, he was 99 per cent accurate (79 of 80 correct) with true pairings, but only 61 per cent correct overall with untrue pairings (49 of 80). Yet when we took the very same photographs and mixed them with an equal number of unfamiliar faces PH was at chance in deciding whether or not each person was one of the members of our research group (8 of 16 and 9 of 16 correct in two separate runs). He had not achieved any overt benefit from the substantial degree of covert recognition that he showed during the learning task.

The parallel with 'automatic' aspects of normal recognition

A number of different ways of thinking about covert recognition have been proposed. These are not necessarily incompatible with each other, but they are often given at different levels of description. I start with the most general, and end up with the more specific.

Let us begin by examining the relation of covert recognition to 'automatic' aspects of normal recognition. For all neurologically normal people, recognition is mandatory (Fodor 1983). We cannot look at a familiar face and decide whether or not to recognize it, no matter how hard we try. The operation of the recognition system proceeds automatically, outside conscious control. This is not to say that errors in recognizing people do not occur in normal people; they certainly do (Hay *et al.* 1991; Young *et al.* 1985). But only a small proportion of these everyday errors reflect the operation of conscious decision mechanisms.

One way of thinking about covert recognition in prosopagnosia is therefore that it continues to reflect the automatic operation of part of the recognition system (Young 1988). There are some grounds for this.

Consider, for example, the associative priming results for PH, shown in Table 11.3. Recall that in this experiment, PH was shown target names to classify as familiar or unfamiliar, and that each of the familiar target names was immediately preceded by a prime that was associatively related to the target, neutral (an unfamiliar person), or unrelated to the target.

In an influential article on associative priming effects in normal people, Posner and Snyder (1975) pointed out that priming could be mediated intentionally, by subjects trying to predict to themselves which target would follow the prime, or automatically, without conscious prediction. If the intentional effect applied, we would expect some cost in the form of slowed responses if the target was not as had been predicted from the prime. Hence, with an intentionally based priming effect, responses to targets preceded by related primes would be facilitated in comparison to responses to targets preceded by neutral primes, but there would also be a characteristic inhibition (i.e. slowing) of responses to targets preceded by unrelated primes, again in comparison to the neutral condition. For a purely automatic effect, we would only expect facilitation from related primes, with no inhibition from unrelated primes.

The form of the associative priming effect found for PH (see Table 11.3) fits Posner and Snyder's (1975) characterization of an automatic effect, because there was facilitation of responses to related targets (related < neutral) without inhibition of responses to unrelated targets (neutral = unrelated).

It is also known that neurologically normal people can show associative priming effects from stimuli whose presentation times are sufficient to allow them to be seen, but too brief for conscious identification (Carr et al. 1982; McCauley et al. 1980). In some ways these form a good analogue of PH's problem, because he knows when he is looking at a face, but lacks any overt sense of whose face it is.

A particularly interesting example of the parallel between findings for normal subjects and prosopagnosic patients comes from Greve and Bauer's (1990) work with LF, the patient investigated in Bauer's (1984) GSR study. Greve and Bauer showed faces to LF for 500 ms each, and then paired each of these faces with a completely novel face. They found that LF showed a preference for the faces shown to him for only 500 ms as being 'more likeable' than the faces he had not seen before, whereas when told he had seen one of the faces before and asked which it was he performed at chance level. An equivalent phenomenon of preference for briefly presented stimuli without overt recognition can be demonstrated in normal subjects (Zajonc 1980).

One very general characterization of covert recognition, then, is that it reflects the continued automatic operation of part of the recognition system. For cases like PH's (de Haan *et al.* 1987*a*) or LF's (Bauer 1984), what seem to be preserved are those aspects of recognition whose operation is relatively automatic, and does not require conscious initiation (Young 1988).

Implicit versus explicit, and related distinctions

It is also possible to draw parallels between covert recognition and phenomena involving implicit memory, which were reviewed by Schacter (1987). This is useful in that it sets findings of covert recognition in a wider theoretical context, and Greve and Bauer's (1990) work shows neatly the benefits of this. But it needs to be done with care, because there are important underlying distinctions to be kept in mind.

A key distinction is between *tasks* and patients' *insight* into their abilities. Here, I use the terms *direct* and *indirect* to refer to tasks designed to test recognition in different ways (see also Humphreys 1981; Reingold and Merikel 1988, 1990). A direct test will immediately inquire about the ability of interest ('Whose face is this?'; 'Which is familiar?'; etc.), whereas in an indirect test the ability in question is introduced as an incidental feature of a task that ostensibly measures something else (effects of familiarity on face matching, effects of different types of face prime on name recognition, etc.). Conversely, I use *overt* and *covert* to refer to patients' insight into their recognition abilities. Overt abilities are ones that the patient knows she or he possesses, whereas covert abilities are found in the absence of acknowledged awareness.

In terms of the findings we have discussed so far, covert recognition of familiar faces is found with indirect tests, whereas the patients fail all direct tests. However, there are important exceptions to this tidy pattern, which make it unsatisfactory simply to equate covert recognition with the use of indirect tests.

The first exception is that not all indirect tests produce evidence of covert recognition. For example, whether PH shows better learning of true than untrue pairings in learning tasks is critically dependent on the type of material to be learned to each face. Young and de Haan (1988) found that he showed better learning of true than untrue names to faces when given the person's full name, but did not show this effect when only first names were used. This shows that covert effects arise at a level of recognition that does not encompass name retrieval, and implies more generally that using an indirect task is not in itself sufficient to produce evidence of covert recognition.

The second exception is that not all direct tests are performed at chance level. This was first noted by Sergent and Poncet (1990). They asked their prosopagnosic patient, PV, to choose which of two names (one correct, the other a distractor belonging to a person of the same gender and occupation) went with a particular face. Her performance (40 of 48 correct) was well above chance, though below that of control subjects (who made no errors). PV herself insisted she was guessing. We have replicated this finding with PH, who also performs this task at an overall level that is well above chance, though obviously impaired (30 of 40, 27 of 40, 26 of 40, and 27 of 40 correct in four separate runs; de Haan *et al.* 1991). Like PV, PH maintains that he is guessing.

Forced-choice decision between two alternative names for a face is a direct test, because it asks about identity ('Which name is correct for the face?'). It is therefore surprising to find above-chance performance, because all other direct tests have been failed by prosopagnosic patients. An important issue, however, concerns whether this forced-choice task elicits covert or overt face recognition abilities. Sergent and Poncet (1990) argued that overt recognition is not involved, because PV insisted she was guessing, she did not know when she had chosen correctly or incorrectly, and was usually just as ready to make a choice between two names even when these were both incorrect for the face shown.

Our findings with PH are the same (de Haan *et al.* 1991). Like Sergent and Poncet (1990), we showed that PH was unaware of the information that allowed him to perform above chance level. When the original task with one correct and one incorrect name alternative was changed to one where both names were incorrect, PH continued to choose a name, oblivious to the fact that no correct answer was possible. In addition, his confidence ratings were the same whether the task included a correct name alternative or not. Therefore, we concluded (like Sergent and Poncet) that forced-choice name decision tasks can show covert recognition effects, even though a direct test is involved, and that PH and PV are comparable in that they both show covert face recognition on this type of task.

It seems that even though forced-choice name decision is a direct test, it allows the patients to utilize covert recognition abilities in some way. Note that this task depends on some form of preserved interaction between input recognition systems for faces and names, as do several of the tasks used to demonstrate covert recognition (see Young and de

Haan 1988). Examples include Bauer's (1984) application of the 'guilty knowledge' test (Table 11.1), and our semantic priming, interference, and learning paradigms (de Haan *et al.* 1987*a*, *b*; Young *et al.* 1988). Because forced-choice name decision involves both face and name inputs, it may tap into this interaction.

It is clear that although contrasts between direct versus indirect tests and overt versus covert abilities can play an important role in helping us initially to characterize patterns of intact and deficient performance, they are not in themselves an adequate explanation. However, neurological, psychological, and computational models have been proposed.

Neurological, psychological, and computational models

Bauer (1984) argued that there are two separate cortico-limbic pathways involved in overt recognition and in orienting responses to emotionally salient stimuli; the ventral route (damaged in prosopagnosia) provides overt recognition, whereas the dorsal route (spared in prosopagnosia) gives the face its emotional significance. This proposal is elegant, and useful in that it can potentially be extended to provide an account of Capgras syndrome (in which people claim that their relatives have been replaced by impostors) as a kind of 'mirror image' of prosopagnosia (the face is recognized, but loses appropriate emotional significance; Ellis and Young 1990), but the nature of the damage to the ventral route needs to be elaborated, in terms of the stage at which overt recognition breaks down.

Tranel and Damasio (1985) suggested that covert recognition arises when 'facial templates' are intact, but the processes required for the 'activation of multimodal associations' from the face are defective. This view was further developed by Tranel and Damasio (1988), who argued that the creation of face records holding information about the physical structure of known faces is intact, and that this is dependent on cortical areas 17, 18, and 19, which were largely preserved for their patients. However, in Tranel and Damasio's (1988) view the face records do not themselves contain any information about the identity of faces. Conscious recognition of identity requires activation of verbal and nonverbal non-face records, which would normally be achieved via the creation of an *amodal convergence zone* linking the face records to non-face records, and capable of 'locking in' to signs of co-occurrent activity in the different sties, and even reconstituting such activity. Disruption of this network of linkages is, in Tranel and Damasio's (1988) model, responsible for the lack of overt recognition and presence of covert recognition effects (mediated via the intact face records) found in prosopagnosia.

This certainly seems to be along the right lines, though I think there are two areas where clarification or slight modification is needed. First, I have argued here that evidence from matching, learning, interference, and associative priming tasks shows that there is covert processing of identity in prosopagnosia. Second, the findings of Bruyer *et al.* (1983), de Haan *et al.* (1987*a*, *b*, 1991), Young *et al.* (1988), Young and de Haan (1988), and Sergent and Poncet (1990) all imply that some multimodal associations are implicated in covert recognition, because in all these reports a salient characteristic of covert face recognition was its ability to interact with name processing. We therefore need to clarify which multimodal associations can and cannot be activated, and why.

Young and de Haan (1988) suggested that in covert recognition the face recognition system may have become disconnected from the cognitive system, but remain able to interact in limited ways with other input recognition systems. This is not inconsistent with Bauer's (1984) or Tranel and Damasio's (1985, 1988) proposals, but in its original formulation it suffered from the problem that Young and de Haan were not able to achieve a precise specification of the nature of the preserved interaction between input recognition systems.

This problem was eliminated in a computer simulation developed by Burton *et al.* (1991). The simulation is based on Burton *et al.*'s (1990) implementation of Bruce and Young's (1986) model of face recognition. The Burton *et al.* (1990) implementation uses a simple interactive activation architecture (cf. McClelland and Rumelhart 1981, 1988). Such models involve a number of distinct pools of units. All the units within a pool are connected to each other with inhibitory links. Units may be connected across pools by excitatory links.

Figure 11.2 shows the overall structure of the Burton *et al.* (1990) model. Following Bruce and Young (1986), Burton *et al.* proposed a number of pools of units corresponding to the following functional distinctions. Face recognition units (FRUs) are representations of the visual characteristics of a known person's face. These units receive input that is assumed to represent the output of visual processing by the perceptual system (structural encoding). Person identity nodes (PINs) are domain- and modality-free gateways into semantic information. They may be accessed through any input domain (face, name, voice, etc.), and provide access to information about that person, coded on semantic information units (SIUs). Name input units (NIUs) represent the same level of abstraction as FRUs, providing a route into the system for the names of known individuals.

Input to the model is made by increasing the activation of an FRU or NIU. The effect of this is that activation is passed along excitatory links

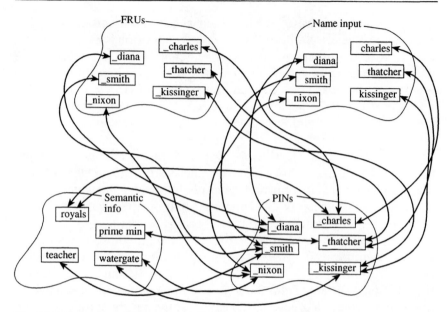

Fig. 11.2 Central architecture of Burton and co-workers' (1990) interactive activation model.

into different pools, thus increasing the activation levels of associated units. In all such models there is also a global decay function that forces units toward a resting activation. Hence, after input to the system, units tend to stabilize when the effect of input activation is balanced by the effect of decay.

In the Burton *et al.* (1990) model, familiarity decisions are taken at the PINs. An arbitrary threshold is set for the pool of PINs, and any unit that reaches the threshold level is taken to be recognized as familiar. Burton *et al.* showed that this conceptualization can simulate the properties of a number of effects in the literature on normal face recognition, including associative priming, repetition priming, and distinctiveness effects.

The mechanism by which associative priming takes place in the Burton *et al.* (1990) model is that after input to a particular FRU (say Prince Charles), the 'Prince Charles' PIN becomes active. As activation at this PIN rises, it in turn passes activation to the relevant SIUs (in this case, 'royal'). Now, as this semantic unit rises in activation, excitatory activation is passed back into the PIN pool, to the 'Princess Diana' PIN, which is connected to some of the same SIUs as the Charles PIN. The consequence of all this is that when the Charles FRU is made more active the Charles PIN will quickly rise above the threshold for a positive familiarity decision, and the Diana PIN will also rise, but stabilize below this threshold. However, on subsequent activation of the Diana FRU, the Diana PIN will quickly rise to threshold, because it is now above its resting level of activation. Hence associative priming effects are found.

It is important to note that in this model associative priming will take place across input domains. Because its mechanism lies in increased activation at the PIN level from the interaction of PINs and SIUs, subsequent input may come from any system that feeds into these PINs. So, for example, if a PIN has previously become active through presentation of a face, then subsequent presentation of a name will also be facilitated, because the appropriate PIN is already above resting activation.

To simulate the associative priming effects observed in PH, Burton *et al.* (1991) followed Young and de Haan (1988) in suggesting that PH's problem must affect the outputs of the FRUs. The functional impairment therefore seems to lie in the connection strengths between the pool of FRUs and the pool of PINs. Although some excitation is passed from an active FRU to its associated PIN, weak connection strengths mean that this activation is small compared to an intact system. The result of this is that the appropriate PIN is active, but below threshold. This activation at the PIN can be passed to the connected SIUs in the normal way, and hence to any associated PIN, though the levels of activation will be smaller. By halving the connection strengths between FRUs and corresponding PINs, Burton *et al.* (1991) were able to show that the system can still pass sufficient activation for associative priming from faces, even though these no longer raise the PINs above the recognition threshold.

This simulation shows that, if approached in the right way, covert recognition may be a more tractable problem than it at first appeared. Of course, there is no claim that a simple simulation of this type solves any of the more fundamental philosophical issues to do with the nature of awareness, but it does allow us to understand how a system that has lost one form of recognition ability can still show preserved priming and other effects.

Breakdown at different levels

One of the points I have already emphasized is that recognition can break down at different levels. This is also demonstrated by work we reported with patient NR (de Haan *et al.* 1992).

NR was unable to recognize familiar people by their faces in most tasks directly demanding recognition, whereas he remained able to recognize the same people by their names. Because of his severe impairment of overt face recognition, the forced-choice familiarity decision task was used as a stringent test for rudimentary overt face recognition abilities that might be missed by more conventional face recognition tasks. Unexpectedly, NR performed well above chance on this task (96 of 128 correct, $z = 5.57$, $p < 0.001$). His performance at choosing the familiar face was much better than the chance-level performance of PH or MS (see Table 11.4).

Exploration of covert recognition for NR mostly produced negative results. However, it was thought that the failure of most of the experiments involving indirect tests to reveal evidence of preserved recognition might be due to the fact that they did not include enough faces for which NR could show recognition in forced choice. This was confirmed in an experiment in which NR demonstrated priming from familiar faces that he had consistently chosen as familiar in all eight trials of a repeated forced-choice test (de Haan *et al.* 1992, experiment 7). A cross-domain self-priming task was used, in which a face prime was presented before a target name. The face could be that of the target ('same person' condition), a neutral (unfamiliar) prime, or an unrelated familiar person. NR's task was to classify the target name as familiar or unfamiliar. His reaction times to familiar target names are shown in Table 11.5, where it can be seen that there was facilitation of responses to the targets when they were preceded by the same person's face, provided it was one of the faces that NR consistently recognized as familiar in the forced-choice task. In contrast, no priming was observed from familiar faces that NR could not reliably discriminate from unfamiliar ones in forced choice (faces that were chosen as familiar four of eight times in the repeated forced-choice test).

NR showed some conscious realization that he chose certain faces consistently as familiar. As the forced-choice familiarity decision test

Table 11.5 Mean reaction times of NR's correct responses to target names (ms) preceded by same person, neutral, and unrelated face primes, (de Haan *et al.* 1992). Reaction times are subdivided according to whether the face primes were consistently recognized as familiar or not recognized in pretest sessions

	Same person	Neutral	Unrelated
Face primes consistently recognized as familiar in pretest	1852	2224	2190
Face primes not recognized in pretest	2273	2101	2250

was repeated more often, he became more sure of himself and commented on the fact that there 'was something with that face', but he was unable to elaborate on this. Although this was not true for all of he faces he recognized in forced-choice familiarity decision tests, and NR certainly did not seem to get any strong feelings of familiarity as such, it is sufficient to lead us to reject the idea that he was relying entirely on covert recognition abilities.

It may thus be better to think of NR's performance on forced-choice face familiarity decision tests as reflecting a very weak degree of overt recognition. Cheesman and Merikle (1985) pointed out with reference to the psychophysical literature that under near-threshold conditions there is a certain region where subjects still perform above chance level, although subjectively they feel they are doing little more than guessing. This may well be analogous to what happened for NR. There were some faces that yielded some form of rudimentary recognition in forced-choice conditions, and could support a degree of facilitation in priming tasks. However, these often remained below or barely above the threshold for overt recognition, leaving NR unable to comment adequately on the choices he was making.

In contrast to PH, NR was above chance at forced-choice recognition of face familiarity (though he was obviously still severely impaired at the task), and only showed priming from faces he could consistently recognize as familiar in forced choice. His consistent performance to certain items on the forced-choice familiarity decision test indicated that NR's deficit might well be better conceptualized as a storage than as an access problem (Shallice 1987, 1988).

De Haan et al. (1992) suggested that NR had suffered degradation of face recognition units. Some of the stored face representations had been completely wiped out at this (face recognition unit) level, and there would be no preserved recognition of these faces. Other representations were sufficiently preserved that they could be recognized as familiar when the choice was between that face and an unfamiliar face, and they could support priming effects.

Clearly, this functional explanation is different from those we have offered for other patients with prosopagnosia we have investigated. We proposed that PH's consistent pattern of preserved recognition of familiar faces on most indirect tests reflected damage to the outputs of otherwise intact face recognition units (Young and de Haan 1988). For MS, we proposed that the consistent absence of preserved recognition of familiar faces reflected higher order perceptual impairment (Newcombe et al. 1989), which would mean that there could be no effective input to face recognition units.

The implication is that there is an underlying hierarchy of possible loci of impairment. In terms of this hierarchy, MS's impairment was centered on a relatively early stage in the system, PH's was relatively late, and NR's lay between. Patterns of preserved and impaired abilities found in cases of prosopagnosia may be complex, but they are not random, and the use of functional models and appropriate experimental techniques has the potential to reveal the underlying order.

Other authors have also advanced similar proposals on the basis of recent work. Etcoff *et al.* (1991) and McNeil and Warrington (1991) both noted that the full range of findings on presence or absence of covert recognition cannot be accounted for simply by proposing that patients who do not show covert recognition have impaired perception; Etcoff *et al.*'s patient did not show covert recognition despite having many well preserved perceptual abilities, and McNeil and Warrington found evidence of less intact perception for their cases with covert recognition. Both Etcoff *et al.* and McNeil and Warrington concluded that brain injury can selectively eliminate stored information about the appearance of familiar faces; in Bruce and Young's (1986) terms this would be equivalent to loss of the face recognition units.

Impairments affecting awareness can also be found at other levels of recognition. One example comes from our work with BD, a post-encephalitic patient who was poor at recognizing people from face, name, or voice. This is a pattern quite unlike prosopagnosia, pointing to a much more 'central' impairment. Yet BD showed evidence of pre-served recognition abilities in learning tasks (Hanley *et al.* 1989).

Even more striking are findings of unawareness of impaired recognition. Young *et al.* (1990) reported the case of a woman with severe and stable face processing impairments, SP, who showed complete lack of insight into her face recognition difficulties. SP was very poor at recognizing familiar faces, yet she was not distressed by this, and maintained that she recognized faces 'as well as before'. She said that she had no problems in recognizing faces in everyday life, in paintings, on the television, in newspapers or magazines, whereas formal testing showed that all of these must have been highly problematic. Even when directly confronted with her failure to recognize photographs of familiar faces, SP could only offer the suggestion that the photograph was a 'poor likeness', or that she had 'no recollection of having seen that person before'.

In contrast to her lack of insight into her face recognition impairment, SP showed adequate insight into other physical and cognitive im-pairments produced by her illness, including poor memory, hemiplegia, and hemianopia. Her lack of insight into her face recognition impairment involved a *deficit-specific anosognosia*. We think that such deficit-specific anosognosias reflect impairment to mechanisms we need in order to monitor our own performance in everyday life (Young *et al.* 1990).

Provoking overt recognition

When we first began working with PH, he seemed to us to be completely unable to achieve overt recognition of familiar faces. De Haan *et al.* (1987*a*) noted that of the hundreds of famous faces they had shown him, only one (Mrs Thatcher) had been spontaneously recognized, and that on only one occasion.

Since then, we have also noted other occasions on which PH has overtly recognized a face during the past few years. There are about a dozen faces he has recognized occasionally, but the only face we have noticed is beginning to be fairly consistently recognized is Mrs Thatcher's (Young and de Haan 1992). It will be interesting to see whether or not her fall from power reverses this trend.

The fact that some faces have been overtly recognized on rare occasions is important, because it indicates that PH's problem cannot be an absolute deficit. If we think of it in terms of impaired links between FRUs and PINs, it makes more sense to see the problem as involving weakened connection strengths (Burton *et al.* 1991) than as a complete disconnection.

The importance of this becomes clear in an extraordinary finding of Sergent and Poncet's (1990) study. They observed that PV could achieve overt recognition of some faces if several members of the same semantic category were presented together. This only happened when PV could determine the category herself. For the categories PV could not determine, she continued to fail to recognize the faces overtly even when the occupational category was pointed out to her. When the same faces were later presented one at a time in random order, PV was again unable to recognize any of them, including those she had recognized when they were placed in appropriate category groupings.

We have been able to replicate this phenomenon of overt recognition provoked by presentation of multiple exemplars of a semantic category with PH (de Haan *et al.* 1991). Table 11.6 shows data from a task in which PH was asked to recognize faces from three broadly defined semantic categories (politicians, television presenters, and comedians) and three narrowly defined categories (the television soap operas 'Neighbours', 'Eastenders', and 'Coronation Street'). There were eight faces from each category. It can be seen that there was a marked

Table 11.6 Number (max. = 8) of correct (+) and incorrect (−) overt identifications by PH in the different conditions of a category presentation task (de Haan *et al.* 1991) involving a pretest with the faces in pseudo-random order, simultaneous presentation of all eight faces from a particular category, and an immediate post-test and delayed post-test (after a two-month interval) with pseudorandom ordering

| | Pretest | | Category presentation | | Post-test | | | |
| | | | | | Immediate | | Delayed | |
	+	−	+	−	+	−	+	−
Broad categories								
Politicians	0	0	0	0	0	0	0	0
TV presenters	0	0	0	0	0	4	0	1
Comedians	2	2	1	0	2	2	1	0
Narrow categories								
'Neighbours'	0	0	1	0	1	0	0	0
'Eastenders'	1	0	6	0	5	0	1	0
'Coronation St'	0	0	1	0	1	1	0	0

improvement in his ability to recognize the 'Eastenders' faces when these were all presented simultaneously (the 'category presentation' condition). There is no reason to think PH was guessing these or deducing them from cues such as age and hairstyle, because there were no misidentifications of the faces in this category. Note also that (in contrast to Sergent and Poncet's 1990 findings) the improvement in overt recognition of these faces transferred to an immediate post-test with the faces presented one at a time in pseudorandom order. The improvement did, though, dissipate across a two-month interval (delayed post-test).

Sergent and Poncet (1990) offered a very similar account to the Burton *et al.* (1991) simulation, suggesting that their demonstration shows that 'neither the facial representations nor the semantic information were critically disturbed in PV, and her prosopagnosia may thus reflect faulty connections between faces and their memories' (p. 1000). They hypo-thesized that the simultaneous presentation of several members of the same category may have temporarily raised the activation level above the appropriate threshold.

The disruption of overt face recognition in prosopagnosia is usually so complete that findings of covert recognition have been a considerable surprise. One cannot fail to be even more impressed by the finding that overt recognition can be provoked under certain conditions, at least for some patients (and some faces). This offers the hope that, given sufficient ingenuity, we may be able to find ways to help at least some of the people who suffer these very disabling conditions. Of course, any effective remedial technique based on such procedures is still a long way off, and will depend on knowing much more about the conditions under which overt recognition cam be provoked and, above all, maintained. But the initial finding is more promising than anything that has emerged from conventional training procedures (e.g. Ellis and Young 1988).

Overview

Work on covert recognition has come a long way in the past few years, from studies that simply demonstrate the existence of these phenomena after brain injury, to investigations intended to probe much more analytically into their nature. It has become clear that awareness of recognition can break down in a number of different ways after brain injury, but that there is an underlying order to these forms of impairment. The challenge for the future is to achieve well specified models that can bring together these observations into a unified theory, and to explore their implications for remediation.

The phenomena of covert recognition present an intriguing challenge to our conceptions of awareness. In particular, they make it hard to accept the commonly held view that the same processes underlie visual analysis and awareness. Were this so, impairments involving the loss of awareness of a particular perceptual quality would always involve the loss of all ability to respond to that quality, regardless of the test used. Studies of covert processing show that this is far from the case.

Pressing this point further, we can see that the existence of covert processing of visual stimuli after brain injury forces up to stop thinking of visual experience as epiphenomenal. Instead, it highlights questions about the purpose of awareness, and what it allows us to do that we could not otherwise achieve. A promising idea is that we need to be aware of something in order to form a judgement or belief about it, and that awareness is indispensable to creatures capable of genuine judgement and belief (Lowe 1992). Certainly, people like PH find that their inability to achieve overt recognition of most familiar faces is socially disabling; in everyday life they act as if they do not recognize people from their faces, despite the extensive covert recognition effects we have demonstrated.

Teuber (1968) likened the concept of agnosia to that of a 'normal percept stripped of its meaning'. However, as Bauer (1984) pointed out, findings of covert recognition show that in some cases the percept has only lost certain aspects of its meaning. These missing aspects are those that are crucial to intentional action.

What are preserved in brain-injured people who show covert recognition are automatic aspects of recognition whose functions include preparing the recognition system for what it is likely to encounter next (Young and de Haan 1988), orientation to stimuli with motivational significance, and arousal responses that set a background emotional tone for any social interaction (Bauer 1984). Thus covert recognition may well exert subtle influences on behaviour, but at the level of intentional actions, the consequences of the failure of overt recognition are overwhelmingly evident. Awareness of recognition is no pointless luxury.

References

Bauer, R. M. (1984). Autonomic recognition of names and faces in prosopagnosia: a neuropsychological application of the guilty knowledge test. *Neuropsychologia*, **22**, 457–69.

Bauer, R. M. (1986). The cognitive psychophysiology of prosopagnosia. In *Aspects of face processing*, (ed. H. D. Ellis, M. A. Jeeves, F. Newcombe, and A. Young), pp. 253–67. Martinus Nijhoff, Dordrecht, Netherlands.

Bauer, R. M. and Verfaellie, M. (1988). Electrodermal discrimination of familiar but not unfamiliar faces in prosopagnosia. *Brain and Cognition*, **8**, 240–52.

Benton, A. L. (1990). Facial recognition 1990. *Cortex*, **26**, 491–9.

Bodamer, J. (1947). Die Prosop-Agnosie. *Archiv für Psychiatrie und Nervenkrankheiten*, **179**, 6–53.

Bruce, V. and Valentine, T. (1986). Semantic priming of familiar faces. *Quarterly Journal of Experimental Psychology*, **38A**, 125–50.

Bruce, V. and Young, A. (1986). Understanding face recognition. *British Journal of Psychology*, **77**, 305–27.

Bruyer, R., Laterre, C., Seron, X., Feyereisen, P., Strypstein, E., Pierrard, E., and Rectem, D. (1983). A case of prosopagnosia with some preserved covert remembrance of familiar faces. *Brain and Cognition*, **2**, 257–84.

Burton, A. M., Bruce, V., and Johnston, R. A. (1990). Understanding face recognition with an interactive activation model. *British Journal of Psychology*, **81**, 361–80.

Burton, A. M., Young, A. W., Bruce, V., Johnston, R. A., and Ellis, A. W. (1991). Understanding covert recognition. *Cognition*, **39**, 129–66.

Carr, T. H., McCauley, C., Sperber, R. D., and Parmelee, C. M. (1982). Words, pictures, and priming: on semantic activation, conscious identification, and the automaticity of information processing. *Journal of Experimental Psychology: Human Perception and Performance*, **8**, 757–77.

Cheesman, J. and Merikle, P. M. (985). Word recognition and consciousness. In *Reading research: advances in theory and practice*, (ed. D. Besner, T. G. Waller, and G. E. Mackinnon), Vol. 5, pp. 311-52. Academic, New York.

Coslett, H. B. and Saffran, E. M. (1989). Evidence for preserved reading in 'pure alexia'. *Brain*, **112**, 327–59.

Damasio, A. R., Damasio, H., and Van Hoesen, G. W. (1982). Prosopagnosia: anatomic basis and behavioral mechanisms. *Neurology*, **32**, 331–41.

Damasio, A. R., Tranel, D., and Damasio, H. (1990). Face agnosia and the neural substrates of memory. *Annual Review of Neuroscience*, **13**, 89–109.

de Haan, E. H. F., Young, A., and Newcombe, F. (1987*a*). Face recognition without awareness. *Cognitive Neuropsychology*, **4**, 385–415.

de Haan, E. H. F., Young, A., and Newcombe, F. (1987*b*). Faces interfere with name classification in a prosopagnosic patient. *Cortex*, **23**, 309–16.

de Haan, E. H. F., Young, A. W., and Newcombe, F. (1991). Covert and overt recognition in prosopagnosia. *Brain*, **114**, 2575–91.

de Haan, E. H. F., Young, A. W., and Newcombe, F. (1992). Neuro-psychological impairment of face recognition units. *Quarterly Journal of Experimental Psychology*, **44A**, 141–75.

De Renzi, E. (1986*a*). Prosopagnosia in two patients with CT scan evidence of damage confined to the right hemisphere. *Neuropsychologia*, **24**, 385–9.

De Renzi, E. (1986*b*). Current issues in prosopagnosia. In *Aspects of face processing*, (ed. H. D. Ellis, M. A. Jeeves, F. Newcombe, and A. Young), pp. 243–52. Martinus Nijhoff, Dordrecht, Netherlands.

Ellis, H. D. and Young, A. W. (1988). Training in face-processing skills for a child with acquired prosopagnosia. *Developmental Neuropsychology*, **4**, 283–94.

Ellis, H. D. and Young, A. W. (1990). Accounting for delusional mis-identifications. *British Journal of Psychiatry*, **157**, 239–48.

Etcoff, N. L., Freeman, R., and Cave, K. R. (1991). Can we lose memories of faces? Content specificity and awareness in a prosopagnosic. *Journal of Cognitive Neuroscience*, **3**, 25–41.

Farah, M. J. (1990). *Visual agnosia: disorders of object recognition and what they tell us about normal vision*. MIT Press, Cambridge, MA.

Fodor, J. (1983). *The modularity of mind*. MIT Press, Cambridge, MA.

Greve, K. W. and Bauer, R. M. (1990). Implicit learning of new faces in proso-pagnosia: an application of the mere-exposure paradigm. *Neuropsychologia*, **28**, 1035–41.

Hanley, J. R., Young, A. W., and Pearson, N. (1989). Defective recognition of familiar people. *Cognitive Neuropsychology*, **6**, 179–210.

Hanley, J. R., Pearson, N., and Young, A. W. (1990). Impaired memory for new visual forms. *Brain*, **113**, 1131–48.

Hay, D. C., Young, A. W., and Ellis, A. W. (1991). Routes through the face recognition system. *Quarterly Journal of Experimental Psychology*, **43A**, 761–91.

Hécaen, H. and Angelergues, R. (1962). Agnosia for faces (prosopagnosia). *Archives of Neurology*, **7**, 92–100.

Humphreys, G. W. (1981). Direct vs. indirect tests of the information available from masked displays: what visual masking does and does not prevent. *British Journal of Psychology*, **72**, 323–30.

Humphreys, G. W., Troscianko, T., Riddoch, M. J., Boucart, M., Donnelly, N., and Harding, G. F. A. (1992). Covert processing in different visual recognition systems. In *The neuropsychology of consciousness*, (ed. A. D. Milner and M. D. Rugg), pp. 39–68. Academic, London.

Landis, T., Cummings, J. L., Christen, L., Bogen, J. E., and Imhof, H.-G. (1986). Are unilateral right posterior cerebral lesions sufficient to cause prosopagnosia? Clinical and radiological findings in six additional patients. *Cortex*, **22**, 243–52.

Lowe, E. J. (1992). Experience and its objects. In *The contents of experience*, (ed. T. Crane). Cambridge University Press.

McCauley, C., Parmelee, C., Sperber, R., and Carr, T. (1980). Early extraction of meaning from pictures and its relation to conscious identification. *Journal of Experimental Psychology: Human Perception and Performance*, **6**, 265–76.

McClelland, J. L. and Rumelhart, D. E. (1981). An interactive activation model of the effect of context in perception, Part 1. An account of basic findings. *Psychological Review*, **88**, 375–406.

McClelland, J. L. and Rumelhart, D. E. (1988). *Explorations in parallel distributed processing*. Bradford, Cambridge, MA.

McNeil, J. E. and Warrington, E. K. (1991). Prosopagnosia: a reclassification. *Quarterly Journal of Experimental Psychology*, **43A**, 267–87.

McNicol, D. (1972). *A primer of signal detection theory*. George Allen & Unwin, London.

Marshall, J. C. and Halligan, P. W. (1988). Blindsight and insight in visuo-spatial neglect. *Nature*, **336**, 766–7.

Meadows, J. C. (1974). The anatomical basis of prosopagnosia. *Journal of Neurology, Neurosurgery, and Psychiatry*, **37**, 489–501.

Nebes, R. D., Martin, D. C., and Horn, L. C. (1984). Sparing of semantic memory in Alzheimer's disease. *Journal of Abnormal Psychology*, **93**, 321–30.

Newcombe, F., Young, A. W., and de Haan, E. H. F. (1989). Prosopagnosia and object agnosia without covert recognition. *Neuropsychologia*, **27**, 179–91.

Pöppel, E., Held, R., and Frost, D. (1973). Residual visual function after brain wounds involving the central visual pathways in man. *Nature*, **243**, 295–6.

Posner, M. I. and Snyder, C. R. R. (1975). Facilitation and inhibition in the processing of signals. In *Attention and performance*, (ed. P. M. A. Rabbitt and S. Dornic), pp. 669–82. Academic, London.

Reingold, E. M. and Merikle, P. M. (1988). Using direct and indirect measures to study perception without awareness. *Perception and Psychophysics*, **44**, 63–75.

Reingold, E. M. and Merikle, P. M. (1990). On the inter-relatedness of theory and measurement in the study of unconscious processing. *Mind and Language*, **5**, 9–28.

Renault, B., Signoret, J. L., Debruille, B., Breton, F., and Bolgert, F. (1989). Brain potentials reveal covert facial recognition in prosopagnosia. *Neuropsychologia*, **27**, 905–12.

Rizzo, M., Hurtig, R., and Damasio, A. R. (1987). The role of scanpaths in facial recognition and learning. *Annals of Neurology*, **22**, 41–5.

Ross, E. D. (1980). Sensory-specific and fractional disorders of recent memory in man, 1. Isolated loss of visual recent memory. *Archives of Neurology*, **37**, 193–200.

Schacter, D. L. (1987). Implicit memory: history and current status. *Journal of Experimental Psychology: Learning, Memory and Cognition*, **13**, 501–18.

Schacter, D. L., McAndrews, M. P., and Moscovitch, M. (1988). Access to consciousness: dissociations between implicit and explicit knowledge in neuropsychological syndromes. In *Thought without language*, (ed. L. Weiskrantz), pp. 242–78. Oxford University Press.

Sergent, J. and Poncet, M. (1990). From covert to overt recognition of faces in a prosopagnosic patient. *Brain*, **113**, 989–1004.

Sergent, J. and Villemure, J.-G. (1989). Prosopagnosia in a right hemispherectomized patient. *Brain*, **112**, 975–95.

Shallice, T. (1987). Impairments of semantic processing: multiple dissociations. In *The cognitive neuropsychology of language*, (ed. M. Coltheart, G. Sartori, and R. Job), pp. 111–27. Lawrence Erlbaum Associates, London.

Shallice, T. (1988). Specialisation within the semantic system. *Cognitive Neuropsychology*, **5**, 133–42.

Shallice, T. and Saffran, E. (1986). Lexical processing in the absence of explicit word identification: evidence from a letter-by-letter reader. *Cognitive Neuropsychology*, **3**, 429–58.

Teuber, H.-L. (1968). Alteration of perception and memory in man. In *Analysis of behavioral change*, (ed. L. Weiskrantz). Harper & Row, New York.

Tranel, D. and Damasio, A. R. (1985). Knowledge without awareness: an autonomic index of facial recognition by prosopagnosics. *Science*, **228**, 1453–4.

Tranel, D. and Damasio, A. R. (1988). Non-conscious face recognition in patients with face agnosia. *Behavioural Brain Research*, **30**, 235–49.

van Zomeren, A. H. and Deelman, B. G. (1978). Long-term recovery of visual reaction time after closed head injury. *Journal of Neurology, Neurosurgery, and Psychiatry*, **41**, 452–7.

Volpe, B. T., Ledoux, J. E., and Gazzaniga, M. S. (1979). Information processing of visual stimuli in an 'extinguished' field. *Nature*, **282**, 722–4.

Warrington, E. K. and Weiskrantz, L. (1968). New method of testing long-term retention with special reference to amnesic patients. *Nature*, **217**, 972–4.

Warrington, E. K. and Weiskrantz, L. (1970). Amnesia: consolidation or retrieval? *Nature*, **228**, 628–30.

Weiskrantz, L. (1986). *Blindsight: a case study and implications*. Oxford University Press.

Weiskrantz, L., Warrington, E. K., Sanders, M. D., and Marshall, J. (1974). Visual capacity in the hemianopic field following a restricted occipital ablation. *Brain*, **97**, 709–28.

Young, A. W. (1988). Functional organization of visual recognition. In *Thought without language*, (ed. L. Weiskrantz), pp. 78–107. Oxford University Press.

Young, A. W. and de Haan, E. H. F. (1988). Boundaries of covert recognition in prosopagnosia. *Cognitive Neuropsychology*, **5**, 317–36.

Young, A. W. and de Haan, E. H. F. (1990). Impairments of visual awareness. *Mind and Language*, **5**, 29–48.

Young, A. W. and de Haan, E. H. F. (1992). Face recognition and awareness after brain injury. In *The neuropsychology of consciousness*, (ed. A. D. Milner and M. D. Rugg), pp. 69–90. Academic, London.

Young, A. W. and Ellis, H. D. (1989). Childhood prosopagnosia. *Brain and Cognition*, **9**, 16–47.

Young, A. W., Hay, D. C., and Ellis, A. W. (1985). The faces that launched a thousand slips: everyday difficulties and errors in recognizing people. *British Journal of Psychology*, **76**, 495–523.

Young, A. W., Ellis, A. W., Flude, B. M., McWeeny, K. H., and Hay, D. C. (1986). Face–name interference. *Journal of Experimental Psychology: Human Perception and Performance*, **12**, 466–75.

Young, A. W., Hellawell, D., and de Haan, E. H. F. (1988). Cross-domain semantic priming in normal subjects and a prosopagnosic patient. *Quarterly Journal of Experimental Psychology*, **40A**, 561–80.

Young, A. W., Newcombe, F., Hellawell, D., and de Haan, E. H. F. (1989). Implicit access to semantic information. *Brain and Cognition*, **11**, 186–209.

Young, A. W., de Haan, E. H. F., and Newcombe, F. (1990). Unawareness of impaired face recognition. *Brain and Cognition*, **14**, 1–18.

Zajonc, R. B. (1980). Feeling and thinking: preferences need no inferences. *American Psychologist*, **35**, 151–75.

12

Covert face recognition without prosopagnosia

Reprinted in slightly modified form from Ellis, H. D., Young, A. W., and Koenken, G. (1993), Covert face recognition without prosopagnosia, *Behavioural Neurology*, **6**, 27–32. With kind permission of co-authors and Professor H. Sagar (Editor, *Behavioural Neurology*).

Summary

An experiment is reported where subjects were presented with familiar or unfamiliar faces for supraliminal durations or for durations individually assessed as being below the threshold for recognition. Their electrodermal responses to each stimulus were measured and the results showed higher peak amplitude skin conductance responses for familiar than for unfamiliar faces, regardless of whether they had been displayed supraliminally or subliminally. A parallel is drawn between elevated skin conductance responses to subliminal stimuli and findings of covert recognition of familiar faces in prosopagnosic patients, some of whom show increased electrodermal activity to previously familiar faces. The supraliminal presentation data also served to replicate similar work by Tranel *et al.* (1985). The results are considered alongside other data indicating the relation between non-conscious, 'automatic' aspects of normal visual information processing and abilities which can be found to be preserved without awareness after brain injury.

Introduction

In recent years there has been much research into the way faces are recognized (see Bruce 1988; Young and Ellis 1989), some of which has centred upon the study of prosopagnosic patients who, by definition, are profoundly unable to recognize previously familiar faces. Instead these patients rely on voice, gait, or clothing to identify people (Bodamer 1947; Ellis and Florence 1991). The reports of prosopagnosic patients include a variety of associated symptoms that imply that there are different types displaying different symptoms. Hécaen (1981) suggested that there were two basic sorts of prosopagnosia; apperceptive (involving distorted or degraded visual input), and mnestic (where there is little or no perceptual problem but a failure to associate the face to stored representations). Damasio et al. (1990) also identify a third subtype which they call 'amnestic' associative prosopagnosia which involves an inability to identify face or voice. They also locate the anatomy of the three types of prosopagnosia. The specificity of the face recognition impairment is apparent from the analysis by Sergent and Signoret (1992a) of a patient, RM, who has obvious perceptual difficulties when viewing faces yet shows an outstanding ability to make fine distinctions among pictures of similar cars.

Bauer (1984) made a remarkable discovery when he found that his prosopagnosic patient LF, with bilateral inferomedial temporal damage following a motorcycle accident, was able to make autonomic discriminations between correct combinations of familiar faces and names compared with incorrect face/name pairings, even though he could not consciously choose which were the correct pairings. Tranel and Damasio (1985) confirmed Bauer's findings by demonstrating that prosopagnosic patients displayed larger skin conductance responses (SCRs) to familiar compared with unfamiliar faces presented in a random sequence. De Haan et al. (1987) and Young et al. (1988) then extended these observations by using behavioural techniques to reveal covert responses to familiar faces in PH, another motorcycle accident victim with posterior cerebral lesions. For example, PH displayed greater ability to learn correct face/name combinations than incorrect ones. Like normal controls, he was faster at deciding whether two photographs were of the same or different people when they were famous; and he showed an associative priming effect such that, for him, preceding a famous name by the face of a professional partner conferred the same latency advantage for declaring the name 'familiar' as that caused by preceding the name by the partner's name. Sergent and Signoret (1992b) have discovered that such implicit access to information about previously known but now unrecognized faces only occurs in prosopagnosic patients without severe perceptual deficits.

The fact that some prosopagnosic patients have displayed covert responses to faces has a number of theoretical ramifications. The one we wish to explore here is the possibility that neurologically intact subjects may also reveal increases in electrodermal activity to familiar faces presented at a level below that which normally produces overt awareness of recognition. This is an important experimental study, not least because the results may help clarify any role of unconscious processing in face recognition; and, in doing so, make us more confident when drawing lessons from studies of prosopagnosic patients for developing a general theory of face recognition.

A similar reasoning led Tranel *et al.* (1985) to examine electrodermal activity in neurologically intact subjects shown, supraliminally, a series of 50 faces, each for 2 s. Eight of the faces were famous (e.g. Ronald Reagan, Bob Hope) and 42 were unknown. Tranel *et al.* found that the famous faces produced larger SCRs than did the unfamiliar ones. The famous faces were rated by other subjects as being more significant than the other faces, which suggested that this significance factor provides signal value to the stimulus face which is reflected in the orienting response as measured by increased autonomic activity.

There is, of course, an obvious difference between the paradigm used by Tranel *et al.* and those used when studying covert recognition by prosopagnosic patients; the latter are not consciously aware that they have been presented with the face of a familiar person. The question then remains as to whether similar autonomic discriminations may be elicited from normal subjects who are shown faces under conditions designed to prevent conscious recognition.

The issue of subliminal perception has a long history and yet still no universally accepted solution. Numerous efforts were made immediately post-war to demonstrate its existence but all too often studies were methodologically flawed. Eventually, in an influential paper. Eriksen (1960) concluded that 'At present there is no convincing evidence that the human organism can discriminate or differentially respond to external stimuli that are at an intensity level too low to elicit a discriminated verbal report' (p. 298). This conclusion from 30 years ago may be seen to be at variance with the subsequent work on covert recognition in prosopagnosics (and, indeed, that on implicit memory in amnesics, e.g. Schacter *et al.* 1988).

A more recent theoretical analysis of subliminal perception by Marcel (1983*a*), however, may be viewed as much more sympathetic. Marcel (1983*b*) had revealed the operation of subliminally presented words upon subsequent word recognition (i.e. priming). On the basis of these and other findings, he was prepared to reject what he termed the 'identity assumption', namely that conscious and non-conscious representations of the same thing are identical. Marcel's position is not universally shared, owing largely to problems in defining thresholds and, therefore, ensuring that subjects do not have at least some opportunity consciously to perceive stimuli intended by the experimenter to be subliminal (see Holender 1986; Cheesman and Merikle 1985).

None the less, the present authors, while mindful of the various methodological pitfalls, were concerned to link work on covert recognition in prosopagnosic patients with face processing by normal subjects. The most direct way to begin to do this, it was felt, would be to investigate autonomic orienting responses to familiar faces presented at a level designed to be subliminal. At the same time it was also considered that the findings of Tranel *et al.* (1985), using supraliminal presentation of familiar and unfamiliar faces, needed to be replicated. So in the following experiment subjects were presented with faces of famous and unknown people at both subliminal and supraliminal levels. For each type of face, SCRs were measured across the palm of the hand.

It is important to note that, when we refer here to faces as being supraliminal or subliminal, this is with respect to the *recognition threshold*. Our interest is in autonomic responses to faces presented for durations too brief to allow them to be recognized. We do not, though, seek to claim that these faces were presented for durations sufficiently brief to prevent their being detected. On some trials subjects may well have known that a face was presented; the important point is that they did not consciously know *whose* face it was. Nor, did it seem, were they able to gain any sense of familiarity from the faces shown on these trials.

This use of the terms supraliminal and subliminal with respect to the recognition threshold is, we believe, appropriate in the present context for two reasons. First, the literature on 'unconscious' priming *does* show consistent effects when the threshold is defined in this way (e.g. McCauley *et al.* 1980). Second, it represents the correct analogue or comparison to prosopagnosia. Prosopagnosic patients know when they are looking at a face, what they no longer know is whose face it is. We sought to create a comparable state in normal people using both brief presentation and pattern masking. This does not mean, of course, that we believe that prosopagnosics experience faces phenomenologically as do normals looking at briefly presented faces that are masked. But instead we wished to explore the possible analogy between the two processes as manifested by changes in the level of autonomic activity.

A similar rationale was provided by Meeres and Graves (1990), who used a paradigm adopted from work with blindsight patients. They found that subjects with normal vision could judge better than chance the location of a circle stimulus followed by a pattern mask even when they reported not having seen it. Meeres and Graves argue that their data may reveal in normal subjects a dissociation between pattern localization and conscious awareness that has the same physiological basis as that involved in blindsight. In the following experiment this is explored using faces as stimuli and skin conductance levels as responses.

Methods

Selection of stimulus slides

From a pool of more than 1000 slides of familiar and unknown faces, all taken from the same source and therefore of uniform quality, 100 slides (50 probably familiar and 50 probably unknown faces) were selected. The familiarity of these faces was then judged by a group of 13 German students on a 6 point scale (0 = completely unknown; 6 = completely familiar). Based on the results of these ratings, the 30 slides with the highest familiarity ratings and the 20 slides with the lowest familiarity ratings were finally selected as stimulus material and partitioned into five series of 10 slides each (three sets of 10 familiar faces, and two sets of 10 unfamiliar faces). These sets were balanced for gender and for the range of professions of the familiar people (i.e. actor, singer, politician). The mean familiarity ratings for the three series of familiar faces were 5.42, 5.49, and 5.52, respectively. For the two sets of unknown faces the ratings were 0.97 and 0.96.

One of the slide series with familiar faces was later used to determine the individual recognition threshold of each subject. The remaining sets of 10 familiar and 10 unknown faces were mixed, which resulted in two series with 20 slides. The sequence of slides within each series was determined at random. Thus there were three series of slides:

(1) series A with 10 slides of familiar faces to determine the individual recognition threshold of each subject;
(2) series B with 20 slides (10 familiar and 10 unknown) for supra-threshold presentation, randomized for each subject;
(3) series C with 20 slides (10 familiar and 10 unknown) for sub-threshold presentation, randomized for each subject.

Four additional slides were used as buffer items which preceded each series of stimulus slides.

Subjects

Twenty-six psychology students aged between 19 and 24 years, from Christian-Albrechts Universität, Kiel, acted as subjects. They were paid for their participation. The first two subjects served as test and training subjects and were discarded from further data analysis. Thus, the final sample consisted of 24 subjects, each of whom was tested individually.

Experimental situation

The subject was seated on a reclining chair in a darkened and sound-proofed laboratory. A screen was placed at a distance of 2 m. The slides were protected from an adjacent room through a window, which meant that any noise produced by the slide projectors could not be heard in the subject's room. Except for the initial information, all instructions were communicated to the subject through an intercom system.

Instructions

All subjects first received general information regarding the experimental procedure (i.e. determination of recognition threshold, supra-liminal and subliminal presentation of slides with familiar and unknown faces). They were told that the goal of the study was the analysis of impressions which were produced by the photographs, and that they would be shown 50 slides with familiar and unknown faces. Some of the slides, they were told, would be presented very briefly, while some others would be shown for a longer duration. Their task, it was explained, would be to judge whether the photograph (not the face of the person) appeared pleasant or unpleasant. This judgement should be made exclusively on the basis of the photograph and not be influenced by the person. The pleasantness judgement should be indicated by lifting the middle finger. This would trigger a light sensitive receiver and be recorded by the computer.

During this explanation, two electrodes for the registration of the SCR were connected to the palm of the hand.

Presentation of stimuli

The projection of the slides was controlled by a computer (Data General Eclipse). One projector presented the stimulus side for a pre-determined time. After an interval of 2 ms a second projector displayed a mask slide containing random facial features on to the same place on the screen for 1 s.

Procedure

The experiment involved three phases. During the first phase the individual recognition threshold was determined. In the second phase, for half of the subjects the slides were presented subliminally; for the remaining half they were shown supraliminally. In the third phase, those subjects who had been shown the subliminal slides were now presented another set of slides supraliminally; and those who had received the supraliminal faces first were now shown the subliminal set. These phases were separated by pauses of 1 min.

Determination of recognition threshold

For each subject the recognition threshold was determined individually by the method of ascending limits. Ten slides with highly familiar faces were used for this task. Each slide was presented at an initial exposure duration of 40 ms, followed almost immediately (after 2 ms) by the mask slide. After a pause of 6.5 s either the same or the next slide was presented, depending on the subject's response. The projection duration was increased in steps of 10 ms until the subject indicated by lifting the index finger that s/he had recognized the person. The name of the person was communicated by the subject via the intercom system. After this response, the computer switched to the next slide. The maximum number of presentations of the same slide was 10. Thus, the final possible projection duration was 130 ms. If the person had not been recognized after the tenth presentation of the slide, the next slide was presented, again starting with a duration of 40 ms.

The individual recognition threshold was defined as the *shortest* exposure duration at which the subject was able to give the name (or some equivalent such as providing unambiguous biographical information) of *any* person correctly.

Our reason for using only ascending series to determine each person's recognition threshold was that we were concerned to ensure that we were measuring the threshold for recognition when subjects did not know which faces to expect (as would be the case in the main series of trials). However, the use of an ascending series can overestimate thresholds if subjects are not always willing to 'guess' at the face's identity, and hold back for a few trials to gain confidence. For this reason, we both encouraged our subjects to guess and used the very conservative procedure of defining the threshold as the shortest duration at which any of the faces was identified correctly. In addition the effectiveness of this procedure was determined in a separate test with seven subjects who were presented faces subliminally (using the same method of calculating individual recognition thresholds). A reward was promised for each correct recognition response. Each subject saw 10 faces of familiar people. Thus, a total of 70 test responses were recorded (seven subjects with 10 slides each). Of those 70 responses, only four were correct recognitions. These correct responses were given to four different slides. We are therefore content to assert that the overwhelming majority of faces presented subliminally in the main experiment could not be identified.

Subliminal presentation

Subliminal presentation was defined as a projection duration which was 10 ms shorter than the shortest threshold for recognizing one of the faces, that is, if a subject gave correct recognition response to slides at projection durations of 70 ms, 60 ms, and 90 ms, the individual recognition threshold was defined as 60 ms and the subliminal projection duration would then be 50 ms.

For the experiment itself, two buffer slides were initially presented, one with a familiar and one with an unknown face. Following these buffer slides the first series of slides was presented (10 familiar faces, and 10 unfamiliar faces, in random order). Almost immediately (2 ms) after the projection of each slide, a mask slide was projected on to the same spot on the screen for 1 s. This was followed by a constant interstimulus interval of 10 s during which skin conductance was recorded.

Supraliminal presentation

Following threshold determination, for half the subjects there was a presentation of subliminal slides, and a pause of 1 min was then inserted. Following this pause, two buffer slides and the 20 slides for the supraliminal projection were presented (10 familiar faces, and 10 unfamiliar faces, in random order). Each slide was presented for 220 ms, again followed by the mask and a pause of 10 s while electrodermal activity (EDA) was recorded. For the other half of the subjects, the subliminal followed the supraliminal presentation condition.

Recording and processing of electrodermal activity

The SCR was registered by two Ag/AgCl 0.7 cm electrodes coated with Beckman electrolyte and placed hypothenar/thenar. They were amplified by a special constant voltage amplifier before the data were transferred to the computer. They were analogue-digital converted with a frequency of 50 Hz and then stored on magnetic tape for later analysis. Before this analysis, the data were digitally filtered to eliminate any noise produced by the pulse.

In the analysis, the following SCR parameters were determined; maximum amplitude of skin conductance, beginning of response, peak latency, and maximum slope of the curve. These parameters were determined by a computer program according to specially devised algorithms. The curve and the parameters were then displayed on a computer screen and visually controlled. In some cases, corrections were applied (e.g. if two peaks occurred and the first was too quick to be a response to the slide, the parameters were semi-automatically corrected, i.e. the second peak was defined as the response and the computer automatically determined the related parameters). Of the 960 responses measured, fewer than 20 per cent occurred after 5 s. All but two peak responses were recorded within 7 s.

Results

The study was designed as a 2 (subliminal v. supraliminal projection) × 2 (familiar v. unknown faces) factorial experiment, with repeated measures on both factors. The data were analysed according to a randomized block model (see Kirk 1968).

ANOVAs were computed with peak amplitude, peak latency, response onset latency, and slope of the curve as dependent variables. The analyses showed a significant effect only for the peak amplitude. For this variable the main effect for familiarity of the face was significant $[F (1, 858) = 8.20; p < 0.001]$.[1] Amplitudes (in μS) for familiar and unknown faces were 3.62 (SD = 3.64) and 3.11 (SD = 3.28), respectively. There was no interaction between familiarity and stimulus condition. For the four experimental conditions the mean peak amplitudes are displayed in Table 12.1.

These results show that only the familiarity of the face, but not the duration for which it was shown, had an influence on the SCR. Thus,

Table 12.1 Peak amplitude EDA (in μS) for familiar and unfamiliar faces presented above (supraliminal) and below (subliminal) the recognition threshold

	Familiar faces	Unfamiliar faces
Subliminal	3.6	3.1
Supraliminal	3.7	3.1

[1] The residual d.f.s were 858 but even if the treatment within-subjects error term is substituted the result is still significant $[F (1, 23) = 8.20; p < 0.05]$.

subjects showed different physiological responses (higher peak amplitudes of EDA) to familiar than to unknown faces, regardless as to whether or not they consciously recognized the faces.

Discussion

The finding that supraliminal face stimuli elicit differential EDA for familiar and unfamiliar faces may be taken as confirmation of the data reported by Tranel et al. (1988). In our study the experimental paradigm, including ratio of famous to unknown faces, stimulus duration, and interstimulus interval were all quite different from that employed by Tranel et al. The fact that our results agree with theirs provides compelling support for the notion that familiar and unfamiliar faces are indeed processed differently (Ellis et al. 1979).

More importantly, the results of this investigation provide support for the idea that, despite not being overtly recognized, familiar faces may elicit a greater SCR than do unfamiliar faces. This finding is entirely consistent with Marcel's (1983a) position regarding the invalidity of the 'identity assumption'. Moreover, it provides yet another useful theoretical bridge between the findings on face recognition from normal and neurologically damaged populations.

Information processing models of face recognition such as Bruce and Young's (1986) have as yet had little to say on the issue of awareness. But evidence of covert recognition in prosopagnosic and other brain-injured patients has already signalled the need to consider awareness at each stage of processing (Young and de Haan 1990, 1991), which has provoked attempts to deal with these issues more systematically both in neuroanatomical (Bauer 1984; Tranel et al. 1985) and computational theories (Burton et al. 1991).

Our results are congruent with Bauer's (1984) view that orienting responses to emotionally significant stimuli and conscious, overt recognition of the same stimuli are mediated by neurologically dissociable mechanisms. Bauer reached this conclusion from consideration of the neuroanatomical pathways likely to be involved, and from the evidence that his prosopagnosic patient showed an increased skin conductance response to faces he did not recognize overtly. The results presented here show a parallel phenomenon in normal subjects, in that elevated skin conductance response can be measured even when overt recognition does not occur.

In fact, there are now a number of lines of evidence pointing toward parallels between the consequences of brain injury and 'automatic' effects which can be elicited under subliminal conditions in normal subjects. For example, Young *et al.* (1988) drew attention to the parallel between the associative priming effects they demonstrated for the prosopagnosic patient PH and associative priming for stimuli presented below the threshold of recognition to normal subjects. Similarly, Greve and Bauer (1990) reported a particularly interesting study in which they demonstrated that patient LF (the same prosopagnosic patient as in Bauer's original SCR study) showed a 'preference' for faces he had seen before but did not overtly recognize as having seen earlier. Again, this type of preference can be found for normal subjects with subliminally presented stimuli (Zajonc 1980).

These parallels between non-conscious aspects of normal and brain-injured performance are not confined to the visual recognition system. For example, the findings of Meeres and Graves (1990), mentioned earlier, indicated that accurate localization can occur without a pattern being detected (a normal analogue of 'blindsight'). Hence these phenomena are not specific to faces, or even to visual recognition, but instead appear to reflect a more general property of visual information processing which will need to be fully mapped out and accounted for in future work. The present data serve to enrich the evidence favouring the idea championed by Marcel (1983*a,b*) that information that is not consciously perceived may, none the less, be processed to a high degree and the results of this activity may become manifest behaviourally or psychophysiologically.

References

Bauer, R. M. (1984). Autonomic recognition of names and faces: a neuro-psychological application of the guilty knowledge test. *Neuropsychologia*, **22**, 457–69.

Bodamer, J. (1947). Die Prosopagnosie. *Archiv für Psychiatrie und Nerven-krankheiten*, **179**, 6–53.

Bruce, V. (1988). *Recognising faces*. Lawrence Erlbaum Associates, Hillsdale, NJ.

Bruce, V. and Young, A. (1986). Understanding face recognition. *British Journal of Psychology*, **77**, 305–27.

Burton, A. M., Young, A. W., Bruce, V., Johnston, R., and Ellis, A. W. (1991). Understanding covert recognition. *Cognition*, **39**, 129–66.

Cheesman, J. and Merikle, P. M. (1985). Word recognition and consciousness. In *Reading research: advances in theory and practice*, V, (ed. D. Besner, T. G. Waller, and G. E. MacKinnon), pp. 311–52. Academic, New York.

Damasio, A. R., Tranel, D., and Damasaio, H. (1990). Face agnosia and the neural substrates of memory. *Annual Review of Neuroscience*, **13**, 89–109.

de Haan, E. H. F., Young, A., and Newcombe, F. (1987). Face recognition without awareness. *Cognitive Neuropsychology*, **4**, 385–415.

Ellis, H. D. and Florence, M. (1991). Bodamer's (1947) paper on prosopagnosia. *Cognitive Neuropsychology*, **7**, 81–105.

Ellis, H. D., Shepherd, J. W., and Davies, G. M. (1979). Identification of familiar and unfamiliar faces from internal and external features: Some implications for theories of face recognition. *Perception*, **8**, 431–9.

Eriksen, C. W. (1960). Discrimination and learning without awareness: a methodological survey and evaluation. *Psychological Review*, **67**, 279–300.

Greve, K. W. and Bauer, R. M. (1990). Implicit learning of new faces in prosopagnosia: an application of the mere-exposure paradigm. *Neuropsychologia*, **28**, 1035–41.

Hécaen, H. (1981). The neuropsychology of face recognition. In *Perceiving and remembering faces*, (ed. G. Davies, H. Ellis, and J. Shepherd), pp. 39–54. Academic Press, London.

Holender, D. (1986). Semantic activation without conscious identification. *Brain and Behavioral Sciences*, **9**, 1–23.

Kirk, N. E. (1968). *Experimental design: procedures for the behavioral sciences.* Brooks/Cole, Monterey.

McCauley, C., Parmalee, C. M., Sperber, R. D., and Carr, T. H. (1980). Early extraction of meaning from pictures and its relation to conscious identification. *Journal of Experimental Psychology: Human Perception and Performance*, **6**, 265–76.

Marcel, A. J. (1983*a*). Conscious and unconscious perception: an approach to the relations between phenomenal experience and perceptual processes. *Cognitive Psychology*, **15**, 238–300.

Marcel, A. J. (1983*b*). Conscious and unconscious perception: experiments on visual masking and word recognition. *Cognitive Psychology*, **15**, 197–237.

Meeres, S. L., and Graves, R. E. (1990). Localization of unseen visual stimuli by humans with normal vision. *Neuropsychologia*, **28**, 1231–7.

Schacter, D. L., McAndrews, M. P., and Moscovitch M. (1988). Access to consciousness: dissociations between implicit and explicit knowledge in neuropsychological syndromes. In *Thought without language*, (ed. L. Weiskrantz), pp. 242–78. Oxford University Press.

Sergent, J., and Signoret J-L. (1992*a*). Varieties of functional deficits in prosopagnosia. *Cerebral Cortex*, **2**, 375–88.

Sergent, J., and Signoret, J.-L. (1992*b*). Implicit access to knowledge derived from unrecognized faces in prosopagnosia. *Cerebral Cortex*, **2**, 389–400.

Tranel, D., and Damasio, A. R. (1985). Knowledge without awareness: an autonomic index of facial recognition by prosopagnosics. *Science*, **228**, 1453–4.

Tranel, D., Fowles, D. C., and Damasio, R. (1985). Electro-dermal discrimination of familiar and unfamiliar faces: a methodology. *Psychophysiology*, **22**, 403–8.

Tranel, D., Fowles, D. C., and Damasio, R. (1988). Non-conscious face recognition in patients with face agnosia. *Behavioural Brain Research*, **30**, 235–49.

Young, A. W., and de Haan, E. H. F. (1990). Impairments of visual awareness. *Mind and Language*, **5**, 29–48.
Young, A. W., and de Haan, E. H. F. (1991). Face recognition and awareness after brain injury. In *The neuropsychology of consciousness*, (ed. A. D. Milner, and M. D. Rugg), pp. 69–90. Academic Press, London.
Young, A. W., and Ellis, H. D. (1989). Semantic processing. In *Handbook of research on face processing*, (ed. A. W. Young, and H. D. Ellis), pp. 1–26. North-Holland, Amsterdam.
Young, A. W., Hellawell, D., and de Haan, E. H. F. (1988). Cross-domain semantic priming in normal subjects and a prosopagnosic patient. *Quarterly Journal of Experimental Psychology*, **40A**, 561–80.
Zajonc, R. B. (1980). Feeling and thinking: preferences need no inferences. *American Psychologist*, **35**, 151–75.

13

Simulating covert recognition

Reprinted in slightly modified form from Burton, A. M., Young, A. W., Bruce, V., Johnston, R., and Ellis, A. W. (1991), Understanding covert recognition, *Cognition*, **39**, 129–66. With kind permission of co-authors and Elsevier Science-NL, Sara Burgerhartstraat 25, 1055 KV Amsterdam, The Netherlands.

Summary

An implementation of Bruce and Young's (1986) functional model of face recognition is used to examine patterns of covert face recognition previously reported in a prosopagnosic patient, PH. Although PH is unable to recognize overtly the faces of people known to him, he shows normal patterns of face processing when tested indirectly. A simple manipulation of one set of connections in the implemented model induces behaviour consistent with patterns of results from PH obtained in semantic priming and interference tasks. We compare this account with previous explanations of covert recognition and demonstrate that the implemented model provides the most natural and parsimonious account available. Two further patients are discussed who show deficits in person perception. The first (MS) is prosopagnosic but shows no covert recognition. The second (ME) is not prosopagnosic, but cannot access semantic information relating to familiar people. The model provides an account of recognition impairments which is sufficiently general also to be useful in describing these patients.

Introduction

A functional model of face recognition

The past decade has seen considerable progress in understanding the processes by which we recognize faces. A number of broadly similar functional models have been proposed which highlight the sequential

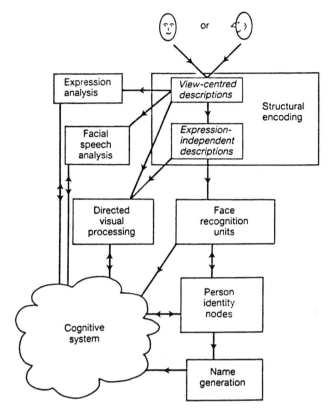

Fig. 13.1 Bruce and Young's (1986) model of face recognition.

nature of the stages involved in identifying people from their faces and the relationship between face recognition and other uses made of facial information (Hay and Young 1982; Bruce and Young 1986; Ellis 1986; Ellis *et al.* 1987*a*). The most complete account is that offered by Bruce and Young (1986), reproduced here as Fig. 13.1. The route shown to the right of the figure represents the processes involved in *identifying* a face. The parallel routes shown to the left show the independent routes (as suggested by evidence reviewed by Bruce and Young 1986) for the processing of facial expression, lip-reading ('facial speech'), and for the deliberate scrutiny of faces in certain tasks involving face matching ('directed visual processing'). In this paper, we are concerned only with the processing of facial identity, and so we will concentrate on the route shown to the right of Fig. 13.1.

After initial structural encoding, the Bruce and Young (1986) model posits three distinct sequential stages involved in identifying a face. The 'face recognition units' (FRUs) store the visual structural descriptions which allow a particular known face to be discriminated from other faces, known or unknown. There is one FRU for each known face, and the model proposes that this unit becomes active when any (recognizable) view of the appropriate face is presented. The activation of an FRU also leads to activation of a 'person identity node', or PIN. These units allow access to semantic information about the individual, for example their occupation, their relationship with the perceiver, and so on. Unlike the FRUs, a PIN may become active as a result of input other than a face. Although not shown in Fig. 13.1, it is assumed that there are other routes into the PIN store, through channels processing someone's voice, written or heard name. The PINs, then, represent the level of classification of a 'person', rather than their particular face. Finally, Bruce and Young propose a stage of 'name generation', which can only occur after activation of an appropriate PIN.

The Bruce and Young (1986) model has proved useful in research on face recognition in a number of ways. First, it provides a framework which gives an account of many empirical findings obtained in experiments with normal adults, or through observations of the patterns of impairment of face processing that may arise as the result of brain injury. This framework has served to point to new research directions in this field and is capable of generating new empirical hypotheses [e.g. see Bruce (1988) and Young and Bruce (1991) for accounts of how this framework has acted to guide research in this area]. It has stood up remarkably well to rigorous experimental test. For example, Brennen *et al.* (1990) induced tip-of-the-tongue states (TOTs) by reading subjects semantic information about familiar people and waiting for occasions when subjects felt the name of the described person was on the 'tip of their tongue'. They argued that presentation of a face should not help to resolve these TOTs, since according to the model there is no direct link between FRUs and the name generation stage. Brennen *et al.*'s (1990) findings supported this counterintuitive prediction.

Although the Bruce and Young (1986) model of face recognition has been useful in guiding new research, it is underspecified in two particular areas which are important for the developments we present here. First, it was assumed by Bruce and Young (1986) that feelings of 'familiarity' to a face arose from the level of the face recognition units themselves; 'When a face is seen, the strength of the recognition unit's signal to the cognitive system will be at a level dependent on the degree of resemblance between its stored structural description and the input provided by structural encoding' (pp. 311–12). This signal was thought to be that used in determining the face's familiarity. However, no clear mechanism for translating such patterns of activation into explicit decisions about the familiarity of the face was described. This was not possible, in part, because of a second element of under-specification in the model. Bruce and Young were unclear about whether the PINs *store* semantic information about people, or *allow access to* this information. Because this was not clearly spelled out it had to be assumed that familiarity decisions were made at the earlier stage of the FRUs. A common error in face recognition is the 'familiar only' error, in which a person is recognized as familiar, but no further information is available (Young *et al*. 1985*a*). If it is maintained that semantic information might be stored *at* the PIN, then clearly a familiarity decision has to be made before this stage of processing.

The lack of specification was thus responsible for the location of familiarity decisions at the FRU level. This in turn made it difficult for the model to accommodate the detailed pattern of effects arising from experiments on priming familiarity decisions. A great deal of the empirical work which has been performed on normal subjects has used the 'face familiarity decision task' introduced by Bruce (1983); for example, see Bruce and Valentine (1985, 1986), Young *et al*. (1985*b*, 1986*a*), Valentine and Bruce (1986), Ellis *et al*. (1987*b*), and Brunas *et al*. (1990). In this task subjects are asked to respond 'yes' or 'no' according to whether they recognize a person's face as familiar. The procedure was developed in order to provide a measure of recognition un-contaminated by the additional (and sometimes difficult) process of name retrieval (Yarmey 1973; Young *et al*. (1985*a*, 1986*b*). Using this task it has been shown that face recognition, like word recognition, gives rise to semantic priming[1] (Bruce and Valentine 1986) and repetition priming[1] effects (Bruce and Valentine 1985; Ellis *et al*. 1987*b*). It was assumed by Bruce and Young (1986) that repetition priming resulted from the direct raising of activation at FRU level through previous exposure, while semantic priming resulted from activation of FRUs in-directly via the PIN/cognitive system. The problem with this assumption is that it fails to account for the different nature of repetition and semantic priming effects. For example, the time courses of these effects are quite different; semantic priming of faces does not survive an inter-vening item (Bruce 1986), while repetition priming remains robust for at least 20 min after first presentation (Ellis 1987*b*). Furthermore, semantic priming crosses input domains; that is, names prime the faces of semantic associates, and faces prime names (Young *et al*. 1988). How-ever, the longer lasting repetition priming effect does not cross input

---

[1] Semantic priming is sometimes referred to as associative priming. Here we use the terms interchangeably. Similarly, repetition priming is sometimes referred to as identity priming, and once again we use these terms interchangeably.

domains. It has been difficult to deal with such findings within the Bruce
and Young (1986) model. Young and Ellis (1989*a*) comment as follows
on this issue;

The problem created by different time courses of semantic priming and
repetition priming effects is that it is thus implausible to attribute both effects to
a common mechanism in the form of increased activation of face recognition
units. This problem is not insuperable, but it will require a more detailed
knowledge of the properties of semantic and repetition priming effects, and
some revision of existing models, before an effective solution can be proposed.
(p. 247).

As we describe below, Burton *et al.* (1990) implemented the Bruce
and Young (1986) model using an interactive activation architecture,
within which it was made explicit that PINs formed modality-
independent *gateways* to semantic information about identity, rather
than themselves containing semantic information. (In fact, this assertion
was not without precedent; see Young *et al.* 1985*a*, p. 517.) If semantic
information is accessed via the PIN, then familiarity decisions could be
taken at PIN level, rather than solely on the basis of activation passed
from FRUs. Burton *et al.* (1990) describe how such an implementation
enables the separation of the locus of effects of semantic and repetition
priming, thus removing one apparent difficulty within the original Bruce
and Young framework. Briefly, semantic priming is taken to affect
activation levels at the PINs, while repetition priming is taken to affect
the strengths of connections between FRUs and PINs. A direct consequence of this is that semantic priming will cross input domains; that
is, names will prime the faces of semantic associates, and faces will
prime names. Burton *et al.* (1990) discuss this proposition (and other
consequences of the characterization of semantic and repetition
priming) at length, and we will return to a more detailed description of
semantic priming below.

In recent years a phenomenon has been reported in the neuropsychological literature which seems to require more radical revision of
the face recognition model. The particular phenomenon of concern here
is that of *covert* recognition of faces by prosopagnosic patients. Here we
review the basic phenomena of prosopagnosia before introducing the
details of covert recognition. We describe how attempts were made to
explain covert recognition in terms of a substantial modification of the
original framework. Finally, we show how an interactive activation
implementation of the original architecture can in fact accommodate
the phenomenon of covert recognition without major modification of
the Bruce and Young model.

Prosopagnosia and covert recognition

Prosopagnosic patients are unable to recognize the faces of familiar people. Even the most familiar faces are affected, such as friends, family, and the patient's own face when seen in a mirror (Hécaen and Angelergues 1962). Prosopagnosic patients remain able to see faces, and can point to the eyes, nose, mouth, and so on. In some cases the processing of expression, age, and sex from facial appearance remains well preserved, even though ability to identify familiar faces overtly is very severely impaired (Bruyer *et al.* 1983; Tranel *et al.* 1988). The condition can occur despite preserved ability to recognize people from non-facial cues, such as their voices or names. These widely reported observations demonstrate that prosopagnosia can involve a problem of face *recognition*, rather than a more general face-processing impairment, and that there need not be any corresponding impairment affecting the patient's knowledge of familiar people.

Prosopagnosia was first identified as a distinct neuropsychological problem by Bodamer (1947). The underlying pathology involves lesions affecting occipito-temporal regions of cerebral cortex. Usually these are bilateral lesions (Meadows 1974; Damasio *et al.* 1982), but several cases involving unilateral lesions of the right cerebral hemisphere have been reported in the more recent literature (e.g. De Renzi 1986; Landis *et al.* 1986; Sergent and Villemure 1989).

Attempts to account for the patterns of deficit found in prosopagnosic patients have focused on the functional nature of the disorder. This trend has occurred in parallel with (and has strongly influenced) the development of detailed functional models of normal face recognition (Hay and Young 1982; Bruce and Young 1986; Ellis 1986; Bruyer 1987; Ellis *et al.* 1987a; Bruce 1988; Young 1988). There is now a body of work which suggests that prosopagnosic symptoms may occur for a variety of reasons, each reflecting breakdown at particular stages in the functional architecture of the recognition system (e.g. Hay and Young 1982; De Renzi 1986; de Haan *et al.* 1987a,b; Young and de Haan 1988; Young *et al.* 1988; Newcombe *et al.* 1989; Sergent and Villemure, 1989; Young and Ellis 1989b; Sergent and Poncet 1990).

Covert recognition represents one of the most challenging findings in the literature on prosopagnosia. Patients with no overt recognition of faces, and who have no more than chance ability to sort familiar from unfamiliar faces, may nevertheless show recognition when tested indirectly. This has now been demonstrated with a number of different types of measure including skin conductance (Bauer 1984; Tranel and Damasio 1985), evoked potentials (Renault *et al.* 1989), eye movements

(Rizzo *et al.* 1987), face-name learning (Bruyer *et al.* 1983; de Haan *et al.* 1987*a,b*; Young and de Haan, 1988; Sergent and Poncet 1990), and matching, priming, and interference techniques derived from experimental psychology (de Haan *et al.* 1987*b*; Young *et al.* 1988).

In order to make sense of the pattern of findings in studies of covert recognition in prosopagnosia, it is useful to draw a distinction between direct and indirect tests of recognition (Young and de Haan 1991). Direct tests will enquire about the ability of interest (e.g. 'whose face is this?', 'which face is familiar?'), whereas in an indirect test the ability in question is introduced as an incidental feature of a task that ostensibly measures something else (e.g. effects of familiarity on face *matching*, effects of different types of face prime on *name* recognition). In demonstrations of covert recognition of familiar faces in prosopagnosia, face recognition is usually tested indirectly. When this is done, the pattern of performance of prosopagnosic patients can show a 'normal' influence of face familiarity, even though performance on direct tests *with the same faces* is at chance level (Young and de Haan 1988; Young *et al.* 1988). These findings are consistent with reports of preserved abilities on indirect tests deriving from a range of neuropsychological conditions (Schacter *et al.* 1988; Young and de Haan 1988). More importantly, they cause us fundamentally to re-examine our conception of at least one form of prosopagnosia, since it is clear that at least some aspects of recognition remain intact, even though there is no awareness of recognition. To account for these effects Schacter *et al.* (1988) have suggested that the problem can be considered one of access to consciousness from the otherwise intact recognition system. In what follows, we shall propose a mechanism for an alternative account; that the recognition system can be damaged in such a way as to preserve covert effects, and yet cause loss of overt recognition. We will show that this is possible without recourse to theorizing about the processes which signal awareness.

It is important to point out that not all prosopagnosic patients show covert recognition (Bauer 1986; Newcombe *et al.* 1989; Sergent and Villemure 1989; Young and Ellis 1989*b*). This observation is, of course, consistent with the view that prosopagnosia as a *symptom* can arise from more than one functionally separable *cause*.

In this paper, we will concentrate particularly on evidence provided by de Haan *et al.* (1987*a,b*) and Young *et al.* (1988). These studies are a result of detailed investigations of one prosopagnosic patient, PH. We will now present a brief case history of this patient and review some of the previous attempts to account for the puzzling effects which his case demonstrates.

PH: Case summary

Because our intention is to examine crucial aspects of PH's performance in tasks involving covert processing of familiar faces, we will summarize pertinent details of his case here. A full description of ophthalmological and neuropsychological assessments is given by de Haan *et al.* (1987*b*).

PH suffered a severe closed head injury in an accident in 1982, when he was 19 years old. His language skills are well preserved (verbal IQ = 91, consistent with his previous education), and he is still able to read without difficulty.

PH's main spontaneous complaint concerns his inability to recognize faces in everyday life. On formal tests he recognized none of 20 highly familiar and 20 moderately familiar faces (de Haan *et al.* 1987*a*) and performed at chance level at discriminating familiar from unfamiliar faces in free choice (18/36; de Haan *et al.* 1987*b*) or forced choice (65/128; Young and de Haan 1988) tasks. Thus he experiences no sense of overt familiarity to well known faces. He is also unable to assign faces overtly to semantic categories (politician, television personality, etc.) at above chance levels (de Haan *et al.* 1987*a,b*). In contrast, he continues to be able to recognize familiar people from their names (de Haan *et al.* 1987*b*; Young and de Haan 1988). It should be noted, though, that PH's recognition of familiar names (118/128) in forced choice is not completely normal, but at 92 per cent correct it is very much better than his chance-level (51 per cent correct) recognition of familiar faces in the equivalent task.

On tests that require him to match views of unfamiliar faces or to identify expressions, PH performs less well than control subjects, but is none the less well above chance level (de Haan *et al.* 1987*b*). However, like several other prosopagnosic patients he experiences severe problems in identifying individual members of other visually homogeneous categories such as cars (3/33) or flowers (0/26) (de Haan *et al.* 1987*b*).

In 'short-term' memory tasks PH's performance is normal for both verbal and non-verbal material, but his performance of 'long-term' memory tasks is impaired. This memory impairment is not typical of other prosopagnosic cases, and it is not considered to be the cause of PH's face recognition problems, since he can recognize most people from their names; that is, he has not forgotten who they are.

Despite his severe impairment of overt face recognition ability, PH shows a remarkable degree of covert access to face identity in indirect tasks. He matches photographs of different views of familiar faces more quickly than photographs of unfamiliar faces (de Haan *et al.* 1987*b*). When taught to associate a name with a photograph, he learns 'true' pairings more readily than 'untrue' pairings (de Haan *et al.* 1987*b*; Young and De Haan 1988). Furthermore in semantic priming and interference tasks, PH shows effects of non-target faces (which he cannot identify overtly) on the processing of target names (de Haan *et al.* 1987*a,b*; Young *et al.* 1988). So, he is faster to recognize a name if it is preceded by the face of a semantic associate; and when asked to decide to which of two semantic categories a name belongs, he is slower if the name is presented simultaneously with the face of a person in the alternative category. In the present paper we demonstrate that it is possible to simulate the last two types of effect (semantic priming and interference from 'unidentified' faces) using an interactive activation model. We will describe these effects in more detail, and present the results of experiments with the simulation.

Previous accounts of covert recognition

Accounting for covert recognition in prosopagnosia has not proved easy. Bauer (1984, 1986) proposed that neurologically dissociable information processing routes are involved in overt recognition and orienting responses to emotionally salient stimuli. Although theoretically elegant, this proposal suffers from the problem that covert recognition effects can be found even to faces of people who seem to have little 'emotional' importance to the patient. Tranel and Damasio (1985) suggested that 'facial templates' are intact in patients who show covert recognition, but that the processes required for the 'activation of multimodal associations' from the face are defective. However, evidence from other studies has shown that if this is the case, then these processes cannot be completely lost. The findings of Bruyer *et al.* (1983), de Haan *et al.* (1987*a,b*), Young *et al.* (1988), Young and de Haan (1988), and Sergent and Poncet (1990) all imply that *some* multimodal associations *are* implicated in covert recognition, since in all of these reports a defining characteristic of covert *face* recognition was its ability to influence *name* processing. In order to account for this fact, Young and de Haan (1988) offered an explanation in terms of the Bruce and Young (1986) model (as shown in Fig. 13.1).

   Young and de Haan (1988) proposed that the patterns of deficit observed in PH could be due to a disconnection of the *outputs* of the FRUs. Figure 13.2 illustrates this proposal; the FRU outputs are highlighted to draw attention to them. Damage to the pathways between FRUs and the cognitive system, and between FRUs and PINs, would prevent overt recognition being achieved despite normal activation at the recognition unit level. Furthermore, damage to the pathway

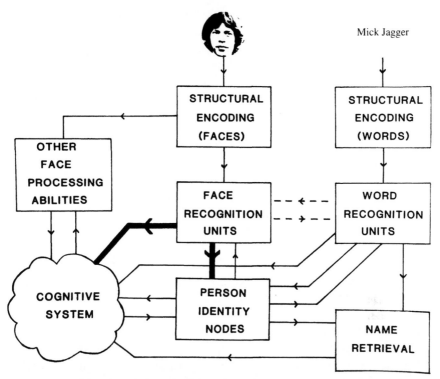

Fig. 13.2 Young and de Haan's (1988) functional model of components involved in face and name recognition. Outputs from FRUs are highlighted to draw attention to the proposed account of PH's deficit.

between FRUs and PINs would also prevent retrieval of any semantic information associated with the presented face. As we discussed above, Bruce and Young (1986) conceive of routes into the PINs through other modalities. So, for example, there will be an analogous 'structural encoding' phase for written names, feeding information into a 'word recognition unit' store which serves the same function as FRUs, but for the written names of people (see Fig. 13.2). If this word/name recognition system is intact, but FRU outputs are eliminated, there should be no deficit in deciding the familiarity of names, or in retrieving appropriate semantic information from names.

This account in terms of disconnected FRUs appears satisfactory in explaining what PH cannot do (i.e. the breakdown of overt recognition of familiar faces). However, as Young and de Haan (1988) noted, it is still necessary to account for how the disconnected face recognition system can influence the word/name recognition system in indirect tasks. To achieve this Young and de Haan (1988) proposed that there is some rudimentary 'semantic' organization in the form of associative links between input systems at the recognition unit level. They argued that it may be useful to build up associations that allow us to recognize Raisa Gorbachev more readily after we have seen Mikhail Gorbachev, or to recognize her photograph in a newspaper more quickly after we have read Mikhail Gorbachev's name. Such associations would serve the purpose of making the recognition system prepared for what it is likely to encounter next. This mechanism would allow semantic priming and interference effects from seen faces, with the patterns of priming and interference reflecting the rudimentary semantic organization present.

Although this proposal has some attractive features, it is not completely satisfactory. In particular, the status of associative links within the input systems must be assumed to be very different from the status of other links in the model (this is represented by the dashed lines in Fig. 13.2). These 'input system organization links' must not serve directly to trigger *firing* of an associated recognition unit. If such a function were possible, prosopagnosic patients could use the FRU to word-recognition-unit links in order to forge a route from face inputs into the cognitive system and the PINs. Young and de Haan (1988) therefore proposed that these links have the effect of lowering the decision thresholds for associated people, and hence produce automatic associative effects without creating alternative routes through the system.

We have seen, then, that attempts have been made to use the Bruce and Young (1986) model to account for covert recognition. However, Young and de Haan's explanation is rather complex, and introduces radically new mechanisms. In the following we will show how the 'IAC' computer implementation of Bruce and Young's (1986) model provides a much simpler account of covert recognition in prosopagnosia. Implementation of this model has led to a clearer characterization of its 'microstructure', and this has suggested an alternative account to that described above. We show how this implementation may be used to understand patterns of recognition in intact and lesioned systems, and demonstrate that it can simulate and thus provide an account of the basic pattern of interaction between face and name input systems observed in cases of prosopagnosia with covert recognition.

The interactive activation model of person recognition

The interactive activation model of person recognition (Burton et al. 1990) is based on Bruce and Young's (1986) functional model described above. It is implemented in the terms of McClelland and Rumelhart (1981), who have used a similar model to study word recognition. This architecture is connectionist in that it comprises units joined by connections of potentially variable strength. However, there are no distributed representations within the simulation – each unit has a discrete referent.

The model comprises a number of distinct pools of units. All the units within a pool are connected to each other with inhibitory links. Units may be connected across pools by excitatory links. Figure 13.3 shows the overall structure of the model. Following Bruce and Young (1986) we propose a number of pools of units corresponding to the following functional distinctions. FRUs become active when the system is presented with any recognizable view of a person's face. In the current simulation, these units receive input which is subsequently passed around the system. This input is arbitrary for the purposes of the demonstrations presented here. However, it is assumed to represent the output of visual processing by the perceptual system (structural encoding). PINs are essentially domain- and modality-free gateways into semantic information. They may be accessed through any input domain (face, name, voice, etc.), and provide access to information about that person. Semantic information units (SIUs) are simply units on which is

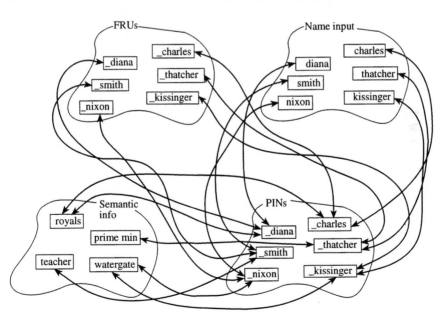

Fig. 13.3 Central architecture of Burton and co-workers' (1990) interactive activation model.

coded particular semantic information. Name input units (NIUs) represent the same level of abstraction as FRUs, providing a route into the system for the names of known individuals. Though not represented in the present implementation, it is assumed that separate clusters of NIUs would be needed for seen or heard names (see Bruce and Young 1986).

The configuration of these clusters is shown in Fig. 13.3. Input to the model is made by exciting the activation of an FRU or a name input unit. Time is modelled here in terms of a number of processing cycles, after each of which activation at units is updated. The effect of this is that activation is passed along excitatory links into different pools, thus increasing the activation levels of associated units. Note that connections are all bidirectional, in keeping with McClelland and Rumelhart's original conception of the interactive activation architecture, and the Bruce and Young (1986) model (see Fig. 13.1). In all such interactive activation models there is also a global decay function which forces units towards a resting activation. After input to the system, units tend to stabilize when the effect of input activation is balanced by the effect of decay. McClelland and Rumelhart (1981, 1988) give details of the equations for governing transfer of activation and decay in these nets, and the Appendix gives the details of the particular parameters used here.

In this model, we propose that familiarity decisions are taken at the PINs. As discussed above, this is a departure from Bruce and Young (1986), who placed familiarity decisions at the interface between FRUs and the cognitive system. As we discussed earlier, this was largely because the relationship between PINs and semantic information was not clearly addressed by Bruce and Young, which forced familiarity decisions to a different locus. These authors thus implied that separate familiarity decision mechanisms must be taken for faces, names, voices, and so forth. However, here the familiarity decision is assumed to be based on 'person familiarity', as the same decision is taken at PINs whether they are activated through either FRU input or NIU input. This now seems to us a more plausible account. In daily life one is often presented with information about a person across more than one modality (e.g. we may see someone's face at the same time as hearing their voice). It would be parsimonious for these various inputs to feed to a single central pool of units at which familiarity judgements can be taken (Burton *et al.* 1990). It is important to note that this conception still allows for the common daily error in which one may recognize a person as familiar, but be unable to retrieve any semantic information about them (Young *et al.* 1985a). We have here explicitly separated PINs and semantic information, and hence in theory it should be possible to access PINs (and hence achieve a sense of familiarity) without accessing semantic information. One situation in which this might occur is if, for some reason, the connections between the PINs and the SIUs were abolished or attenuated. We will develop this idea in detail below.

The mechanism for decisions in the present model, unlike standard logogen models, is comparison of activation of units against a *constant* threshold. So, in familiarity decision, an arbitrary threshold is set for the pool of PINs, and any unit which reaches the threshold level is taken to be recognized as familiar. Note that this proposal has nothing to say about the *phenomenal experience* of awareness. We simply characterize a *familiarity judgement* as occurring when a PIN crosses a threshold. We do not offer any account of introspective awareness here.

Burton *et al.* (1990) have shown that this (Fig. 13.3) conceptualization can account for a number of effects in the literature on normal face recognition, including semantic (associative) priming, repetition (identity) priming, and distinctiveness effects. The different time courses of semantic and repetition priming are explained by proposing that semantic priming affects activation levels at the PINs while repetition affects the strength of the connections between FRUs and PINs.

The mechanism by which semantic priming takes place is of particular importance here, and so we will describe it using an illustrative example from the architecture shown in Fig. 13.3. After input to a particular FRU (say Prince Charles), the 'Prince Charles' PIN becomes active. As activation at this unit rises, it in turn passes activation, along the excitatory links to the relevant semantic information units (say, 'royal'). Now, as this unit rises in activation, excitatory activation is passed back into the PIN pool, to the 'Princess Diana' PIN, which is connected to some of the same semantic information units as 'Prince Charles'. Hence, it is possible for several units within the same pool to rise in activation level, even though all units within a pool actually inhibit each other. During the scenario presented here, the Charles PIN will quickly rise above the threshold for a positive familiarity decision. However, because there is some cost involved in passing information, the Diana PIN will rise, but stabilize below this threshold. Now, on subsequent activation of the 'Diana' FRU, the 'Diana' PIN will quickly rise to threshold. Because the 'Diana' PIN is already above its resting activation, it will take a shorter time to reach threshold than if it started at rest. This is the model of semantic priming. When we come to describe experiments with the model, we will present data from exactly this scenario (see Fig. 13.4 in the following).

It is important to note that in this model semantic priming will take place across input domains. Because its mechanism is the excitation of PINs, subsequent input may come from any system which feeds into these PINs. So, for example, if a PIN has previously become active through presentation of a face, then subsequent presentation of a name will also be facilitated, since the appropriate PIN is already above resting activation. Cross-domain semantic priming of this type is found for normal subjects, as well as in some prosopagnosics (Young *et al.* 1988). We will present demonstrations of these effects below, and a more detailed analysis of semantic and other priming effects is given by Burton *et al.* (1990).

Implementation

The model as described here was developed using McClelland and Rumelhart's (1988) 'IAC' (interactive activation and competition) program. This is a small software environment for exploration of connectionist models. In the Appendix we present a detailed list of the parameters associated with the current implementation, in order that readers may replicate these simulations.

As a simplifying assumption in the model, all excitatory links have the same weight. Similarly, all inhibitory links have the same weight, though this is smaller than the excitatory links (see Appendix). The assumption of equality of weights does not correspond to the real situation. We are taking connection strength as an analogue of 'degree of association' within the system. However, there will almost certainly be faces that are better known than others (i.e. by analogy, will have stronger con- nections between FRU and PIN), and there will also be varying degrees of association between PINs and SIUs (e.g. 'Prince Charles is a member of the royal family' will be a strong link, whereas 'Prince Charles studied in Cambridge' will be a weak link for most people). However, the commitment to equality of connection strengths within the imple- mented model serves to simplify the assumptions made here. In short, we aim to show that the behaviour exhibited by the model is a conse- quence of a *general* architecture, and not due to local manipulation of particular parameters.

Finally, note that this is not a simulation of learning. Unlike many connectionist models (see, for example, Hinton and Anderson 1981; McClelland *et al.* 1986; Rumelhart *et al.* 1986), we do not modify the values of connection strengths in the simulations presented here.[1] Instead the model is at present intended to implement a particular state

---

[1] A version incorporating a learning rule was subsequently developed by Burton (1994).

of the face recognition system. As such, it has the same status as many other functional models, though as we will show below it allows for examination of a number of hypotheses which are hidden from view in unimplemented systems.

Our account of covert recognition

We now turn to the simulation of effects observed in the prosopagnosic patient, PH. We begin by noting that PH can match different views of faces (de Haan *et al.* 1987*b*, tasks 1 and 2) and that he shows an advantage in reaction time (RT) for matching different views of familiar over unfamiliar faces, despite the fact that he denies recognizing any of the faces. The pattern of faster matching of familiar than unfamiliar faces is also found for normal subjects (Young *et al.* 1986*c*) and, like normal subjects, PH only shows this phenomenon of faster matching of familiar faces when the match must be based on the face's internal features (eyes, nose, mouth) as opposed to external features (hair, face shape, chin) (Young *et al.* 1985*c*, experiment 1; de Haan *et al.* 1987*b*, task 2).

As has been noted in previous studies, these effects of familiarity in face-matching tasks provide evidence that there is no gross impairment affecting the structural encoding of seen faces (including configural processing) sufficiently to prevent recognition by PH, and that FRUs themselves remain intact (de Haan et al. 1987*b*; Young and de Haan 1988). Any impairment for PH cannot be located at this level.

In terms of the Burton *et al.* (1990) implementation of the Bruce and Young (1986) model, we therefore propose that the functional impairment lies in the *connection strengths* between the pool of FRUs and the pool of PINs. We propose that PH suffers attenuated connection strengths between these two pools. Hence, while *some* excitation is passed from an active FRU to its associated PIN, the weak connection strengths mean that this activation is small compared to an intact system. The result of this is that the appropriate PIN is active, but below threshold. This activation at the PIN can be passed to the connected SIUs in the normal way, and subsequently on to any associated PIN. The only difference between this and the intact system is that the levels of activation will be smaller.

We make this proposal to account for the fact that despite being unable to recognize faces overtly, PH displays some effects which are affected by structure deep in the face recognition system. A plausible account of these effects is that some activation is passed into this system, but that this is sufficiently attenuated to destroy the ability to make overt judgements of familiarity. To demonstrate that this is a plausible account, we now consider and simulate two of these effects; semantic priming and interference from 'unrecognized' faces.

Semantic priming

We will begin the exploration with an account of covert recognition in prosopagnosic patients as demonstrated by semantic priming from 'unrecognized' faces. In normal subjects, presentation of the face of a familiar person as a prime stimulus facilitates a subsequent familiarity decision to the target face of a close semantic associate. So, for example, it is known that subjects are faster to respond positively to Oliver Hardy's face if it has been preceded by Stan Laurel's face, than if it has been preceded by an unrelated familiar face (e.g. Ronald Reagan) or by an unfamiliar face (Bruce and Valentine 1986).

Semantic priming effects have been shown to cross stimulus input domains (Young *et al.* 1988). That is, Oliver Hardy's *face* primes recognition latency for Stan Laurel's *name*. This cross-domain semantic priming effect provides a technique for examining covert recognition in prosopagnosia, since it allows the influence of a face prime to be investigated in the task of making familiarity decisions to name targets. Although PH is unable to recognize face primes overtly, he can readily identify most name targets, and thus carry out the task. Young *et al.* (1988) reported that prior presentation of (for example) Eric Morecambe's face facilitated PH's recognition of Ernie Wise's name (these being a famous English comedy duo).

Young *et al.* (1988, experiment 4) studied cross-domain (face prime and name target) and within-domain (name prime and name target) semantic priming of name recognition by PH. Although PH could not recognize face primes overtly but could recognize name primes overtly, the priming effect was equivalent across the different prime domains. In both cases there was facilitation of responses to targets preceded by related primes, and no significant inhibition from unrelated primes. Thus, presence or absence of overt recognition of the primes did not modify semantic priming. Although PH's reaction times were slower than those of normal subjects, the *pattern* of his performance across conditions remained the same (i.e. facilitation of responses to targets preceded by related primes, and equivalent cross-domain and within-domain effects; Young *et al.* 1988).

Figure 13.4 shows the effects of cross-domain and within-domain semantic priming in the intact Burton *et al.* (1990) model. These data come from a small net of 18 people (each with an FRU, PIN, and NIU) and 9 SIUs. Figure 13.4(a) shows the effect of a related face prime on name recognition. Fig. 13.4(b) shows the effect of a related name prime on name recognition, and Fig. 13.4(c) shows the unprimed name recognition cycle. We have previously shown that unprimed (equivalent to 'neutral condition' here) and unrelated prime conditions produce almost identical patterns of activation (Figs 3 and 5 in Burton *et al.* 1990). We therefore present only one of these controls in the diagrams given here.

The diagrams show activation at two PINs. In fig. 13.4(a) input is made to an FRU (Prince Charles), and the model is allowed to run for 80 cycles with this FRU activated to its maximum level. During this time, the Prince Charles PIN increases in activation until stabilizing at a particular value. Furthermore, the PIN of a semantic associate also rises in activation, through the route described above. What is happening here is that activation at the 'Charles' PIN is passing activation to the 'royal' SIU, which is in turn passing activation to the 'Diana' PIN. Both PINs tend to stabilize after a number of cycles, though the semantic associate achieves a lower activation level than the prime itself. So, in this case, the 'Charles' PIN crosses the (arbitrarily set) threshold for a positive familiarity decision to be taken. While the 'Diana' PIN becomes active, it remains below this threshold.

The system is then given a 'rest period' of 20 cycles in which it is allowed to run with no external input; that is, the FRU activation is discontinued. This corresponds to the 'inter-stimulus interval' used in experimental studies. During this time, units tend to decay. Note that the 'Charles' PIN quickly drops below threshold. In this case, the 'Diana' PIN continues to rise by a small amount, although if given more cycles it too would begin to decay (see Burton *et al.* 1990).

During the final 80-cycle period, the NIU for 'Diana' is activated. As the 'Diana' PIN remains above its resting position, the time taken for it to reach threshold is shorter than would normally be the case. To see this, Fig. 13.4(c) shows the effect of activating the 'Diana' NIU with no previous priming. In the primed case, the name 'Diana' produces a familiarity decision after around 10 cycles, whereas in the unprimed condition it requires over 20 cycles. Of course we do not intend these thresholds to have any special meaning – they are chosen arbitrarily. For this reason Burton *et al.* (1990) discuss the fact that the model may make only ordinal predictions. However, the point of interest is that *wherever a threshold is set* the primed condition produces an advantage over the unprimed.

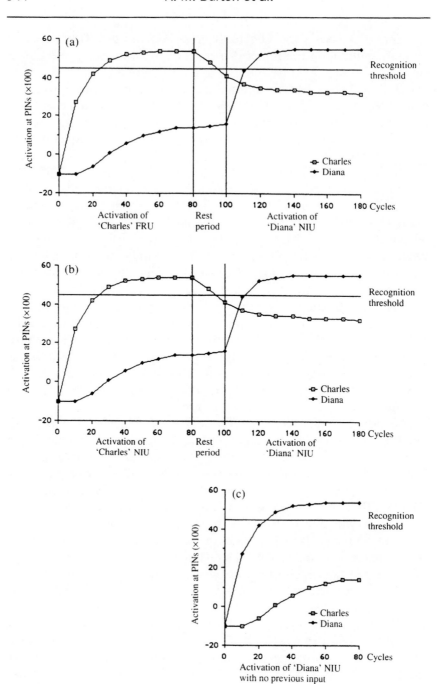

We should note here that this effect is not due to our choice of the number of cycles for which the model is allowed to run. We have chosen to illustrate an 80-cycle presentation and a 20-cycle inter-stimulus interval (ISI) in order to demonstrate the fact that the units tend to stabilize. Figure 13.4(a) shows that priming would exist over much shorter presentation times, and over all longer presentation times. Furthermore, the effect exists over a very large range of ISIs, including zero ISI. Given sufficiently large ISI, both active units will decay to resting activation (hence eliminating priming), though this takes many hundreds of cycles (Burton *et al.* 1990).

Figure 13.4(b) shows the effects of a name prime ('Charles') on subsequent activation in response to a related name ('Diana'). This is equivalent to within-domain semantic priming. As is found for normal subjects, the effect is closely comparable to that observed following a face prime (Fig. 13.4(a); cross-domain semantic priming). Having demonstrated these effects in the intact net, we now turn to the simulation of PH.

We mentioned earlier that our view of PH is that the FRU–PIN links have been affected by his brain injury. Figure 13.5 shows a replication of the experiments shown in Fig. 13.4, but this time the connection strengths between all FRUs and PINs have been halved to represent our conception of PH's impairment. In Fig. 13.5(a) activation of the 'Charles' FRU does not cause the 'Charles' PIN to reach the threshold for familiarity. However, both it and the semantic associate (Diana) PINs are active (above resting position) at the end of the rest period. This means that subsequent presentation of the 'Diana' NIU causes the 'Diana' PIN to rise more quickly to threshold than would usually be the case. For comparison, Fig. 13.5(c) shows the rise in activity of the 'Diana' PIN when the 'Diana' NIU is activated, but there has been no previous priming. Once again, we see that there is an advantage for a primed person.

In this way we can account for the semantic priming observed in PH. Although the patient is unable to reach threshold recognition at the PIN level for a presented face, these PIN units are nevertheless active. This activity can be passed around the system and produce the semantic priming effects on name recognition observed in empirical studies.

Fig. 13.4 Activation of PINs after input to FRUs and NIUs in the intact net, showing the effect of semantic priming. (a) Cross-domain semantic priming; the 'Charles' FRU is activated for 80 cycles, followed by a 20-cycle rest period, followed by activation of the 'Diana' NIU for 80 cycles. (b) Within-domain semantic priming; from a name prime ('Charles') to a second name input ('Diana'). (c) An 'unprimed' comparison in which the 'Diana' NIU is activated with no previous input.

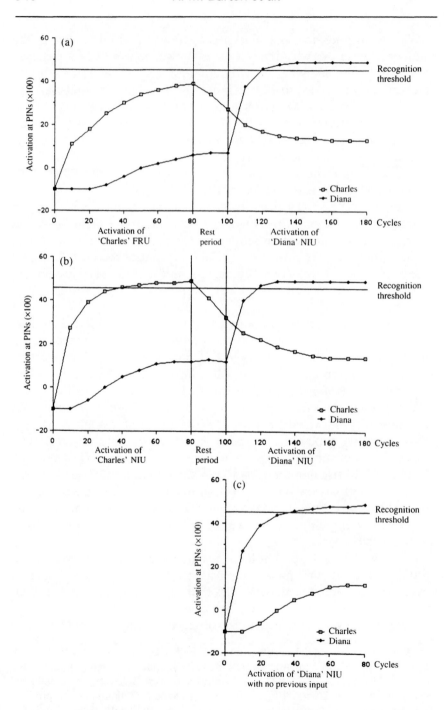

Fig. 13.5 Activation at PINs after input to FRUs and NIUs in the simulation of PH. (a) Effect of 80 cycles input to the 'Charles' FRU, followed by a 20-cycle rest, followed by 80 cycles input to the 'Diana' NIU. This corresponds to cross-domain semantic priming. (b) Effect of 80 cycles activation of the 'Charles' NIU, followed by 20 cycles rest, followed by 80 cycles activation of the 'Diana' NIU; corresponding to within-domain semantic priming. (c) Effect of activating the 'Diana' NIU with no previous input, to provide an 'unprimed' comparison.

Figure 13.5(b) shows the effect of name-to-name (within-domain) semantic priming in the simulation of PH. It can be seen that the effect of priming (i.e. the comparison with Fig. 13.5(c)) is present whether the prime is an (unrecognized) face or a (recognized) name. This is the pattern observed in data from PH. Of course the main effect of *prime type* noted by Young *et al.* (1988) is not reflected in the simulation. The empirical data for PH show that, in general, names which have been primed by other names are recognized faster than names which have been primed by faces. However, as Young *et al.* (1988) note, this may simply reflect the order in which PH was given the different blocks of trials. In addition, the present model does not attempt to simulate the configural processing necessary for FRUs or NIUs to become active in the first place. The important point to note is that priming delivers an *advantage* to name recognition whether the prime is a name or a face, and that this can happen for primes which remain below the threshold for recognition at the PIN level. In these ways the simulation provides a close parallel to the findings with PH.

An interesting (and unintended) emergent property of this simulation is that comparing Figs 13.4(c) and 13.5(c) shows a general deficit in the attenuated model. Despite the fact that the only connection strengths to have been weakened are those between FRUs and PINs, the 'lesioned' model takes longer to reach a familiarity judgement to a *name* input than the intact model. This is a consequence of the fact that all links are bidirectional. When a PIN becomes active through name input, it will pass activation on to the FRU (and vice versa). This in turn passes activation back to the PIN, and these units tend mutually to increase each other's activation level. So, wherever links are attenuated in this model, there will be a general decrease in performance throughout the system. In fact, this decrease in performance is also shown by PH (compared to controls). Of course, there are many reasons why a patient with neurological damage may show a general slowing of RT, but the results described here provide one possible mechanism for the effect. What is lost is the facility for related units to bolster each other's activation in the system.

Finally, we should note that for the same reasons that it can simulate PH's preserved semantic priming from faces that do not reach recognition threshold, the Burton *et al.* (1990) model provides a general account of semantic priming under conditions in which stimuli do not reach threshold for normal subjects, such as when visual masking is introduced before overt recognition has occurred (e.g. McCauley *et al.* 1980; Carr *et al.* 1982). The parallel between these findings and those obtained for PH had been made by Young *et al.* (1988), so it is reassuring that a similar account can be given.

Interference effects

In common with normal subjects, PH shows interference from distractor faces onto the semantic classification of simultaneously presented target names (de Haan *et al.* 1987*a,b*). The paradigm for this investigation comes from Young *et al.* (1986*d*). If subjects are asked to make a semantic decision about the names of familiar people (e.g. 'is this a politician or a pop star?') there is an inhibitory effect when the name is presented simultaneously with the face of someone in the opposite semantic group. So, the decision that the name 'Mick Jagger' is that of a pop star is made more quickly when the name is presented on its own, or when it is accompanied by the face of another pop star, than when it is presented simultaneously with the face of Neil Kinnock (a politician).

The same effect was observed in PH (de Haan *et al.* 1987*a,b*), even though his performance at explicitly classifying face stimuli into semantic categories was very poor. Once again, this suggests that this particular case of prosopagnosia has its roots deeper than any inability to extract configural information. The face recognition system is being activated in a way that invalidates this option.

In the following simulation we have copied the experimental design of Young *et al.* (1986*d*; experiment 2) and of de Haan *et al.* (1987*b*, task 3). The net is presented with the name of a person (i.e. the NIU is activated). This is done in one of four conditions:

(1) name input together with the face of the person whose name it is (equivalent to Young *et al.*'s 'same person' condition);

(2) name input alone (Young *et al.*'s 'name only' condition);

(3) name input together with the face of a person from the same category (Young *et al.*'s 'related' condition);

(4) name input together with the face of a person from the opposite category (Young *et al.*'s 'unrelated' condition).

For this simulation, a net was assembled containing 18 people, nine of whom were linked to one SIU (say 'pop star'); and the remaining nine to a second SIU (say 'politician'). Both Young *et al.* (1986*d*) and de Haan *et al.* (1987*b*) found no significant differences between RTs in the first three conditions, but the unrelated face presentation caused a decrement in performance.

In order to simulate these experiments, it is necessary this time to examine the semantic information units rather than the PINs. By analogy with the person familiarity task (which is assumed to have its locus at the PINs) it seems reasonable to propose that the categorization decision occurs due to the appropriate semantic unit reaching some threshold value. Figure 13.6 shows the activation of the SIU associated with the *name* input, for each of the four conditions. This is in keeping with the experiments we are simulating, as the experimental task is to make a semantic judgement to the presented name. Figure 13.6(a) is for the intact net, while Fig. 13.6(b) shows effects of the net in which FRU–PIN links have half the normal weight. For comparison, the RT means (in ms) for normal subjects (Young *et al.* 1986*d*, experiment 2) and for PH (de Haan *et al.* 1987*b*, task 3) are presented in Table 13.1.

In both Fig. 13.6(a) and (b), it can be seen that presentation of an unrelated face in conjunction with the target name provides the slowest route to any threshold one cares to set. This is consistent with the data in Table 13.1. None of the remaining three conditions showed significant differences in empirical work. However, it is clear in Fig. 13.6 that for the simulation there is a trend for the name only (no distractor) condition to be slower than the related name and same person conditions. This pattern is observed in Table 13.1, though the differences are not statistically significant. There is also a non-significant trend in the empirical data for the same person condition to produce faster responses than the related face condition. This is not found to be the case in the simulation presented here. Of course, it is not strictly appropriate to compare a non-significant trend from empirical data with output from the model. (Though note that the levels of activation from the same person and related face conditions are similar, and in fact cross in experiments from the model; see Fig. 13.6). We therefore do not take this difference to be fatal for the model. In fact, any possible facilitative effects from related or same face conditions will depend crucially on the semantic associativity between people. So, for example, in the real situation, famous people will have many SIUs, some of these shared within groups, and some unique. We cannot hope to capture such richness in a simple model of the type used above. However, the situation is clearer in the inhibitory case; when the system is presented

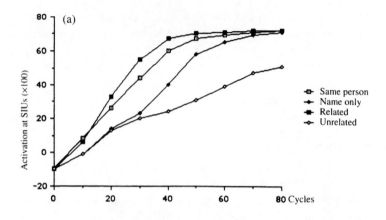

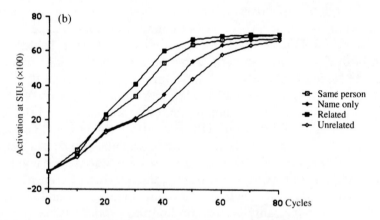

Fig. 13.6 Activation at SIUs after input to FRUs and NIUs. The traces shown are the activations for the SIU associated with name input in each of the four conditions. (a) Data from the intact net. (b) Repetition of the same experiment with the simulation of PH.

Table 13.1 Mean reaction times (ms) for name classification with different types of face distractors by normal subjects (Young *et al.* 1986, experiment 2), and PH (de Haan *et al.* 1987*b*, task 3)

Type of face distractor	Same person	None	Related	Unrelated
Normal subjects	789	821	815	875
PH	1502	1565	1560	1714

with inputs which do not share SIUs in common, the within pool inhibition built into IAC models will ensure that these SIUs will rise slower than if no competing stimulus were present.

We have now shown that it is possible to simulate empirical findings on face–name interference for PH and normal subjects without modification of the architecture used to simulate cross-domain and within-domain semantic priming. For interference, though, there is a noticeable difference in the sizes of effects over the intact and 'lesioned' nets. In the simulation of PH, the interference from an unrelated face distractor appears to be smaller than in the intact net; this is because the 'distractor' face has a smaller influence at PIN level due to attenuated FRU–PIN links. This discrepancy in the size of the effect is not observed in the original data. However, as mentioned above, it is impossible to make accurate comparisons of size of effect in the simulations presented here; instead we are limited to ordinal predictions. This is partly because we do not know the nature of the mapping between 'cycles' in the model and RT data from subjects (other than that it is monotonic). The ordinal prediction concerning relative difficulty of the different conditions (the unrelated condition will be most difficult both for normals and PH) *is* verified in experimental data.

Other effects from the study of PH

Our characterization of PH's deficit raises an interesting possibility. Given the combinative effects of name and face input on person recognition (shown in the model of interference), might it be the case that name input can aid *face* recognition in a prosopagnosic patient? In a further series of experiments with PH, de Haan *et al.* (1991a; see also Young and de Haan 1992) have observed an increased level of performance in face identification due to processing of a name. PH was simultaneously presented with a face and two names, one of these being the correct name for the face. When asked to choose the correct name in a forced-choice task, PH was able to perform above chance, though far from perfectly (30/40, 27/40, 26/40, and 27/40 correct in four separate runs). The same effect has recently been reported by Sergent and Poncet (1990) with another prosopagnosic patient, PV. In this case, PV chose the correct name in 40/48 trials, though once again her performance was below that of control subjects (who made no errors). Interestingly, neither PH nor PV reported any awareness of scoring above chance in this task. The presentation of names did not induce *overt* recognition of the faces.

This pattern appears to have an analogue in the IAC model. When presented with two names and a face simultaneously (i.e. when two NIUs and one FRU are activated), the PIN receiving input from two sources (name and face) rises faster, and stabilizes at a higher level of activation than the PIN receiving input from a name only. This occurs both in the 'lesioned' and intact model. We might postulate that in a forced-choice test the subject would choose the person whose PIN has the highest level of activation, or the PIN which is the first to reach threshold. Note that this proposal is independent of the processes which signal awareness, as the NIU–PIN links are unlesioned, and therefore name input is able to produce activation levels for a familiarity judgement at the PINs. The presence of the 'unrecognized' face simply contributes to this process.

Limits of the simulation of PH

While we have provided an account of some covert recognition effects in normals and PH, we must make clear that there are certain effects that are inaccessible with a model of the present type. In particular, we cannot address the issues of attention or learning using this model.

The problem of attention arises with respect to the interference studies reported above. In the Young *et al.* (1986*d*, experiment 2) procedure, normal subjects are presented simultaneously with a face and a name, and asked to make a semantic judgement to the name only. However, given that both the name and face are recognizable, how is the subject to discriminate between an SIU which has been stimulated through face input and an SIU which has been stimulated through name input? This discrimination is necessary in order to make the correct response. Given that the two stimuli are spatially separated, and present throughout any given trial, a simple solution would be to assert that active *routes* through the system are available for inspection by some homuncular process. However, this is hardly satisfactory without explication of the homuncular process itself.

In fact, this is a general problem for all interference tasks. It has been the topic of much research into the Stroop effect (Stroop 1935). One possible solution is to modulate one pathway into the SIUs through attentional control (Logan 1980). In an attempt to implement such modulation, Cohen *et al.* (1990) introduce specific 'task demand' units into a connectionist model of human performance on the Stroop task. While this approach may provide a solution, the IAC model presented above has no such facility. In order to be clear about the range of phenomena which this model can address, we should point out that we are not in a position to provide an account of selective attention here. Amongst other things, a model incorporating such an account would need to contain representations of spatial location to form the basis of this selective attentional capacity.

Phenomena associated with learning are also at present inaccessible using this model. A number of studies of covert recognition have used a learning paradigm. For instance, de Haan *et al.* (1987*b*, task 5) examined PH's facility to learn associations between faces and semantic categories. This study was based on a paradigm due to Bruyer *et al.* (1983) which requires the patient to examine a number of faces of familiar people, and try to learn an occupation for each. The stimuli are manipulated such that half the associations are veridical and half non-veridical. So in one condition PH was shown the face of Paul Newman, and told that this was the face of an actor. In the second condition he was shown (for example) Geoffrey Boycott's face (an English cricketer), and told that this was a quiz show host. De Haan *et al.* (1987*b*) showed an advantage for learning veridical associations.

Couched in interactive activation terms, this result seems to be due to the fact that learning can take advantage of existing, though attenuated, connections between FRUs and PINs. We postulate that forming a new pathway is more trouble than using an existing one. Although the present model allows the possibility of some learning through modification of connection strengths (see Burton *et al.* 1990), it does not specify a mechanism for the creation of new units or links. There is therefore no account of learning in the normal course of events. This problem is in fact a general one, common to all current functional accounts of face recognition (e.g. Bruce and Young 1986). We are currently exploring ways of introducing such a facility into the model.[2] In the meantime, we can only note that findings with learning tasks are not inconsistent with the general architecture of our model (de Haan *et al.* 1987*b*; Young and de Haan 1988; Sergent and Poncet 1990) but cannot be directly simulated by it in its present form.

Prosopagnosia without covert recognition

PH's covert recognition abilities are not typical of *all* cases of prosopagnosia. Whilst several patients showing covert recognition of familiar faces have been reported, there are now also a number of reports in the literature of prosopagnosic patients who do *not* show these effects

[2]See Burton (1994).

(Bauer 1986; Newcombe *et al.* 1989; Sergent and Villemure 1989; Young and Ellis 1989b). We will now briefly discuss one of these patients, MS (studied by Newcombe *et al.* 1989), in terms of the functional model presented here.

MS contracted a febrile illness in 1970, at the age of 23, and was given a presumptive diagnosis of herpes encephalitis. He has normal visual acuity, and is able to read without difficulty. However, his colour vision is severely impaired, and there is evidence of some impairment in semantic memory, particularly for living things (Young *et al.* 1989). Newcombe and Ratcliff (1974) and Ratcliff and Newcombe (1982) provide a full case description of this patient.

MS is completely unable to recognize familiar faces, scoring 0/20 on tests of both highly familiar and moderately familiar faces (Newcombe *et al.* 1989). He is also poor on matching photographs of unknown people, with a score of 33/54 on the Benton test of facial recognition (Newcombe *et al.* 1989). MS also suffers from object agnosia, recognizing only 8/36 line drawings of familiar objects (Ratcliff and Newcombe 1982).

Newcombe *et al.* (1989) showed that there is no evidence of covert recognition in MS. Unlike PH, he shows no effect of face-to-name semantic priming, though name-to-name semantic priming continues to exist. Furthermore, in a learning task, MS shows no evidence of an advantage for learning 'true' name–face associations over 'false' associations.

In the terms of the model presented here, MS shows no evidence of activation at the PIN level as a result of face input. This could arise for at least three reasons:

(1) the FRU–PIN links have been abolished, or at least more severely attenuated than is the case for PH;

(2) the FRUs themselves are in some way damaged, preventing output being passed along the links to PINs;

(3) the *input* to the FRUs is damaged; that is, the configural processing leading to FRU activation has been impaired.

Explanation 1 would lead to the pattern observed in this patient. As there are no (or only severely attenuated) links between FRU and PIN, activation at FRUs would not be passed to PINs, and so a face input would be unable to cause a rise in activation of a PIN necessary for a familiarity decision. In PH, we assume that there is *some* (sub-threshold) activation passed to a PIN; however, in MS, there is no activation passed to these units from FRUs. There will therefore be no face-to-name semantic priming. In this case, however, there will be preserved name-to-name priming, proceeding through the normal route.

Explanations 2 and 3 also imply that there is no activity at FRUs to be passed along (possibly intact) links to PINs. Once again, a simulation of this patient in which no activation reaches the PINs should show an intact name-to-name semantic priming effect, but no face-to-name semantic priming, and, of course, no overt recognition of faces.

Disrupted configural processing (explanation 3) would be consistent with MS's general object agnosia, and may provide the most natural account of his particular deficit. Given his poor performance in matching faces in different views, it seems likely that the deficit occurs in the system feeding input to FRUs. This account, in terms of higher order perceptual impairment, was the explanation given by Newcombe *et al.* (1989).

Other neurological deficits of person recognition

We have shown how Burton *et al.*'s (1990) interactive activation implementation of the Bruce and Young (1986) functional model of face recognition can provide the basis for a principled account of the impairments underlying different forms of prosopagnosia, and the otherwise puzzling phenomenon of covert recognition. However, if the approach is to be of general utility, it should also be able to encompass other forms of neuropsychological deficit affecting person recognition.

One of the interesting features of functional models is that they can be used to predict the existence of types of neuropsychological deficit which have not previously been observed. A clear example of this arises from the present model. Consider what would happen if the connection strengths between the pool of PINs and the pool of SIUs were reduced. If these links have attenuated strength, then the model would predict intact ability to perform the person familiarity task, whether this is carried out to face or name input, but attenuation of performance in retrieving any semantic information. So, the SIUs will not reach the activation threshold necessary for a semantic decision to be made. The resulting deficit will thus be a domain-independent impairment of access to identity-specific semantic information, with a preserved sense of familiarity. It should be noted that this is quite different from prosopagnosia, since prosopagnosia primarily affects only one input domain (faces), and prosopagnosic patients experience no overt sense of a face's familiarity.

Exactly this predicted pattern of preserved familiarity and impaired access to semantic information has been found in a patient, ME, studied by de Haan *et al.* (1991*b*). ME has high IQ (verbal IQ 120; performance IQ 125), normal short-term memory, language comprehension, and visuoperceptual abilities. However, she has severely impaired long-term memory. ME is able accurately to rate pictures of faces as familiar or not, scoring similarly to controls on familiarity ratings to a line-up of high-familiar, low-familiar, and unfamiliar faces. Similar results hold for her familiarity ratings of names; once again her performance on a name line-up echoes that of controls. The implication of this, couched in terms of the interactive activation model (and in terms of Bruce and Young 1986), is that the system linking FRUs, NIUs, and PINs is intact.

In contrast to this well preserved ability to make familiarity decisions, ME is unable to retrieve semantic information about familiar people from either names or faces. Occasionally she is able to retrieve a broad occupational category such as 'politician' (de Haan *et al.* 1991*b*). However, her performance in accessing appropriate identity-specific semantic information is considerably below that of control subjects.

The case of ME provides further evidence for the modifications of the Bruce and Young (1986) model made by Burton *et al.* (1990). Our characterization of her deficit (i.e. attenuated PIN–SIU links) implies that she should be able to *match* names to faces, despite being unable to retrieve semantic information from either input. This is because the same PIN will rise in response to each input. De Haan *et al.* (1991*b*) chose 26 famous people whom ME was able to categorize as familiar, but about whom she was unable to retrieve any semantic information. She was shown each face, and simultaneously presented orally with three names, one being correct, one being the name of a celebrity from the same occupational category, and one being the name of an unrelated person. ME was very accurate on this task of matching names to faces, scoring 23/26 correct. From this we may conclude that the functional locus of ME's deficit must lie after the point where the face and name recognition systems converge (i.e. the PINs). So, this case provides support for both of our modifications to Bruce and Young's model:

(1) that familiarity decisions are taken at PINs; and
(2) PINs provide gateways to semantic information, rather than storing semantic information themselves.

In addition to re-describing the functional complaint of this patient, the present model has the advantage that it can also make empirical predictions concerning phenomena one might well not think to test – for example, our account of ME's impairment implies that SIUs are active (i.e. above resting state) but below threshold. Thus, for reasons similar to those used above for PH, ME should show some semantic priming both in within-domain and cross-domain variants of semantic priming tasks using the familiarity decision paradigm. It will not necessarily be of the same size as for normal subjects, as the amount of activation passing between PIN and SIU and back to associated PIN will be small. However, it should exist, even if in attenuated form. The ability to make predictions of this type is a powerful feature of the present model.

Discussion and conclusions

We have shown how a model, couched in interactive activation terms, can be used to provide an explanation for different effects observed in patients with impaired recognition of familiar people, both in prosopagnosic and other forms. We have presented demonstrations of observed effects, and proposed possible mechanisms for these. We have also used the model to make empirical predictions about these patients, demonstrating that it has predictive, as well as descriptive, capabilities.

This model provides an advance over previous work in this area. For example, it demonstrates how apparently similar functional deficits can occur for a variety of reasons. So, it is clear that the term prosopagnosia refers not to a single complaint, but to a number of possible deficits, at different locations, each of which lead to different but predictable patterns of behaviour. This much is in fact evident from the empirical papers on which we have drawn, and from the Bruce and Young (1986) functional model. However, the use of a computer implementation has allowed us to progress further in exploring the functional system than did the original unimplemented version. The Bruce and Young (1986) model does not have the same range of predictive power as the present IAC account. As with any modelling exercise, the process of implementation forces one to be explicit about the nature of the elements with which one is dealing. For example, it is not sufficient to specify that FRUs are linked to PINs; instead one must specify exactly what is the nature of these links. For this reason, the unimplemented version could not have predicted the nature of the cross-domain priming effect, or the complex patterns of rising activation in the interference tasks described above.

As we have shown, a simple modification of the Burton et al. (1990) model, involving attenuation of the FRU–PIN connections, can provide an effective simulation of the semantic priming and interference effects from 'unrecognized' faces observed in one form of prosopagnosia. Our account of this form of prosopagnosia has similarities to that offered by

Young and de Haan (1988), in so far as it places emphasis on defective output from intact FRUs, but it also has considerable advantages over Young and de Haan's (1988) account. Not the least of these is, again, that because it involves a computer implementation, we can demonstrate that it has the properties claimed. In addition, it is simpler than Young and de Haan's (1988) account, because all of the necessary properties are achieved without postulating any modification to the basic architecture. In particular, we have demonstrated that the problematic FRU–NIU links proposed by Young and de Haan are unnecessary.

To avoid becoming overenthusiastic, though, we should be clear about the status of the model presented here. It is clearly a functional model, which has its location at the same level of abstraction as standard box and arrow models of cognition. The fact that we have used one form of connectionism (interactive activation) to implement the model does not commit us to any statement about the neurological hardware in which cognition is implemented. The physical instantiation of a lesion can be a loss of connections between neurones. Such a lesion may have the functional effect of attenuating the information passed from one functional location to another. We suggest, then, that the characterization of prosopagnosia as presented here is not implausible given neurological constraints.

We also need to be clear that, although our simulation takes much of the enigma from covert recognition, and shows how the phenomena involved have their place in the operation of normal or disordered systems organized in the way we have described, it is not intended as a solution to more 'philosophical' questions concerning the nature of awareness. Characterizing PH's deficit as a loss of awareness of recognition (de Haan *et al.* 1987*b*; Young and de Haan 1990) remains an adequate description; all we have done here is to reveal something of what might be the underlying mechanism. We do not claim to have solved the problem of what 'awareness' is. Our computer is not 'aware' of 'recognizing' a face just because it passes an arbitrary threshold.

In future work we aim to extend the model to take account of different effects in face recognition. We have mentioned the need to model the learning of faces, and there is also a need for a name output mechanism to be added. There is considerable evidence accruing that naming is a specialized task, more difficult than retrieval of semantic information, and subject to specific deficit (Young *et al.* 1985*a*, 1986*b*; Hanley and Cowell 1988; Flude *et al.* 1989; Brennen *et al.* 1990). The model presented here incorporates only name *input* units, and has nothing to say about the process of name *retrieval*. For this reason it is unable to address such issues as the relative difficulty of name retrieval (compared to retrieval of other semantic information; e.g. Johnston and Bruce 1990; Young *et al.* 1985*a*) or TOT states induced on naming (e.g. Hanley and Cowell 1988; Brennen *et al.* 1990). In current work we are examining how the model presented here might be developed to provide a framework for investigations in these areas (Burton and Bruce 1992).

Appendix

All simulations reported here were run using McClelland and Rumelhart's (1988) interactive activation and competition program IAC. Update functions are given by McClelland and Rumelhart (1988, p. 13). The global parameters were set as follows in all cases:

Maximum activation	1.0
Minimum activation	−0.2
Resting activation	−0.1
Decay rate	0.1
Estr (strength of external input)	0.4
Alpha (strength of excitatory input)	0.1
Gamma (strength of inhibitory input)	0.1

In each of the simulations, excitatory connections had weight 1.0, while inhibitory connections had weight −0.1. In the simulation of PH, excitatory connections between FRU and PIN were reduced to 0.5, while all other connections remained unchanged.

- *References*

Bauer, R. M. (1984). Autonomic recognition of names and faces in prosopagnosia: a neuropsycholgogical application of the guilty knowledge test. *Neuropsychologia*, **22**, 457–69.

Bauer, R. M. (1986). The cognitive psychophysiology of prosopagnosia. In *Aspects of face processing*, (ed. H. D. Ellis, M. A. Jeeves, F. Newcombe, and A. Young), pp. 253–67. Martinus Nijhoff, Dordrecht.

Bodamer, J. (1947). Die Prosop-Agnosie. *Archiv für Psychiatrie und Nervenkrankheiten*, **179**, 6–53.

Brennen, T. J., Baguley, T., Bright, J., and Bruce, V. (1990). Resolving semantically induced tip of the tongue states for proper nouns. *Memory and Cognition*, **18**, 339–47.

Bruce, V. (1983). Recognising faces. *Philosophical Transactions of the Royal Society*, **B302**, 423–36.

Bruce, V. (1986). Recognising familiar faces. In *Aspects of face processing*, (ed. H. D. Ellis, M. A. Jeeves, F. Newcombe, and A. Young), pp. 107–17. Martinus Nijhoff, Dordrecht.

Bruce, V. (1988). *Recognising faces*. Lawrence Erlbaum, London.

Bruce, V. and Valentine, T. (1985). Identity priming in the recognition of familiar faces. *British Journal of Psychology*, **76**, 373–83.

Bruce, V. and Valentine, T. (1986). Semantic priming of familiar faces. *Quarterly Journal of Experimental Psychology*, **38A**, 125–50.

Bruce, V. and Young, A. (1986). Understanding face recognition. *British Journal of Psychology*, **77**, 305–27.

Brunas, J., Young, A. W., and Ellis, A. W. (1990). Repetition priming from incomplete faces: evidence for part to whole completion. *British Journal of Psychology*, **81**, 43–56.

Bruyer, R. (1987). *Les mécanismes de reconnaissance de visages*. Presses Universitaries de Grenoble.

Bruyer, R., Laterre, C., Seron, X., Feyereisen, P., Strypstein, E., Pierrard, E., and Rectem, D. (1983). A case of prosopagnosia with some preserved covert remembrance of familiar faces. *Brain and Cognition*, **2**, 257–84.

Burton, A. M. (1994). Learning new faces in an interactive activation and competition model. *Visual Cognition*, **1**, 313–48.

Burton, A. M. and Bruce, V. (1992). I recognise your face but I can't remember your name: a simple explanation? *British Journal of Psychology*, **83**, 45–60.

Burton, A. M., Bruce, V., and Johnston, R. A. (1990). Understanding face recognition with an interactive activation model. *British Journal of Psychology*, **81**, 361–80.

Carr, T. H., McCauley, C., Sperber, R. D., and Parmelee, C. M. (1982). Words, pictures and priming: on semantic activation, conscious identification, and the automaticity of information processing. *Journal of Experimental Psychology: Human Perception and Performance*, **8**, 757–77.

Cohen, J. D., Dunbar, K., and McClelland, J. L. (1990). On the control of automatic processes: a parallel distributed processing account of the Stroop effect. *Psychological Review*. **97**, 332–61.

Damasio, A. R., Damasio, H., and Van Hoesen, G. W. (1982). Prosopagnosia: anatomic basis and behavioural mechanisms. *Neurology*, **32**, 331–41.

de Haan, E. H. F., Young, A. W., and Newcombe, F. (1987a). Faces interfere with name classification in a prosopagnosic patient. *Cortex*, **23**, 309–16.

de Haan, E. H. F., Young, A. W., and Newcombe, F. (1987b). Face recognition without awareness. *Cognitive Neuropsychology*, **4**, 385–415.

de Haan, E. H. F., Young, A. W., and Newcombe, F. (1991a). Covert and overt recognition in prosopagnosia. *Brain*, **114**, 2575–91.

de Haan, E. H. F., Young, A. W., and Newcombe, F. (1991b). A dissociation between the sense of familiarity and access to semantic information concerning familiar people. *European Journal of Cognitive Psychology*, **3**, 51–67.

De Renzi, E. (1986). Current issues in prosopagnosia. In *Aspects of face processing*, (ed. H. D. Ellis, M. A. Jeeves, F. Newcombe, and A. Young), pp. 243–52. Martinus Nijhoff, Dordrecht.

Ellis, H. D. (1986). Processes underlying face recognition. In *The neuropsychology of face perception and facial expression*, (ed. R. Bruyer), pp. 1–27. Lawrence Erlbaum, Hillsdale, NJ.

Ellis, A. W., Young, A. W., and Hay, D. C. (1987a). Modelling the recognition of faces and words. In *Modelling cognition*, (ed. P. E. Morris), pp. 269–97. Wiley, London.

Ellis, A. W., Young, A. W., Flude, B. M., and Hay, D. C. (1987b). Repetition priming of face recognition. *Quarterly Journal of Experimental Psychology*, **39A**, 193–210.

Flude, B. M., Ellis, A. W., and Kay, J. (1989). Face processing and name retrieval in an anomic aphasic: names are stored separately from semantic information about familiar people. *Brain and Cognition*, **11**, 60–72.

Hanley, J. R. and Cowell, E. (1988). The effects of different types of retrieval cues on the recall of names of famous faces. *Memory and Cognition*, **16**, 545–55.

Hay, D. C. and Young, A. W. (1982). The human face. In *Normality and pathology in cognitive functions*, (ed. A. W. Ellis), pp. 173–202. Academic Press, London.

Hécaen, H. and Angelergues, R. (1962). Agnosia for faces (prosopagnosia). *Archives of Neurology*, **7**, 92–100.

Hinton, G. E. and Anderson, J. A. (1981). *Parallel models of associative memory*. Lawrence Erlbaum, Hillsdale, NJ.

Johnston, R. A. and Bruce, V. (1990). Lost properties: retrieval differences between name codes and semantic codes for familiar people. *Psychological Research*, **52**, 62–7.

Landis, T., Cummings, J. G., Christen, L., Bogen, J. E., and Imhof, H. G. (1986). Are unilateral right posterior cerebral lesions sufficient to cause prosopagnosia? Clinical and radiological findings in six additional patients. *Cortex*, **22**, 243–52.

Logan, G. D. (1980). Attention and automaticity in Stroop and priming tasks: theory and data. *Cognitive Psychology*, **12**, 523–53.

McCauley, C., Parmelee, C., Sperber, R., and Carr, T. (1980). Early extraction of meaning from pictures and its relation to conscious identification. *Journal of Experimental Psychology: Human Perception and Performance*, **6**, 265–76.

McClelland, J. L. and Rumelhart, D. E. (1988). *Explorations in parallel distributed processing*. Bradford, Cambridge, MA.

McClelland, J. L. and Rumelhart, D. E. (1981). An interactive activation model of the effect of context in perception, Part 1. An account of basic findings. *Psychological Review*, **88**, 375–406.

McClelland, J. L., Rumelhart, D. E., and the PDP Research Group (1986). *Parallel distributed processing: explorations in the in microstructure of cognition. Vol II: Applications*. Bradford, Cambridge, MA.

McWeeny, K. H., Young, A. W., Hay, D. C., and Ellis, A. W. (1987). Putting names to faces. *British Journal of Psychology*, **78**, 143–9.

Meadows, J. C. (1974). The anatomical basis of prosopagnosia. *Journal of Neurology. Neurosurgery, and Psychiatry*, **37**, 489–501.

Newcombe, F. and Ratcliff, G. (1974). Agnosia: a disorder of object recognition. In *Les syndromes de disconnexion calleuse chez l'homme*, (ed. F. Michel and B, Schott), pp. 317–41. Colloque Internationale de Lyon.

Newcombe, F., Young, A. W., and de Haan, E. H. F. (1989). Prosopagnosia and object agnosia without covert recognition. *Neuropsychologia*, **27**, 179–91.

Ratcliff, G. and Newcombe, F. (1982). Object recognition: some deductions from the clinical evidence. In *Normality and pathology in cognitive function*, (ed. A. W. Ellis), pp. 147–71. Academic, London.

Renault, B., Signoret, J. L., DeBruille, B., Breton, F., and Bolgert, F. (1989). Brain potentials reveal covert facial recognition in prosopagnosia. *Neuropsychologica*, **27**, 905–12.

Rizzo, M., Hurtig, R., and Damasio, A. R. (1987). The role of scanpaths in facial recognition and learning. *Annals of Neurology*, **22**, 41–5.

Rumelhart, D. E., McClelland, J. L., and the PDP Research Group (1986). *Parallel distributed processing: explorations in the microstructure of cognition, Vol. I: Foundations*. Bradford, Cambridge, MA.

Schacter, D. L., McAndrews, M. P., and Moscovitch, M. (1988). Access to consciousness: dissociations between implicit and explicit knowledge in neuropsychological syndromes. In *Thought without language*, (ed. L. Weiskrantz), pp. 242–78. Oxford University Press.

Sergent, J. and Poncet, M. (1990). From covert to overt recognition of faces in a prosopagnosic patient. *Brain*, **113**, 989–1004.

Sergent, J. and Villemure, J.-G. (1989). Prosopagnosia in a right hemispherectomized patient. *Brain*, **112**, 975–95.

Stroop. J. R. (1935). Studies of interference in serial verbal reactions. *Journal of Experimental Psychology*, **18**, 643–62.

Tranel, D. and Damasio, A. R. (1985). Knowledge without awareness: an autonomic index of facial recognition by prosopagnosics. *Science*, **228**, 1453–4.

Tranel, D., Damasio, A. R., and Damasio, H. (1988). Intact recognition of facial expression, gender and age in patients with impaired recognition of face identity. *Neurology*, **38**, 690–6.

Valentine, T. and Bruce, V. (1986). Recognising familiar faces: the role of distinctiveness and familiarity. *Canadian Journal of Psychology*, **40**, 300–5.

Yarmey, A. D. (1973). I recognise your face but I can't remember your name: further evidence on the tip-of-the-tongue phenomenon. *Memory and Cognition*, **1**, 287–90.

Young, A. W. (1988). Functional organization of visual recognition. In *Thought without language*, (ed. L. Weiskrantz), pp. 78–107. Oxford University Press.

Young, A. W. and Bruce, V. (1991). Perceptual categories and the computation of 'grandmother'. *European Journal of Cognitive Psychology*, **3**, 5–49.

Young, A. W. and de Haan, E. H. F. (1988). Boundaries of covert recognition in prosopagnosia. *Cognitive Neuropsychology*, **5**, 317–36.

Young, A. W. and de Haan, E. H. F. (1990). Impairments of visual awareness. *Mind and Language*, **5**, 29–48.

Young, A. W. and de Haan, E. H. F. (1992). Face recognition and awareness after brain injury. In *The neuropsychology of consciousness*, (ed. A. D. Milner and M. Rugg), pp. 69–90. Academic, London.

Young. A. W. and Ellis, H. D. (1989*a*). Semantic processing. In *Handbook of research on face processing*, (ed. A. W. Young and H. D. Ellis), pp. 235–62. North-Holland, Amsterdam.

Young, A. W., Hay, D. C., and Ellis, A. W. (1985a). The faces that launched a thousand slips: everyday difficulties and errors in recognising people. *British Journal of Psychology*, **76**, 495–523.

Young, A. W., Hay, D. C., McWeeny, K. H., Ellis, A. W. and Barry, C. (1985b). Familiarity decisions for faces presented to the left and right cerebral hemispheres. *Brain and Cognition*, **4**, 439–50.

Young, A. W., Hay, D. C., McWeeny, K. H., Flude, B. M., and Ellis, A. W. (1985c). Matching familiar and unfamiliar faces on internal and external features. *Perception*, **14**, 737–46.

Young, A. W., McWeeny, K. H., Hay, D. C., and Ellis, A. W. (1986a). Access to identity-specific semantic codes from familiar faces. *Quarterly Journal of Experimental Psychology*, **38A**, 271–95.

Young, A. W., McWeeny, K. H., Ellis, A. W., and Hay, D. C. (1986b). Naming and categorising faces and written names. *Quarterly Journal of Experimental Psychology*, **38A**, 297–318.

Young, A. W., McWeeny, K. H., Hay, D. C., and Ellis, A. W. (1986c). Matching familiar and unfamiliar faces on identity and expression. *Psychological Research*, **48**, 63–8.

Young, A. W., Ellis, A. W., Flude, B. M., McWeeny, K. H., and Hay, D. C. (1986d). Face–name interference. *Journal of Experimental Psychology: Human Perception and Performance*, **12**, 466–75.

Young, A. W., Hellawell, D., and de Haan, E. H. F. (1988). Cross-domain semantic priming in normal subjects and a prosopagnosic patient. *Quarterly Journal of Experimental Psychology*, **40A**, 561–80.

Young, A. W., Newcombe, F., Hellawell, D., and de Haan, E. H. F. (1989). Implicit access to semantic information. *Brain and Cognition*, **11**, 186–209.

14

Consciousness

Reprinted in abridged form from Young, A. W. and Block, N. (1996), Consciousness, in *Unsolved mysteries of the mind: tutorial essays in cognition*, (ed. V. Bruce), pp. 149–79, Hove, East Sussex. Erlbaum (UK) Taylor and Francis. With kind permission of Professor N. Block and Psychology Press (Erlbaum UK, Taylor and Francis).

Summary

Consciousness remains the greatest unsolved mystery of the mind. At present, we have no idea how to get a fully satisfying account. None the less, some modest progress has been made in identifying different aspects of the problem, marshalling pertinent data, and exploring the feasibility of different types of solution. So all is not hopeless. In fact, many contemporary discussions in philosophy, psychology, and neuroscience share a widespread perception that we are at last starting to get somewhere with this very difficult topic.

The explanatory gap

How it is that anything so remarkable as a state of consciousness comes about as a result of irritating nervous tissue, is just as unaccountable as the appearance of Djin when Aladdin rubbed his lamp.

So said T. H. Huxley in 1866. This explanatory gap (Levine 1983) is still with us. Advances in neuroscience have not given us an account of subjective experience – what it is like to see red, have a pain, or just to be awake.

For example, it has been known for many years that wakefulness and arousal are influenced by the brainstem reticular formation, and especially noradrenergic neurones in the locus coeruleus. These and many other facts about sleep and wakefulness are presented in text-books of physiological psychology (Carlson 1991). In essence, we know that when we are awake, it is because neurotransmitters are sprinkled into the synapses of huge numbers of neurones in the cerebral cortex by ascending pathways with very widespread projections. Similarly, doctors are able to distinguish different levels of perturbation of consciousness, ranging from delirium through stupor and coma to brain death, and they know many of the neuroanatomical correlates of such states (Bates and Cartlidge 1994). These facts certainly point us to the view that consciousness is a product of brain activity, because it is clear that it is intimately linked to the underlying anatomy and biochemistry. For this reason, we can reject the Cartesian view that consciousness does not have a physical basis; instead, it is undoubtedly a product of what our brains are doing at the time. However, the explanatory gap remains; the anatomical and biochemical facts seem to tell us nothing about what it *feels* like to be conscious. Worse, it is hard to even imagine future work in neuroscience that would close this gap.

What we would like is a theory that links the activity of cortical neurones to consciousness, or at least to some aspect of consciousness. Then we could understand what it feels like to be us in terms of a combination of our understanding of the functions of cortical neurones and the modulatory influences of neurotransmitters.

Many philosophers and neuroscientists believe that the explanatory gap will close and then disappear as our knowledge of brain function increases (Flanagan 1992). However, at present the gap remains dauntingly large.

A neurobiological theory

To take a closer look into this chasm, let's buy the story that what we must do is to marry our knowledge of the modulatory properties of neurotransmitter systems to an account of how cortical neurones mediate at least one aspect of consciousness. For this purpose, we can select visual awareness as the aspect of consciousness we will explore, because the anatomy of the visual system has been studied extensively and a detailed account of visual awareness has been offered by Crick and Koch (1990).

Crick and Koch (1990) are quite clear in their enterprise; they recognize that our awareness of the things we see forms an important aspect of consciousness, they claim that it requires a scientific explanation, and they consider that the problem can only be solved by an explanation at the neural level. To this end, they seek to define what unusual features might be characteristic of the activity of neurones in the cerebral cortex concerned with vision when we are conscious of seeing something.

This seems like a reasonable start. We know that consciousness is not simply a consequence of *any* neuronal activity because there are plenty of things the neurones in our central nervous systems do that seem to be independent of consciousness, like adjusting the size of the eye's pupil to the prevailing illumination, or which carry on automatically but can be subject to occasional conscious intervention, like breathing. In general, these automatic activities do not require the activity of neurones in the cerebral cortex. Even for the cerebral cortex, though, neuronal activity is not in itself sufficient to produce consciousness; studies of the brain's electrical activity show that when we are in deep sleep, cortical neurones still do something, but that something is different from how they function when we are awake (Carlson 1991). Conversely, we know that when cortical neurones are damaged, loss of sensation can result. In the case of vision, damage to the visual cortex creates a region of apparent blindness which can be mapped and related precisely to the area of damaged cortical tissue (Kolb and Whishaw 1990).

Putting these facts together it is clear that intact visual cortex is necessary for normal visual experience, but that normal visual experience only happens when cortical neurones are working in a certain way.

Anatomical studies of the visual system have revealed a startlingly intricate arrangement, involving distinct areas in the cerebral cortex and several parallel cortical and subcortical visual pathways (Weiskrantz 1990; Zeki 1993). In general, it seems that the task of seeing is devolved to separate processing streams containing components that have become specialized for particular purposes, responding selectively to wavelength (needed for colour perception), orientation (for perception of form and space), temporal change (movement), and so on. This holds not only for basic aspects of vision, such as the perception of lightness and orientation, but also for higher order visual abilities involved in the perception and recognition of complex shapes, such as faces (Perrett *et al.* 1992).

These specialist areas in the brain have been shaped by evolution, and during evolution specialization can carry costs as well as benefits. Hence, the optimal balance of costs and benefits is likely to allow scope for some cross-talk between specialist areas, and we would not expect the kind of discrete components found in a human-engineered product like a radio.

The presence of functional specialization has led neurophysiologists to propose that the brain must somehow coordinate activity within and between these different specialist regions to achieve an integrated percept; this is known as the binding problem. Crick and Koch (1990, p. 269) put it like this:

If you are currently paying attention to a friend discussing some point with you, neurons in area MT that respond to the motion of his face, neurons in area V4 that respond to its hue, neurons in auditory cortex that respond to the words coming from his face and possibly the memory traces associated with recognition of the face all have to be 'bound' together, to carry a common label identifying them as neurons that jointly generate the perception of that specific face.

The solution proposed by Crick and Koch is that binding is achieved through a degree of synchronization of the firing of the neurones involved so that 'neurons in different parts of cortex responding to the currently perceived object fire action potentials at about the same time' (Crick and Koch 1990, p. 270). In particular, they note evidence of synchronous firing of some neurones in the cat's cerebral cortex, with frequencies in the 40–70 Hz range. This synchronized activity is, in Crick and Koch's view (1990, p. 272), how binding takes place:

We suggest that one of the functions of consciousness is to present the result of various underlying computations and that this involves an attentional mechanism that temporarily binds the relevant neurons together by synchronizing their spikes in 40 Hz oscillations. These oscillations do not themselves encode additional information, except in so far as they join together some of the existing information into a coherent percept. We shall call this form of awareness 'working awareness'.

Although it is obviously speculative, this is an ambitious attempt to tie visual awareness to a particular feature of cortical activity. Right or wrong, it therefore has much to commend it, because it is detailed, clear, and potentially falsifiable. Moreover, the same general approach has been adopted in other cases where there is an apparent need to bind together different parts of the visual scene that belong with each other, as in shape recognition (Hummel and Biederman 1992), and it has even been suggested that synchronized oscillations can usefully be incorporated into models of language understanding and human reasoning (Shastri and Ajjanagadde 1993). This wide applicability of the idea of dynamic binding through synchronized oscillation is consistent with Crick and Koch's view that it may prove to be a quite general feature of consciousness. But how much can this approach explain?

Crick and Koch's claim is that a solution to the binding problem will provide a basis for understanding visual awareness. There is some plausibility to the idea that binding and consciousness might be intimately related, because the binding problem gains its force from the discrepancy between the subjective unity of visual experience (on which, more later) and the apparently fragmented nature of visual processing pathways in the brain. For example, when we see a moving blue square, the movement, colour, and shape are represented in different cortical areas and pathways, yet we experience them as attributes of a single object. However, we have a suspicion that looking for a direct solution to this neat trick in the form of a binding agent may prove as misleading as searching the brain for the little screen on which the visual picture is assembled and displayed.

For the sake of the argument, though, we will set aside the insidious possibility that there is actually no distinguishable binding mechanism. This allows us to focus on the hypothesis that the neural basis of binding is to be found in phase-locked 40 Hz neural oscillations. Let us suppose that this is indeed true. But how does a 40 Hz neural oscillation explain, as Nagel (1974) put it, what it is like to be us? What is so special about a 40 Hz oscillation as opposed to some other physical state?

To see the force of this point, one needs only to consider the implications of the fact that binding through synchronized activity is already being incorporated into some computer simulations (Hummel and Biederman 1992; Shastri and Ajjanagadde 1993). Does this mean that building some form of binding machinery into its program makes the computer conscious? We suspect not, but in the absence of any convincing reason to settle the argument either way, it has to be conceded that binding in itself offers an incomplete account.

Because of this incompleteness, one can ask why couldn't there be weird green space creatures with brains just like ours in their physical and functional properties, including their 40 Hz oscillation patterns, whose owners' experiences were very unlike ours, or who were zombies with no subjective experiences at all? We don't have to suppose that there really could be creatures with brains just like ours who have different experiences or no experiences to ask for an account of why not. But no one has a clue about how to answer these questions.

To be fair to Crick and Koch, they did not set out to solve this particular problem. Instead, they argue that several topics are best set aside at the moment, and they include among these the problem of qualia (whether my experience of red is the same as yours, what it feels like to be me, etc.). But unless this problem is addressed, the explanatory gap remains. Even though we might reasonably feel that Crick and Koch's hypothesis has the potential to reduce the gap a little bit, we have not been given compelling reasons to expect that in future a large number of similar small reductions will suffice to eliminate it.

Perspectives from philosophy

We gain some perspective on the explanatory gap if we contrast the issue of the physical and functional basis of consciousness with the issue of the physical and functional basis of thought. In the case of thought, we do have theoretical proposals about what thought is, or at least what human thought might be, in scientific terms. Cognitive scientists have had some success in explaining some features of thought processes in terms of the notions of representation and computation. There are many disagreements among cognitive scientists; especially notable is the disagreement between connectionists and classical 'language of thought' theorists (Ramsey *et al* 1991). However, the notable fact is that in the case of thought, we actually have more than one substantive research programme and their proponents are busy fighting it out, comparing which research programme handles which phenomena best.

It is true that some philosophers have expressed concern that an approach that views the mind as the embodiment of a computer program, instead of grounding its explanations securely in biology, is at best incomplete and quite possibly doomed to failure (Searle 1984). We share some of these concerns, but remain impressed by the achievements of the segment of cognitive science that is oriented around the computer model of the mind (Johnson-Laird 1988). Cognitive science can provide a platform from which to work towards a neurobiology of thought. But in the case of consciousness, we have nothing worthy of being called an equivalent research programme. Researchers are stumped.

Needless to say, philosophers have taken many different attitudes towards this problem, but four of them stand out. First, there is *eliminativism*, the view that consciousness as it is commonly understood involves a set of conceptual confusions in our everyday beliefs, and hence simply does not exist (Dennett 1988). So there is nothing for there to be an explanatory gap about. Second, we have various forms of *reductionism*, notably functionalism and physicalism. According to these views, there is such a thing as consciousness, but there is no singular explanatory gap; that is, there are no mysteries concerning the physical basis of consciousness that differ in kind from run of the mill unsolved scientific problems about the physical and functional basis of liquidity, inheritance, or computation. On this view, there is an explanatory gap, but it is unremarkable. A third view is what Flanagan (1992) calls the new mysterianism. Its most extreme form is *transcendentalism* (White 1991), the view that consciousness is simply not a natural phenomenon and is not explainable in terms of science at all. A less extreme form of new mysterianism is that of McGinn (1991), which concedes that consciousness is a natural phenomenon but emphasizes *our* problem in understanding the physical basis of consciousness. McGinn argues that there are physical properties of our brains that do in fact explain consciousness, but although this explanation might be available to some other type of being, it is cognitively closed off to us; just as we can understand the motor system of a cockroach even though the cockroach cannot, so a superior being might be able to understand the physical explanation of human consciousness, but humans cannot. A fourth view that has no well known name (Flanagan 1992; Nagel 1974; Searle 1992), holds that although there may be important differences between a naturalistic explanation of consciousness and naturalistic explanations of other phenomena, there is no convincing reason to regard consciousness as non-natural or unexplainable in naturalistic terms. This view is suggested by Nagel's remark that we are like the person ignorant of relativity theory who is told that matter is a form of energy but who does not have the concepts necessary to appreciate how. The explanatory gap exists because we lack the scientific concepts. But future theory may provide those concepts.

Forms of consciousness

The wide range of opinions held by those who have written about consciousness reflect the difficulty of the topic and our current scientific ignorance. However, we also think that they represent a degree of confusion, best epitomized by the widely adopted assumption that there is a single phenomenon denoted by 'consciousness' that requires a unitary explanation. This assumption allows discussions of consciousness to proceed as if everyone is talking about the same thing. This has rightly been considered unwise (Allport 1988), and our view is that, like many complex phenomena, consciousness involves different aspects which will need to be accounted for in different ways. We thus reject the idea that one should seek *the* solution to *the* problem of consciousness; instead, it is essential to be clear about which aspect of consciousness each putative solution is meant to cover.

As a start, we will distinguish some different phenomena that terms like 'consciousness' and 'awareness' (we regard these as approximate synonyms) are used to designate:

1. *Phenomenal consciousness*: the experience of seeing, hearing, feeling pain, etc.
2. *Access consciousness*: a mental state is access conscious if you can think about it, report its content, and use it to guide action. Access

consciousness applies most directly to occurrent states, but we can extend the notion to memories. In this extended sense, we are access conscious when recognizing an object or a face or remembering a past event

3. *Monitoring and self-consciousness*: this would include thinking about one's own actions and their effects, and monitoring perceptual information for discrepancies with current plans and hypotheses. Self-consciousness also involves the possession of a concept of the self and the ability to use this concept in thinking about oneself. It is possible to distinguish monitoring from self-consciousness (for example, not all monitoring seems to involve consciousness of self), but we have kept them together here because much of self-consciousness involves monitoring what one is doing.

This list is grounded in the distinctions made by Block (1991). Of course, we recognize that there are also different forms of consciousness *within* each of these different categories. It seems obvious enough that the phenomenal awareness involved in seeing something is not like phenomenal awareness of hearing or touch, and even within vision the phenomenal 'feel' of colour, shape, and other visual attributes can be quite different. Similarly, remembering what you did on your holidays last year is a different experience to recognizing that an object is a table, even though both are considered forms of access consciousness because they involve bringing stored knowledge to mind, and access to the content of one's thought is different from access to the content of one's pain. Likewise, monitoring the process of stopping your car at a red traffic light need not involve the same skills as monitoring the course of a conversation.

So any complete explanation is going to need to be able both to account for different forms of consciousness and to account for each of the variants within each form. Clearly, it is going to look quite complicated, but we should not be deterred by complications if they are needed to establish the true state of affairs.

So far, we have mainly been talking about phenomenal consciousness. But the other concepts of consciousness, (access consciousness, monitoring consciousness, and self-consciousness) bear a special relationship to phenomenal consciousness. One could imagine phenomenal consciousness (e.g. the sensation of seeing red) without access consciousness, monitoring, or self-consciousness. For example, many people have had the experience of noticing a loud noise and *at the same time* realizing that the noise has been going on for some time and that they had been hearing it for some time. So the experience of a loud

noise took place for a time without the reasoning system having access
to the content of that experience, and without any thought to the effect
that one was having that experience. But it is harder to imagine any of
these without some form of phenomenal consciousness. Perhaps we can
imagine a zombie who has access consciousness without phenomenal
consciousness. But it is hard to imagine how we non-zombies could be in
such a situation. This makes it easy for eliminativists or reductionists
about phenomenal consciousness to tacitly slide from phenomenal
consciousness to one or another of these other concepts, which are more
clearly functional in nature.

We have said that access consciousness and monitoring consciousness
are more clearly functional in nature. That is to say they are constituted
by information-processing relations and so are obviously in the domain
of current cognitive theories. Phenomenal consciousness, by contrast, is
not self-evidently a cognitive phenomenon at all.

There are important differences between access consciousness and
phenomenal consciousness that must be acknowledged. The type of
consciousness depends on the type of content; a phenomenally conscious state must have phenomenal content, and an access-conscious
state must have representational content. Access consciousness is
therefore a functional notion, but phenomenal consciousness is not.
Whereas access consciousness applies to state tokens, or rather tokens
at times, phenomenal consciousness is best thought of as a feature of
state types. Let us explain. The following inscription, 'teeth', which you
have just read, contains five letter tokens, but of only three letter types.
There is a token of the type bath in many houses, but the type bath itself
is an abstract object that doesn't exist anywhere in space–time. Here is
why access is a matter of tokens at times: a single token state might be
access conscious at one time but not another, because of changes in
information flow in the system, just as your keys are accessible at some
times but not others (e.g. when you lose them). The type is neither
access conscious or not; access consciousness is a feature of tokens. By
contrast, there is such a thing as a phenomenally conscious type or kind
of state. For example, the feel of pain is a phenomenally conscious type
or kind of state. Every pain must have that feel.

In distinguishing a number of different concepts of consciousness, we
are claiming that for serious thinking we need this kind of conceptual
clarification. There are two notable sorts of trouble that writers get into
by not making these distinctions; both involve conflating different forms
of consciousness. One is to be found in Jaynes (1976) and Dennett
(1991), who allege that consciousness is a cultural construction; Jaynes
even gives its invention a date between the events reported in the

Odyssey and the *Iliad*. Of course, certain aspects of consciousness do indeed show clear evidence of being culturally constructed; especially some features of self-consciousness (Neisser 1988). However, Jaynes (1976) and Dennett (1991) seem to be talking about phenomenal consciousness; but, with no disrespect to the ancient Greeks, if one accepts the distinctions we have described, consciousness could not have been *invented* by anyone. If there is such a thing as phenomenal consciousness, it has been around for a very long time as a basic biological feature of us. What Jaynes and Dennett ought to be saying is that there is no such thing as phenomenal consciousness as distinct from the other consciousnesses. They ought to be reductionists or eliminativists about consciousness. The conflation is especially apparent in Jaynes (1976), where 'consciousness' in the sense in which it is supposed to have been invented by the Greeks is something like a *theory* of consciousness in roughly the phenomenal sense.

A second type of problem of conflation has nothing to do with reductionism or eliminativism. Consider, for example, Searle's (1992) reasoning about a function of consciousness. Searle mentions Penfield's description of epilepsy patients suffering absence (*petit mal*) seizures who are apparently 'totally unconscious', but none the less continue their activities of walking or driving home or playing a piano piece, but in an inflexible and uncreative way. Searle says that the lack of consciousness explains the lack of flexibility and creativity, and so one of the functions of consciousness is to add powers of flexibility and creativity. Searle is talking about the function of *phenomenal consciousness*, but he gives no reason to think that people suffering absence seizures lack *that* kind of consciousness. For example, Searle describes the epileptic walker as threading his way through the crowd. Isn't there something it is like for him to see, say, a street corner, at which he knows to turn right? What is most obviously deficient in these patients is not phenomenal consciousness, but monitoring and self-consciousness. When Penfield said that the patients are totally unconscious, he appears to have had some sort of monitoring consciousness in mind, not phenomenal consciousness.

Selective impairments of consciousness

We have shown that distinguishing different types of consciousness can help in discussing theoretical issues. However, we also claim that these distinctions have direct empirical importance. Specifically, different types of brain injury can lead to impairments that affect one or other of the forms of consciousness we have outlined, often in highly selective ways. The existence of these selective impairments of consciousness suggests that they are implemented by different neural mechanisms, and strongly supports the utility of the underlying distinctions.

A wide range of neuropsychological impairments can be considered relevant (Milner and Rugg 1992; Schacter *et al.* 1988; Young and de Haan 1990). Here, we will look at some examples of problems affecting phenomenal consciousness, access consciousness, and monitoring and self-consciousness.

Phenomenal consciousness

A consequence of brain injury involving the primary visual cortex, area V1, can be a loss of vision for part of the visual field, known as a scotoma. To test for a visual field defect the person is usually asked to report what he or she sees when stimuli are presented at different locations in the visual field. Notice that vision is tested by asking about phenomenal consciousness, and that this is lost for stimuli presented within the scotoma. Such work has shown that there is an orderly mapping of the area of lost vision onto the damaged region of visual cortex.

The fact that the loss of phenomenal visual consciousness can be restricted to an area corresponding to the damaged region of visual cortex is in itself of considerable interest, as it so clearly highlights the role of visual cortex in the creation of phenomenal visual experience. However, what has really captured the attention off neuroscientists and philosophers has been the demonstration of accurate responses to visual stimuli presented within the scotoma (Pöppel *et al.* 1973; Weiskrantz 1986, 1990; Weiskrantz *et al.* 1974). These accurate responses are usually elicited with tasks in which the patient is encouraged to 'guess' what has been presented. Weiskrantz's term 'blindsight' neatly sums up the paradoxical result of accurate responses to stimuli that people insist they do not 'see', and for which there is no phenomenal visual experience.

Weiskrantz *et al.* (1974) showed that their patient, DB, could point to where he guessed a flash of light had been presented, and that he could discriminate the orientation of stimuli presented within his scotoma. By asking DB to guess whether a presented stimulus was a sine-wave grating of vertical dark and light bars they were able to determine his visual acuity (in terms of the narrowest grating that could be detected). Gratings with bar widths of 1.5′ could be detected in the sighted part of his field of vision, and a rather less fine but still impressive 1.9′ in the 'blind' field.

Later studies have confirmed and extended the original findings. In particular, DB could detect the presence or absence of a light stimulus even when it was introduced or extinguished quite slowly; he could readily distinguish static from moving stimuli; and more detailed testing of acuity in the scotoma showed that (unlike normal vision) it increased as the stimuli were moved to positions further away from fixation.

As well as using forced-choice guessing, blindsight phenomena can be demonstrated by very different methods; Weiskrantz (1986, 1990) gives authoritative reviews. For example, it is possible to demonstrate automatic reactions in the form of skin conductance changes (Zihl *et al.* 1980) or altered pupil diameter (Weiskrantz 1990). Several studies have also demonstrated interactions between stimuli presented in the blind and sighted parts of the visual field. Pizzamiglio *et al.* (1984) noted that a full-field rotating disc produced a larger subjective tilt than did stimulation of one visual hemifield alone, for both normal and hemianopic subjects. Marzi *et al.* (1986) found that bilateral light flashes produced faster reaction times to detect a flash than did a single unilateral stimulus, even when one of the bilateral flashes fell in a hemianopic area of the visual field, from which a single flash would not have been detected.

Some of the most tantalizing findings were noted by Torjussen (1976, 1978), who found that patients with right hemianopias reported seeing a circle when it was presented so as to fall half in the blind and half in the sighted region, but they reported seeing a semicircle if this was presented in the sighted region, and nothing if a semicircle was presented in the blind right visual field. Torjussen's findings are particularly significant because they show that the interaction between the stimuli in the blind and sighted parts of the visual field can affect what people report that they see in the blind region. Notice that presenting a semicircle in the blind field alone was insufficient for it to be perceived, but essentially the same stimulus was reported as having been seen when it formed part of a complete figure that extended into the sighted field.

Studies of blindsight, then, strongly suggest that the processing of visual stimuli can take place even when there is no phenomenal awareness of seeing them. Although accurate visual processing is involved, the pathways mediating these effects do not have the same sensitivity as normal vision. It has been widely speculated that the non-conscious visual processing found in blindsight is mediated subcortically, but detailed study of the visual pathways underlying these effects has shown clear involvement of cerebral cortex outside the primary visual area V1 (Cowey and Stoerig 1991, 1992). This can happen because the primary visual pathway through area V1 is not the only visual pathway with cortical projections; there are other pathways that bypass V1. Hence, visual areas outside V1 can be involved in visual functions without corresponding visual experience.

Work on achromatopsia is also relevant. Achromatopsic patients experience the world in shades of grey, or in less severe cases, colours can look very washed out (Meadows 1974). This is quite different to the forms of colour-blindness produced by deficiencies in one of the three types of cone receptor in the retina, for which there is still experience of colour but certain colours are not discriminated from each other. Instead, severe achromatopsias produced by cortical injury are described by the patients themselves in terms that suggest they are experienced as more like watching black and white television. Hence, achromatopsia provides an interesting example of loss of one aspect of visual experience – colour.

The full details of the mechanisms underlying human colour vision are not known, but some of their essential features have been established. The retina contains three types of cone, each of which is maximally sensitive to light of a different wavelength. Outputs from these three types of cone are converted into colour-opponent signals, and a separate luminance (brightness) response.

This arrangement means that we are more sensitive to light of certain wavelengths than others, and the shape of the function relating light sensitivity to wavelength for normal daytime vision has distinct peaks which, because of the opponent cone mechanisms, do not correspond to the sensitivity peaks of the cones themselves. Heywood et al. (1991) therefore measured this spectral sensitivity function for an achromatopsic patient who has no experience of colour, MS. Their study followed up previous observations of preserved behavioural responses to wavelength for this patient (Mollon et al. 1980). In Heywood et al.'s (1991) test, MS described all the stimuli he saw as 'dim white' or 'grey', despite the differences in wavelength. Similarly, other work established that MS could not match or name colours, and performed at random when asked to arrange colour patches by hue. However, although MS showed a general overall loss of sensitivity, Heywood et al. (1991) found that he showed maximal sensitivity to the same wavelengths as a normal observer. This demonstrates the presence of opponent cone mechanisms despite the complete loss of colour experience.

There is a striking difference between the absence of colour experience for MS and the preservation of opponent cone mechanisms shown in his spectral sensitivity function. This difference is highlighted by the fact that MS was also able to detect boundaries defined by a change in wavelength, which would look like a change in colour to a normal observer. MS could do this even when the colours on each side of the boundary were of matched brightness (Heywood *et al.* 1991). Thus, he was able to distinguish whether or not a series of hues was in the correct chromatic order as long as the adjacent colour patches abutted one another. If a small (5 mm) gap was introduced between each colour patch, his performance deteriorated to chance level. Heywood *et al.* (1991) account for this by suggesting that the salience of any chromatic border will depend on the contrast between the hues on each side of the border; a random series of adjacent colour patches will have some very sharp borders (where very different hues abut each other) and some that are less sharp, whereas for an ordered series there should be no variation in the salience of each border.

In cases of achromatopsia, then, there is evidence that some aspects of colour processing mechanisms continue to function. However, although some of the cortical mechanisms that show sensitivity to different wavelengths still operate, there is no subjective experience of colour.

Memory and recognition without access consciousness

Access consciousness is involved when we remember something that happened in the past, or recognize a familiar object or face. Amnesic patients, who often cannot remember what they were doing a few hours ago, are therefore experiencing a dense impairment of access consciousness. In such cases, performance in direct tests of memory can be at chance. Direct tests would include recalling the items from a list learned earlier, picking them out from a list of previously learned items and new distractors, and so on. Following Warrington and Weiskrantz (1968, 1970), however, many studies have documented preserved memory in amnesia if memory is tested indirectly, through priming effects.

Warrington and Weiskrantz (1968, 1970) asked amnesic patients to identify fragmented pictures or words, and showed that subsequent identification of the same stimuli was facilitated. In other words, it becomes easier to recognize a fragmented picture of an object if you have already had to recognize the same object before. This type of finding holds as much for amnesics as for normal people, and it can be obtained for amnesic patients even when they fail to remember having taken part in any previous testing sessions. Such findings seem to arise when amnesics' memories are tested indirectly, in terms of the facilitation of subsequent recognition of the same stimuli (Schacter 1987). As we have noted, direct tests, such as asking whether or not items were among those previously shown, lead to very poor performance. Hence amnesics show a form of memory without access consciousness, in which their performance can be affected by previous experiences they completely fail to remember overtly. Access consciousness of a content, you will recall, is a matter of a representation of its content being 'inferentially promiscuous', that is, freely available as a premise in reasoning, and in the consequent utility of these contents in guiding action and speech. The amnesic patients just mentioned have memory representations that affect their responses when they encounter the fragmented stimuli again, but not so as to produce access consciousness.

The key point here is that in amnesia the central difficulty need not be with memory *per se*, as priming effects clearly involve a form of remembering. Rather, the problem lies in being able to deploy the remembered information in reasoning, guiding action, and reporting; in other words, it does look like a failure of access consciousness. Of course, there is also a failure of monitoring consciousness, because the patient does not know he or she has any memory of the event, but the failures of access and monitoring are distinct. What is not clear, though, is whether access consciousness, which is so conspicuously lacking in amnesia, depends on a different memory system to that involved in priming effects on indirect tests, or whether it involves adding something to what are essentially the same memory traces.

An even more circumscribed deficit of access consciousness can be found in prosopagnosia, an uncommon neurological deficit affecting the recognition of familiar faces. Although prosopagnosic patients no longer recognize familiar faces overtly, there is substantial evidence of covert recognition from physiological and behavioural measures (Bruyer 1991; Young and de Haan 1992; Young 1994).

Findings of covert recognition in prosopagnosia show responses based on the unique identities of familiar faces, even though overt recognition of these faces is not achieved. Prosopagnosia can thus be considered a selective deficit of access consciousness, in which access to information about the identities of familiar faces is lost. The phenomenal experience of familiarity is also lost, though the phenomenal experience of seeing a face remains, and there may even be relatively good preservation of other aspects of face perception, such as the perception of sex or emotional expression (Bruyer *et al.* 1983). However, recognition of identity only seems to take place at a non-conscious level.

Observations of covert recognition in prosopagnosia fit naturally into a model in which activation must cross some form of threshold before it can result in access consciousness. This can be simulated quite simply with an interactive activation model in which excitation can be passed continuously from one functional unit to another, but a separate threshold is set to determine any explicit output. As a minimum, access consciousness requires an explicit representation.

Burton *et al.* (1990) had proposed a simulation of this type that could encompass several findings related to normal face recognition. It was then easy to demonstrate that the prosopagnosic pattern of preserved priming effects without explicit classification of face inputs could be simulated with this model by halving the connection strengths between two of its pools of functional units (Burton *et al.* 1991). This makes the finding of this pattern in some cases of prosopagnosia much less mysterious.

We can thus understand one way in which covert responses can be preserved when there is no overt discrimination, and this seems highly relevant to understanding access consciousness. However, although it represents a step forward, this type of simulation should not be mistaken for a full solution to the problem of understanding access consciousness. What has actually been established so far is only that this is one form of possible mechanism, not that it is the only or the correct answer. Further, explaining access consciousness is not the same as explaining phenomenal consciousness. As we noted earlier, zombies aside, it is hard to imagine access consciousness without phenomenal consciousness. But what reason do we have to think that the units in a computer program become phenomenally conscious when their activation passes whatever threshold is necessary for access? The fact that we do not know whether they do or not shows that an understanding of access consciousness does not necessarily involve an understanding of phenomenal consciousness.

Monitoring and self consciousness

Problems in self-consciousness seem to arise after frontal lobe lesions, when patients may engage in socially inappropriate behaviours without apparent concern or embarrassment (Damasio *et al.* 1990; Stuss 1991), but these are poorly understood. Rather more progress has been made in understanding monitoring problems that lead to unawareness of impairment (anosognosia).

The classic observations of unawareness of impairment were made by Von Monakow (1885) and Anton (1899), whose patients denied their own blindness or deafness. Subsequent reports have mostly concentrated on denial of blindness, now known as Anton's syndrome. Most emphasize that the patients are unaware of their blindness, behave as if they can see, and may even confabulate visual experiences (Raney and Nielsen 1942; Redlich and Dorsey 1945). There are, however, some cases in which insight is achieved. Raney and Nielsen (1942) described a woman who, after a year of apparent lack of insight into her problems, exclaimed 'My God, I am blind! Just to think, I have lost my eyesight!'.

As well as blindness and deafness, a wide range of types of impairment can be subject to anosognosia (McGlynn and Schacter 1989). An important observation is that patients with more than one deficit may be unaware of one impairment but perfectly well aware of others. Von Monakow (1885) had noted that his patient complained of other problems, even though he was not aware of his visual impairment. Anton (1899) made similar observations, and suggested that unawareness of impairment of a particular function is caused by a disorder at the highest levels of organisation of *that* function.

This position has been further developed by Bisiach *et al.* (1986), who demonstrated dissociations between anosognosia for hemiplegia and anosognosia for hemianopia. Paralysis to one side of the body (hemiplegia) and blindness for half the field of vision (hemianopia) are relatively common consequences of brain injury. The fact that patients can show awareness of their hemiplegias but not their hemianopias, and vice versa, shows that anosognosia does not result from a general change in the patient's monitoring abilities or of access consciousness of perceptual states, but can be specific to particular disabilities. Bisiach *et al.* (1986, p. 480) concluded that 'monitoring of the internal working is not secured in the nervous system by a general, superordinate organ, but is decentralized and apportioned to the different functional blocks to which it refers'.

Note that monitoring problems need not be restricted to deficits of phenomenal consciousness; for example, unawareness of visual recognition impairments has also been noted. A detailed description of a case involving unawareness of impaired face recognition, SP, is given by Young *et al.* (1990).

Unawareness of impairment, then, does not result from any overall change in the patient's ability to monitor or access. Like other impairments of consciousness, monitoring problems can be highly selective.

Unity or disunity of conscious experience

The neuropsychological impairments we have discussed fit neatly against our distinctions between phenomenal consciousness, access consciousness, and monitoring and self-consciousness. In blindsight, there is no phenomenal consciousness of stimuli projected to the blind field; there is also no access to those perceptual contents and no monitoring of the contents (until the patient hears his or her own guesses). The same is true for achromatopsia, showing that defects of consciousness can exist in very restricted aspects of experience. Proso-pagnosia is primarily a defect of access consciousness, but the phenomenal feel of familiarity is also missing. None the less, proso-pagnosics often show information about the faces they have seen when tested indirectly. In amnesia, there is impaired access to memories of things that happened in the past, but the influence of representations of these events is evident in indirect measures. Anosognosia can also be a highly selective defect confined to monitoring a particular form of access or phenomenal consciousness.

The main point, then, is that these defects of consciousness are highly selective. Phenomenal, access, and monitoring consciousness function well in one domain, but can be defective in another domain.

One thrust of such findings is to highlight the danger of thinking that the subjective unity of conscious experience implies that a unitary brain system is involved. Many discussions of conscious experience begin by emphasizing its subjective unity and continuity (James 1890), and some have argued that materialist theories cannot account for this unity (Tallis 1991). The hidden agenda is that subjective unity is then taken to imply that there is a place in the brain where everything is put together; Dennett and Kinsbourne (1992) label this the Cartesian Theatre, because Descartes had proposed that integration requires a single interface between mind and brain. This conception lurks behind many contemporary accounts of consciousness, although few neuroscientists now accept Descartes' proposed locus for the interface of the pineal gland.

The Cartesian Theatre fits with what is for many people a compelling intuition. At present, we do not know that it is definitely wrong, and it remains possible to argue that the types of neuropsychological dis-sociation we have described reflect disconnection of different functional modules from a single, central conscious mechanism (Schacter 1987; Young and de Haan 1990). However, the weight of evidence now makes this look unlikely. So many different types of dissociation are being revealed that one has to wonder whether it isn't the subjective unity of conscious phenomena that is illusory. Even if there were multiple conscious mechanisms, why shouldn't they have a subjective 'feel' of being unified in their operation?

Another hypothesis is that the contents of consciousness correspond to the information that is made available to executive mechanisms to coordinate and integrate what would otherwise be independent pro-cessing streams (Baars 1988; Morris and Hampson 1983). This could include the feedback of information that these executive mechanisms need to continue to make available to themselves, as well as information

from perceptual, memory, and monitoring systems. From this perspective, the different types of loss of conscious awareness caused by
brain injuries are much less of a surprise (Morris 1992). However, the
principal assumption of a single locus for consciousness remains; both
Baars (1988) and Morris and Hampson (1983) think that there is only a
single executive system.

A major problem is that these approaches tend to drop the issue of
explaining phenomenal consciousness. Even if there is a single
executive system, which if true would certainly be pertinent to understanding access consciousness, what exactly does it have to do with
phenomenal consciousness? These theorists start out trying to explain
phenomenal consciousness, but they run the risk of ending up with no
place for it.

A related argument to the approach linking consciousness to
executive mechanisms is used by Damasio (1992, p. 208), who points out
that 'the rejection of *one* biologically impossible Cartesian Theater does
not amount to rejecting the sense of *one* self doing the experiencing',
and argues that a satisfactory model of consciousness 'should indicate
how the dis-integrated fragments operate to produce the integrated
self'. Again, there is an attempt to account for subjective unity by
arguing that there is indeed a high degree of unity, but it is imposed late
in the system.

Marcel (1993) offers reasons to doubt even this. He draws attention to
dissociative phenomena in anosognosia which have potentially important implications. First, as has been noted by Bisiach and Geminiani
(1991), there can be inconsistencies between denial as evidenced in
actions and verbal reports. For example, a patient with left-sided
paralysis following a right hemisphere stroke may bemoan his or her
paralysis but keep trying to get out of bed and walk, whereas another
patient denies having any deficit on verbal interrogation but makes no
attempt to get out of bed. In the one case, a verbally acknowledged
deficit does not seem to constrain behaviour, whereas in the other
behaviour is constrained even though there is no verbal acknowledge-
ment. Which are we to take as reflecting the patient's 'real' insight, when
words and actions are inconsistent with each other?

A second type of dissociation noted by Marcel (1993) reflects the use
of a first-person or third-person perspective. It is standard practice in
investigations of anosognosia to ask the patient directly about his or her
disabilities; 'Can you walk?', 'Can you tie your shoes?', and so on. But
Marcel (1993) reports that when he and Tegnér asked anosognosic
patients with paralysis affecting one side of the body to rate how well
the examiner could perform each activity – 'if I [the questioner] were in

your [the patient's] current condition' – much better insight into the implications of the paralysis could be obtained.

Marcel (1993) points out that such phenomena are reminiscent of hypnosis and other dissociative states; part of the patient's mind seems to know the relevant facts, but another part doesn't. However, it is unlikely that they arise after brain injury for purely psychodynamic reasons. For example, denial of paralysis is more common after brain injury affecting the right cerebral hemisphere, which creates paralysis of the left side of the body, than after brain injury affecting the left cerebral hemisphere and consequent right-sided paralysis (Bisich and Geminiani 1991). So it is unlikely that denial of paralysis only reflects an emotional reaction; for a right-handed person paralysis of the right hand is potentially much more upsetting, but it is left-sided paralysis that is usually denied. Even more strikingly, it is known that failure to acknowledge left-sided paralysis (anosognosia for hemiplegia) is often associated with a more general failure to respond to the left side of space (known as unilateral neglect), and that temporary remission of both problems can be obtained after stimulation of the vestibular system through irrigation of the canals of the left outer ear with cold water (Cappa *et al.* 1987). This procedure generates a reflex response which involves eye and head turning in the direction of the stimulated ear, but the exact mechanism by which it leads to remission of unilateral neglect and anosognosia is not understood in detail. However, such findings again point one away from psychodynamic interpretations.

Dissociative phenomena in neuropsychology need not be restricted to anosognosia; they may also be fairly common for delusions caused by brain injury. Consider, for example, the Capgras delusion, which involves the bizarre conviction that one's relatives have been replaced by impostors (Ellis and de Pauw 1994). This delusion can arise in a variety of pathological settings, which include damage to temporo-parietal and frontal areas of the right cerebral hemisphere (Alexander *et al.* 1979; Lewis 1987; Spier 1992). Although violence against the impostors is noted in some Capgras patients (Silva *et al.* 1992), this is much less frequent when the delusions have a clear organic basis (Malloy *et al.* 1992). In fact, while Capgras patients complain that their relatives have been replaced, a number do not otherwise act in accordance with this belief, showing neither violence nor aggression to the impostors, and failing to report the matter to the police or to initiate any search for their 'original' relatives. Notice that this is not just a motor versus verbal dissociation; telephoning the police station would be just as much a verbal action as stating that your husband is an impostor.

The thrust of such examples is to undermine the idea of a unified self overseeing what we do. If different aspects of our behaviour can be so inconsistent, we can infer that our sense of self is built on a coalescence that can be disrupted under unusual or pathological circumstances. The intuition of a unified consciousness is so directly tied to a first-person perspective that, without a unified self, the case for unified consciousness collapses.

Consciousness and evolution

The fact that consciousness is so intimately related to what our nervous systems are doing has led many people to conclude that a biologically based account will be needed. Searle (1992, p. 90) has made the point eloquently:

Consciousness, in short, is a biological feature of human and certain animal brains. It is caused by neurobiological processes and is as much a part of the natural world order as any other biological features such as photosynthesis, digestion, or mitosis.

This line of reasoning leads naturally to questions about the evolutionary background to consciousness, but these are not easy to answer. Not every behaviour is affected directly by natural selection, and there are many possibilities for emergent properties or unintended consequences of behaviours whose utility or survival value was initially related to quite different purposes. To illustrate this, Searle (1992, p. 106) uses the example of alpine skiing:

The spread of skiing has been simply phenomenal; and the sacrifices that people are willing to make in money, comfort, and time for the sake of a few hours on a ski slope is at least pretty good evidence that they derive satisfactions from it that are inherent to their biological nature. But it's simply not the case that we were selected by evolution for our predilection for alpine skiing.

Despite these difficulties, Searle (1992) argues that there are evolutionary advantages to consciousness. We have already discussed his argument that consciousness gives us flexibility and creativity, based on the lack of these during attacks of absence (*petit mal*) epilepsy. However, we noted that this line of reasoning seems to work better for monitoring and access consciousness than for phenomenal consciousness.

In general, it seems to us that different forms of consciousness serve different purposes. Phenomenal consciousness and access consciousness are likely to be intimately linked to intentional actions; patients who show blindsight in laboratory tasks don't respond to objects located in their blind field in everyday life, and prosopagnosic patients who show covert recognition effects in the laboratory do not act as if they recognize people from their faces.

To see why certain types of consciousness have become linked to intentional actions, one needs to consider the delicate balance between speed of response and flexibility of response. Perceptual systems have evolved to create representations of external events that can permit effective action in the world that an organism inhabits. Fast responses are best made by dedicated, relatively inflexible systems. Flexibility of response requires more sophisticated representations of events, which take longer to compute. These costs of flexibility become especially marked when time is spent not only in constructing an adequate representation, but also in weighing up possible alternative actions. An obvious way to balance the competing demands of flexibility and speed is therefore to allow many actions to run off under automatic control, and to involve conscious mechanisms which can allow greater choice only when these are needed. This is a particularly convenient solution for the nervous system, in which many actions (like breathing) can be safely left under automatic pilot much of the time, and only require occasional conscious intervention (if you are about to stick your head underwater, etc.).

A compelling demonstration of this comes from the dissociation of action and conscious perception found in the elegant work of Milner, Goodale, and their colleagues (Goodale and Milner 1992; Goodale et al. 1991; Milner et al. 1991). They have made a very thorough investigation of a neuropsychological case, patient DF, with severely impaired shape perception. When DF was asked to make judgements about the orientation or size of an object, she performed very poorly. However, when DF was asked to put her hand into a slot she immediately oriented it correctly, and she shaped her fingers appropriately for the size of an object she was about to pick up (Goodale and Milner 1992; Goodale et al. 1991). In general, DF could make accurate responses to tasks that involved a well practised everyday movement that can be run off without conscious control (putting your hand into something, or picking something up), whereas inaccurate responses arose in tasks that need continual conscious intervention.

Other forms of consciousness, such as monitoring and self-consciousness, may well be more intimately linked to different purposes, including trouble-shooting and the prediction of the social behaviour of others. In discussing possible functions of consciousness, we therefore need to keep clear which form of consciousness might have which type of function.

One way forward may be to adopt an evolutionary approach, the most detailed of which has been offered by Humphrey (1992, 1994). Humphrey (1992) argues that, in evolutionary terms, the first function of sensations was to mediate affective responses to stimulation occurring at the body surface, because an animal 'that had the means to sort out the good from the bad—approaching or letting in the good, avoiding or blocking the bad—would have been at a biological advantage' (Humphrey 1992, p. 142). He says, then, that sensation evolved to allow something to be done about the stimulus, and that this was originally done at the point of stimulation; the animal both detected and responded to the stimulus with the same bit of its skin, much as we still do if we wiggle a toe when it itches. Humphrey (1992) claims that this fundamental coupling of sensation, affect, and action plans is maintained even for more highly developed senses, like vision, which seem subjectively to carry information about the world beyond the body. According to Humphrey, this is achieved through the construction of internal feedback loops to substitute for overt actions; in his view, feeling a particular sensation corresponds to issuing whatever instructions are required to create the appropriate outgoing signal from the brain.

At present, we find it easier to imagine how this idea can fit bodily sensations than external senses like hearing or vision. However, it has to be remembered that eyes evolved by grouping together light-sensitive receptor cells which were originally at the body surface (Gregory 1972), and that the advantage of hearing or vision is simply that they extend one's capacity to respond outwards, to encompass stimuli beyond those that are in direct contact with the surface of the body. So Humphrey's (1992) claim that a general solution to the problems of phenomenal consciousness is possible should not be dismissed lightly. Moreover, even if his approach does prove only to work for bodily sensations (pain, itching, and so on), accounting successfully for how these feel would in itself be a major step forward, justifying Humphrey's (1992, p. 219) optimistic conclusion:

A seeming miracle? No, as close to a real miracle as anything that ever happened. The twist may be that it takes only a relatively simple scientific theory to explain it.

References

Alexander, M. P., Stuss, D. T., and Benson, D. F. (1979). Capgras syndrome: a reduplicative phenomenon. *Neurology*, **29**, 334–9.
Allport, A. (1988). What concept of consciousness? In *Consciousness in*

contemporary science, (ed. A. J. Marcel and E. Bisiach), pp. 159–82. Oxford University Press.

Anton, G. (1899). Ueber die Selbstwahrnemung der Herderkrankungen des Gehirns durch den Kranken bei Rindenblindheit und Rindentaubheit. *Archiv für Psychiatrie und Nervenkrankheiten*, **32**, 86–127.

Baars, B. J. (1988). *A cognitive theory of consciousness*. Cambridge University Press.

Bates, D. and Cartlidge, N. (1994). Disorders of consciousness. In *The neurological boundaries of reality*, (ed. E. M. R. Critchley), pp. 383–99. Farrand, London.

Bisiach, E. and Geminiani, G. (1991). Anosognosia related to hemiplegia and hemianopia. In *Awareness of deficit after brain injury: clinical and theoretical issues*, (ed. G. P. Prigatano and D. L. Schacter), pp. 17–39. Oxford University Press.

Bisiach, E., Vallar, G., Perani, D., Papagno, C., and Berti, A. (1986). Unawareness of disease following lesions of the right hemisphere: anosognosia for hemiplegia and anosognosia for hemianopia. *Neuropsychologia*, **24**, 471–82.

Block, N. (1991). Evidence against epiphenomenalism. *Behavioural and Brain Sciences*, **14**, 670–2.

Bruyer, R. (1991). Covert face recognition in prosopagnosia: a review. *Brain and Cognition*, **15**, 223–35.

Bruyer, R., Laterre, C., Seron, X., Feyereisen, P., Strypstein, E., Pierrard, E., and Rectem, D. (1983). A case of prosopagnosia with some preserved covert remembrance of familiar faces. *Brain and Cognition*, **2**, 257–84.

Burton, A. M., Bruce, V., and Johnston, R. A. (1990). Understanding face recognition with an interactive activation model. *British Journal of Psychology*, **81**, 361–80.

Burton, A. M., Young, A. W., Bruce, V., Johnston, R., and Ellis, A. W. (1991). Understanding covert recognition. *Cognition*, **39**, 129–66.

Cappa, S. F., Sterzi, R., Vallar, G., and Bisiach, E. (1987). Remission of hemineglect and anosognosia after vestibular stimulation. *Neuropsychologia*, **25**, 775–82.

Carlson, N. R. (1991). *Physiology of behavior*, 4th edn. Allyn & Bacon, Boston.

Cowey, A. and Stoerig, P. (1991). The neurobiology of blindsight. *Trends in Neurosciences*, **14**, 140–5.

Cowey, A. and Stoerig, P. (1992). Reflections on blindsight. In *The neuropsychology of consciousness*, (ed. A. D. Milner and M. D. Rugg), pp. 11–37. Academic, London.

Crick, F. and Koch, C. (1990). Towards a neurobiological theory of consciousness. *Seminars in The Neurosciences*, **2**, 263–75.

Damasio, A. R. (1992). The selfless consciousness. *Behavioral and Brain Sciences*, **15**, 208–9.

Damasio, A. R., Tranel, D., and Damasio, H. (1990). Individuals with sociopathic behavior caused by frontal damage fail to respond autonomically to social stimuli. *Behavioural Brain Research*, **41**, 81–94.

Dennett, D. C. (1988). Quining qualia. In *Consciousness in contemporary science*, (ed. A. J. Marcel and E. Bisiach), pp. 42–77. Oxford University Press.

Dennett, D. C. (1991). *Consciousness explained*. Allen Lane, Penguin, Harmondsworth.

Dennett, D. C. and Kinsbourne, M. (1992). Time and the observer: the where and when of consciousness in the brain. *Behavioral and Brain Sciences*, **15**, 183–201.

Ellis, H. D. and de Pauw, K. W. (1994). The cognitive neuropsychiatric origins of the Capgras delusion. In *The neuropsychology of schizophrenia*, (ed. A. S. David and J. C. Cutting), pp. 317–35. Lawrence Erlbaum, Hove, UK.

Flanagan, O. (1992). *Consciousness reconsidered*. MIT Press, Cambridge, MA.

Goodale, M. A. and Milner, A. D. (1992). Separate visual pathways for perception and action. *Trends in Neurosciences*, **15**, 20–5.

Goodale, M. A., Milner, A. D., Jakobson, L. S., and Carey, D. P. (1991). A neurological dissociation between perceiving objects and grasping them. *Nature*, **349**, 154–6.

Gregory, R. L. (1972). *Eye and brain: the psychology of seeing*, 2nd edn. World University Library, London.

Heywood, C. A., Cowey, A., and Newcombe, F. (1991). Chromatic discrimination in a cortically colour blind observer. *European Journal of Neuroscience*, **3**, 802–12.

Hummel, J. E. and Biederman, I. (1992). Dynamic binding in a neural network for shape recognition. *Psychological Review*, **99**, 480–517.

Humphrey, N. (1992). *A history of the mind*. Chatto & Windus, London.

Humphrey, N. (1994). The private world of consciousness. *New Scientist*, 8 January, 23–5.

James, W. (1890). *The principles of psychology, Vol. 1*. Dover, New York. [1950 reprint of original edition published by Henry Holt & Co.]

Jaynes, J. (1976). *The origin of consciousness in the breakdown of the bicameral mind*. Houghton-Mifflin, Boston.

Johnson-Laird, P. N. (1988). *The computer and the mind: an introduction to cognitive science*. Fontana, London.

Kolb, B. and Whishaw, I. Q. (1990). *Fundamentals of human neuropsychology*, 3rd edn. W. H. Freeman, New York.

Levine, J. (1983). Materialism and qualia: the explanatory gap. *Pacific Philosophical Quarterly*, **64**, 354–61.

Lewis, S. W. (1987). Brain imaging in a case of Capgras syndrome. *British Journal of Psychiatry*, **150**, 117–21.

McGinn, C. (1991). *The problem of consciousness*. Blackwell, Oxford.

McGlynn, S. and Schacter, D. L. (1989). Unawareness of deficits in neuropsychological syndromes. *Journal of Clinical and Experimental Neuropsychology*, **11**, 143–205.

Malloy, P., Cimino, C., and Westlake, R. (1992). Differential diagnosis of primary and secondary Capgras delusions. *Neuropsychiatry, Neuropsychology, and Behavioral Neurology*, **5**, 83–96.

Marcel, A. J. (1993). Slippage in the unity of consciousness. In Ciba Foundation Symposium No. 174, *Experimental and theoretical studies of consciousness*. Wiley, Chichester, UK.

Marzi, C. A., Tassinari, G., Agliotti, S., and Lutzemberger, L. (1986). Spatial summation across the vertical meridian in hemianopics: a test of blindsight. *Neuropsychologia*, **24**, 749–58.

Meadows, J. C. (1974). Disturbed perception of colours associated with localized cerebral lesions. *Brain*, **97**, 615–32.

Milner, A. D. and Rugg, M. D. (eds) (1992). *The neuropsychology of consciousness*. Academic, London.

Milner, A. D., Perrett, D. I., Johnston, R. S., Benson, P. J., Jordan, T. R., Heeley, D. W., *et al.* (1991). Perception and action in 'visual form agnosia'. *Brain*, **114**, 405–28.

Mollon, J. D., Newcombe, F., Polden. P. G., and Ratcliff, G. (1980). On the presence of three cone mechanisms in a case of total achromatopsia. In *Colour vision deficiencies, V*, (ed. G. Verriest), pp. 130–5. Hilger, Bristol, UK.

Morris, P. E. (1992). Cognition and consciousness. *The Psychologist: Bulletin of the British Psychological Society*, **5**, 3–8.

Morris, P. E. and Hampson, P. J. (1983). *Imagery and consciousness*. Academic, London.

Nagel, T. (1974). What is it like to be a bat? *Philosophical Review*, **83**, 435–50.

Neisser, U. (1988). Five kinds of self-knowledge. *Philosophical Psychology*, **1**, 35–59.

Perrett, D. I., Hietanen, J. K., Oram, M. W., and Benson, P. J. (1992). Organization and functions of cells responsive to faces in the temporal cortex. *Philosophical Transactions of the Royal Society, London*, **B335**, 23–30.

Pizzamiglio, L., Antonucci, G., and Francia, A. (1984). Response of the cortically blind hemifields to a moving visual scene. *Cortex*, **20**, 89–99.

Pöppel, E., Held, R., and Frost, D. (1973). Residual visual function after brain wounds involving the central visual pathways in man. *Nature*, **243**, 295–6.

Ramsey, W., Stich, S., and Rumelhart, D. (eds) (1991). *Philosophy and connectionist theory*. Lawrence Erlbaum, Hillsdale, NJ.

Raney, A. A. and Nielsen, J. M. (1942). Denial of blindness (Anton's symptom). *Bulletin of Los Angeles Neurological Society*,1 **7**, 150–1.

Redlich, F. C. and Dorsey, J. F. (1945). Denial of blindness by patients with cerebral disease. *Archives of Neurology and Psychiatry*, **53**, 407–17.

Schacter, D. L. (1987). Implicit memory: history and current status. *Journal of Experimental Psychology: Learning, Memory, and Cognition*, **13**, 501–18.

Schacter, D. L., McAndrews, M. P., and Moscovitch, M. (1988). Access to consciousness: dissociations between implicit and explicit knowledge in neuropsychological syndromes. In *Thought without language*, (ed. L. Weiskrantz), pp. 242–78. Oxford University Press.

Searle, J. (1984). *Minds, brains and science: the 1984 Reith lectures*. British Broadcasting Corporation, London.

Searle, J. R. (1992). *The rediscovery of the mind*. MIT Press, Cambridge, MA.

Shastri, L. and Ajjanagadde, V. (1993). From simple associations to systematic reasoning: a connectionist representation of rules, variables and dynamic bindings using temporal synchrony. *Behavioral and Brain Sciences*, **16**, 417–51.

Silva, J. A., Leong, G. B., and Weinstock, R. (1992). The dangerousness of persons with misidentification syndromes. *Bulletin of the American Academy of Psychiatry Law*, **20**, 77–86.

Spier, S. A. (1992). Capgras syndrome and the delusions of misidentification. *Psychiatric Annals*, **22**, 279–85.

Stuss, D. T. (1991). Disturbance of self-awareness after frontal system damage. In *Awareness of deficit after brain injury: clinical and theoretical issues*, (ed. G. P. Prigatano and D. L. Schacter), pp. 63–83. Oxford University Press.

Tallis, R. (1991). A critique of neuromythology. In *The pursuit of mind*, (ed. R. Tallis and H. Robinson), pp. 86–109. Carcanet, Manchester, UK.

Torjussen, T. (1976). Residual function in cortically blind hemifields. *Scandinavian Journal of Psychology*, **17**, 320–2.

Torjussen, T. (1978). Visual processing in cortically blind hemifields. *Neuropsychologia*, **16**, 15–21.

Von Monakow, C. (1885). Experimentelle und pathologisch-anatomische Untersuchungen Über die Beziehungen der sogenannten Sehsphäre zu den infracorticalen Opticuscentren und zum N. opticus. *Archiv für Psychiatrie aund Nervenkrankheiten*, **16**, 151–99.

Warrington, E. K. and Weiskrantz, L. (1968). New method of testing long-term retention with special reference to amnesic patients. *Nature*, **217**, 972–4.

Warrington, E. K. and Weiskrantz, L. (1970). Amnesia: consolidation or retrieval? *Nature*, **228**, 628–30.

Weiskrantz, L. (1986). *Blindsight: a case study and implications*. Oxford University Press.

Weiskrantz, L. (1990). The Ferrier lecture, 1989. Outlooks for blindsight: explicit methodologies for implicit processes. *Proceedings of the Royal Society, London*, **B239**, 247–78.

Weiskrantz, L., Warrington, E. K., Sanders, M. D., and Marshall, J. (1974). Visual capacity in the hemianopic field following a restricted occipital ablation. *Brain*, **97**, 709–28.

White, S. (1991). *The unity of the self*. MIT Press, Cambridge, MA.

Young, A. W. (1994). Conscious and nonconscious recognition of familiar faces. In *Attention and Performance*, *XV* (ed. C. Umiltà and M. Moscovitch), pp. 153–78. Bradford Books/MIT Press, Cambridge, MA.

Young, A. W. and de Haan, E. H. F. (1990). Impairments of visual awareness. *Mind & Language*, **5**, 29–48.

Young, A. W. and de Haan, E. H. F. (1992). Face recognition and awareness after brain injury. In *The neuropsychology of consciousness*, (ed. A. D. Milner and M. D. Rugg), pp. 69–90. Academic, London.

Young, A. W., de Haan, E. H. F., and Newcombe, F. (1990). Unawareness of impaired face recognition. *Brain and Cognition*, **14**, 1–18.

Zeki, S. (1993). *A vision of the brain*. Blackwell, Oxford.

Zihl, J., Tretter, F., and Singer, W. (1980). Phasic electrodermal responses after visual stimulation in the cortically blind hemifield. *Behavioural Brain Research*, **1**, 197–203.

AUTHOR INDEX

SUBJECT INDEX